THIS HOUSE OF NOBLE DEEDS

ARTHUR H. AUFSES, JR., and
BARBARA J. NISS

THIS HOUSE
OF NOBLE DEEDS

The Mount Sinai Hospital, 1852–2002

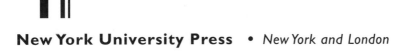

New York University Press • *New York and London*

NEW YORK UNIVERSITY PRESS
New York and London

© 2002 by New York University

Library of Congress Cataloging-in-Publication Data
Aufses, Arthur H.
This house of noble deeds : Mount Sinai Hospital, 1852–2002 /
Arthur H. Aufses, Jr., and Barbara Niss.
p. ; cm.
Includes bibliographical references and index.
ISBN 0-8147-0500-6 (cloth : alk. paper)
1. Mount Sinai Hospital (New York, N.Y.)—History.
2. Hospitals—New York (State)—New York—History.
[DNLM: 1. Mount Sinai Hospital (New York, N.Y.)
2. Hospitals—history—New York City.
3. Medical Staff, Hospital—New York City. WX 11 AN7 A918t 2002]
I. Title: Mount Sinai Hospital, 1852–2002. II. Niss, Barbara. III. Title.
RA982.N5 M814 2002
362.1'1'097471—dc21   2002009291

New York University Press books are printed on acid-free paper,
and their binding materials are chosen for strength and durability.

Manufactured in the United States of America

10 9 8 7 6 5 4 3 2 1

Contents

Preface and Acknowledgments

The tradition of an academic institution is based on the particular and frequently unique characters of the men [*sic*] who make up its community of scholars. Long before it became a medical school Mount Sinai was, besides being a hospital, an academic institution dedicated to teaching and research. The unusual aura of The Mount Sinai Hospital was based upon this uniqueness.[1]

It is the men and women of The Mount Sinai Hospital, their unique characters, and especially their accomplishments, that this book celebrates. Nowhere is the expression "We stand on the shoulders of giants" more true than at Mount Sinai. The 150th anniversary of the Hospital, in 2002, provides an ideal opportunity to honor those who established the clinical reputation of The Mount Sinai Hospital of New York and paved the way for the academic health center of today.

The goal of this book is to describe the scientific contributions of the staff of The Mount Sinai Hospital over the past 150 years. This is not a history of the institution, per se. In 1952, two publications heralded the one-hundredth anniversary of the Hospital. *The First 100 Years of the Mount Sinai Hospital of New York: 1852–1952*, by Joseph Hirsh and Beka Doherty, detailed the expansion and development of the institution in the context of the growth and changes occurring in New York and in medicine.[2] In November 1952, the *American Journal of Medicine*[3] reprinted a dozen seminal articles by members of the staff and made reference to a number of others. Other than our own Levy Library reprint collection, there is no other compendium of the important works produced by the staff. We hope that this volume will help to fill that void.

By whatever criteria one wishes to use—bed complement, size, reputation of its staff, or scientific productivity—Mount Sinai ranks among the elite institutions of the world. From its earliest days and throughout the first half-century of its existence, the reputation of the Hospital was essentially a reflection of the clinical repute of a distinguished staff of outstanding physicians, selected by the lay board from the schools and hospitals of New York City. Many of these physicians had been part of a major migration of clinicians from European centers of learning that took place in the middle of the nineteenth century; these professionals came to the United States to establish their careers in the more liberal environment of the New World.

But clinicians alone would never have been able to sustain the reputation of the institution. It is to the credit of the institutional leadership at all levels—lay board, medical and nursing staff, and administration—that as medicine evolved, the Hospital not only kept up with the changing milieu but continuously positioned itself at the front edge of scientific progress.[4] As laboratory science developed in the early part of the twentieth century, the laboratories were placed in the hands of highly skilled specialists in laboratory medicine. In 1944, when it became apparent that clinical teaching had reached a level that could no longer be sustained by an all-voluntary faculty, the trustees decided to begin appointing salaried physicians as chiefs of service. And when it became apparent that a stand-alone hospital could not keep up with the rapid progress of science in the second half of the twentieth century, the Hospital's leadership was almost unanimous in agreeing to found a medical school, not only to keep up with the science of medicine but also to enable the Hospital to continue to attract the best and the brightest of medical school graduates to the many clinical training programs of the Hospital and then, later, to retain the best of them on the staff, because excellence in patient care was, and remains, of paramount importance.

Over the past 150 years, the institution's progress appears to fall into clearly defined periods: 1855 to 1893, when the first laboratory was created; 1893 to 1926, when the now multiple laboratories were placed in the hands of full-time specialists; 1926 to 1944, when the first full-time chiefs were appointed to the two divisions of the Medical Service and the full-time "system" began; 1944 to 1963, when the charter for the Medical School was obtained; and 1963 to the present, during which time the Medical Center reached its current state of maturity. While a chronological history emphasizing those periods would get across the intellectual vibrancy of the institution, we chose to tell this story on a departmental basis. This gave us the opportunity not only to present the scientific productivity of the members of each specialty group but also to trace the development of the departments and the various training programs, which now number more than seventy and which train more than eight hundred residents and fellows each year. Still, this approach tends to obscure the richness of the interaction of the departments with the laboratories and with one another, and the workings of the institution as a whole.

There are many facets of Mount Sinai that cannot be adequately represented in a volume that has been deliberately kept within a size limitation. While the exact number can never be ascertained, considerably more than 250,000 papers and books have been published over the years by Mount Sinai staff. We have attempted to highlight those that we deemed most significant—those on the many syndromes, diseases, and other "firsts" that have come from Mount Sinai—and we hope that none have been forgotten. We have taken the additional step of creating a Web site, www.mountsinaihistory.org, to serve as an adjunct to this volume. The site will contain annotated citations to works that we have uncovered but could not include in the print edition, as well as more inclusive biographical and pictorial information relating to Mount Sinai physicians and scientists. We thank the staff of Mount Sinai's Janet W. and Gustave L. Levy Library for their help with the Web site.

Another area that cannot be covered adequately is that of the many trainees who have left Mount Sinai and gone on to great success in their chosen fields. It is a duty dear to the hearts of the physicians who have served Mount Sinai over the years to teach young doctors and scientists, and many consider this group of trainees to be part of their legacy to medicine. Unfortunately, there is not enough space to list all those who have studied here, and the risk of inadvertently omitting even a few has caused us to exclude such lists altogether.

Another omission is the history of the founding of the Mount Sinai School of Medicine and its effect on the Hospital. In the interest of space, we have left the story of the School, the basic science departments, and the Departments of Genetics, Health Policy, and Community and Preventive Medicine for another time. We hope to produce a publication on these topics in 2003, for the fortieth anniversary of the School. We have also omitted the history of the Department of Nursing because two comprehensive books have already been written that document the monumental contributions the Mount Sinai nurses have made to patient care in peace time and in two wars, bringing distinction to themselves and to the Hospital.[5]

Finally, every institution has a culture of its own; Mount Sinai is no exception. When word of the writing of this volume circulated, many people volunteered anecdotes and stories. We decided to include as many stories as possible, but these have had to take second place to our original goal of telling the scientific tale of the Hospital. We have tried to get across the feel of the institution in the chapter "The Years of the Giants," but we recognize that this does not do justice to the institution, or to the rich treasure trove of material available.

We have been incredibly fortunate in obtaining help from individuals in every department, and we would like to acknowledge them here: Raymond Miller, in Anesthesiology; Paul Kirschner and Robert Litwak, in Cardiothoracic Surgery; Jack Klatell and Leo Stern, Jr., in Dentistry; Leslie Libow and Robert Butler, in Geriatrics; J. Lester Gabrilove, Scott Friedman, George Atweh, Alvin Teirstein, David Sachar, Janice Gabrilove, Peter Gorevic, Sherman Kupfer, Lloyd Mayer, Mary Klotman, and Valentin Fuster, in Medicine; Edward Bottone, in Microbiology; Douglas Altchek, in Dermatology; Louis Lapid, Nathan Kase, and Carmel Cohen, in OB/GYN; Seymour Gendelman, in Neurology; Ira Eliasoph, in Ophthalmology; Patricia Wells in Otolaryngology; Robert Siffert, in Orthopaedics; Steven Geller, in Pathology; Donald Gribetz, in Pediatrics; Marvin Stein, in Psychiatry; Sidney Silverstone (deceased),in Radiation Oncology; Jack Rabinowitz, in Radiology; and Kristjan Ragnarsson, in Rehabilitation Medicine. Some have provided extensive written expositions about their departments, others helpful advice and information. Additionally, each department's chapter has been read by the respective chairperson, and many have provided thoughtful comments and corrections. If there are errors or omissions in this book, they are ours; if there is value, we thank those who helped us.

Over the years, a number of departmental histories have been written, most of them published in *The Mount Sinai Journal of Medicine*. With the help of the original authors, we have expanded these articles to meet the goals of this volume. We are therefore indebted to Sherman Kupfer, M.D., Editor of the *Journal*, for blanket permission to reproduce these revised articles.

This book also could not have been written were it not for Dr. Albert S. Lyons, Emeritus Clinical Professor of Surgery, who in the early 1960s had the prescience to convince the Trustees and administration of the Hospital to set aside money and space to develop an institutional archive. Not only was Al Lyons our only archivist for many years, gathering material that might have been lost; he also created a library of oral history tapes that today contains more than eighty-five interviews with physicians, administrators, and trustees of the institution. In the 1980s, he again took the initiative in securing the appointment of a professional archivist to carry on his work. All those interested in the history of Mount Sinai are truly in his debt.

Early on in the preparation of the book, Lily Saint, Joshua Richter, and Quynh-Nhu Thi Pham (Mount Sinai School of Medicine, 2002) were of great assistance in researching the history of the Department of Surgery. Alicia Cohen (Mount Sinai School of Medicine, 2004) prepared the chapter on the Department of Geriatrics. A major contributor to our efforts has been Kristin Wilson. Working with us for sixteen months on a full-time basis, she took on major responsibilities for a number of the chapters, conducting research and interviews and writing the first drafts. Her efforts on our behalf have made an enormous difference in our ability to produce the work on time. Harriet Aufses read, and reread, every revision of every section; her comments were invaluable.

Clearly we have benefited from the help of many who have supported us, sustained us, and pointed us in directions we never knew existed. Among these, we must number the leadership of the Hospital who have allowed us to devote our resources to this work. John W. Rowe, M.D., CEO and President of the Medical Center from 1988 to 2000, and Barry Freedman, President of The Mount Sinai Hospital, encouraged and sponsored our efforts to go ahead with this project. Gary Rosenberg, Ph.D., Senior Vice President of the Medical Center, has been an invaluable resource. We also owe thanks to Nathan Kase, M.D., Dean of the Mount Sinai School of Medicine from 1987 to 1997 and currently interim CEO and President of the Medical Center and interim Dean of the Medical School, and Arthur Rubenstein, M.D., Dean of the School from 1997 to 2001, for their understanding of our inability to include the history of the School in this project. We are indebted to New York University Press and to its very talented staff. The assistance we have received from Eric Zinner, Editor-in-Chief, Emily Park, Editorial Assistant, and Despina Papazoglou Gimbel, Managing Editor, has been vital to our ability to have the publication ready for our anniversary year.

We have tried to determine when something was truly a first and have investigated many claims for priority. We have attempted to give credit when due and to highlight work that has been forgotten by the passing of time. While we may not claim total impartiality, we have tried to exercise diligence and fairness. We regret that, due to space constraints, the story often leaps from one Chief to the next, leaving out many who dedicated their lives to furthering both medical science and Mount Sinai. Their legacy lies not in these pages but in the people whose lives they have touched and made better.

Introduction

The Mount Sinai Hospital: An Overview

ON JANUARY 15, 1852, nine men representing various Hebrew charitable organizations came together to establish the Jews' Hospital in
New York to offer free medical care to indigent Hebrews in the City
who were not able to provide for themselves during their illnesses. This
was the beginning of the Mount Sinai Hospital.[1]

Sampson Simson was unquestionably the father of Mount Sinai. He
was the first president of the Board of Directors; he gave the land on
which the first hospital was built; and he personally assumed many of
the financial burdens of the young institution. When he resigned in February 1855 at the age of seventy-five, the other Directors sent a delega-
tion to his home in Yonkers to beg him to reconsider, to no avail.

With the founding of the organization, its leadership began a fund-
raising effort to secure enough money to erect a hospital building. But,
as costs mounted, it was the bequest of Judah Touro for $20,000 that re-
ally ensured the timely completion of the venture. Ground was broken
for the Hospital in the fall of 1853. A year and a half later, on May 17,
1855, the Jews' Hospital was officially dedicated with a religious cere-
mony; it opened to patients on June 5.

This first hospital was located on West 28th Street between 7th and
8th Avenues and extended through to 27th Street. That area of the City
in the mid-1850s was still rural, and vegetable gardens grew next to the
Hospital. The building accommodated forty-five patients initially, but
additions were built during the Civil War to house Union soldiers. The
Hospital offered almost exclusively ward service—as did all hospitals
at this time—but a small section was set aside for paying patients.

Quality patient care was the goal of these first Hospital Directors.
(The title Director was changed in 1917 to Trustee, allowing the Superintendent to take his modern title of Director of The Mount Sinai Hospital.) To meet this goal, the Directors hired a Superintendent to run the

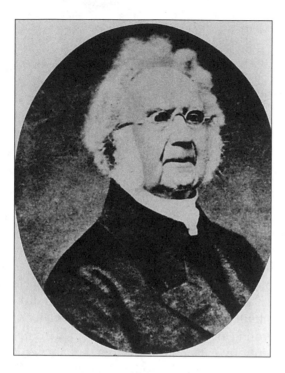

Sampson Simson, first
President of the Jews'
Hospital, later
The Mount Sinai Hospital.

daily operations of the Hospital. (Later a Matron was added to run the household end of the institution.) A pharmacy of some kind was established from the beginning, although it is unclear from the records whether a pharmacist was hired and on what basis. The Directors also sought to assemble a staff of respected and dedicated doctors. These efforts were rewarded as physicians such as Valentine and Alexander Mott, Benjamin McCready, Thomas Markoe, Willard Parker, and Israel Moses signed on early as Consulting and Attending Staff. The Resident Attending Physician, who provided the day-to-day medical care at the Hospital, was Mark Blumenthal, the physician for the Portuguese Synagogue congregation. (He and Israel Moses were the only Jewish physicians on the first staff.) Although Blumenthal maintained a private practice, he had appointed hours at the Hospital and was continually on call. For this, he received $250 the first year, and $500 in subsequent years.

With only a forty-five-bed capacity, the Hospital was quickly and continuously full. Intended originally as a purely sectarian institution, the Jews' Hospital never turned away emergency patients, regardless of creed. In the first year of its existence, the Hospital admitted 216 patients, only five of whom were born in this country. The largest group, numbering 110, was from Germany. The Hospital was a completely charitable enterprise; the Directors relied on gifts from friends and members of the Hospital Society, as well as on payments from the City, to provide enough to subsidize the care.

The 1860s were hectic years for the Hospital on 28th Street. The City was racked with violent riots in 1863 when citizens protested the draft procedure for the Union Army. Ironically, the injured rioters were taken in and treated at the Hospital alongside wounded Union soldiers, whom the Hospital cared for in large numbers.

These turbulent years at the Hospital proved two things: the Hospital was clearly no longer sectarian, and it needed to move. The Directors feared that, if they retained the limiting name of Jews' Hospital, the Hospital would be considered ineligible for State support. So, in 1866, the charter of the Hospital was amended by an Act of the State Legislature that designated as the new name The Mount Sinai Hospital. Also, by the 1860s, the downtown location was much too small for the needs of the Hospital, and the area had become very industrial. In 1868, a steam boiler exploded in a factory adjacent to the Hospital, shaking the

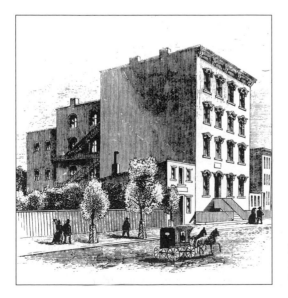

First hospital building, 1855–1872, located at West 28th Street.

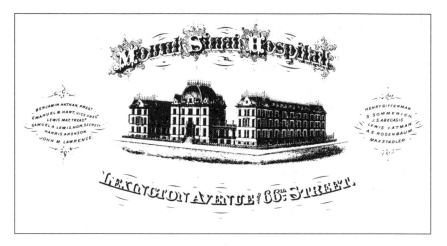

Mount Sinai Hospital buildings, 1872–1904.

building and breaking some windows. The Directors were spurred to action. On October 6, 1868, the City granted The Mount Sinai Hospital a ninety-nine-year lease for property on Lexington Avenue, between 66th and 67th streets. For the sum of $1.00, the Hospital had acquired the land for its second home. A new building fund-raising campaign was begun.

THE SECOND MOUNT SINAI HOSPITAL, 1872–1904

When The Mount Sinai Hospital moved into its new home on Lexington Avenue in 1872, the Directors were sure their new neighborhood would provide them with all the quietness, fresh air, and sunlight they knew a hospital required. The area was open, the street unpaved; they were indeed on the fringes of the City and hoped to remain so.

The Hospital was dedicated on May 29, 1872. It had 120 beds and had cost $335,000 to build. There was no electricity in the building (it was lit with gas) but a telephone system was installed in 1882. A steam whistle, and later a gong, would sound to announce the arrival of a member of the Consulting Staff. A synagogue was part of the original building; a separate operating room, however, was added only after a few years had passed. This speaks to the priorities and realities of the institution during this period.

This second home of Mount Sinai saw the beginnings of many aspects of the modern institution that are now taken for granted: the Out-Patient Department (OPD) was established in 1875; in 1895, a Pharmacist was first officially listed in the Annual Report, although a Hospital Pharmacy had long existed; the Medical Board was created in 1872 and at its first meeting urged the formation of a House Staff; in 1881, The Mount Sinai Hospital Training School for Nurses was established, ushering in professional nursing care to a hospital previously served by untrained male and female attendants. (In 1928 the name of the school was changed to The Mount Sinai Hospital School of Nursing.) In these last two events can be seen the beginning of Mount Sinai's commitment to education, although teaching was still not considered an official part of Sinai's mission.

No firm date can be given to mark when research began at Mount Sinai. In 1867, a microscope was purchased for the use of the staff, but this may have been for diagnostic use only. It was another twenty-six years before a laboratory was set up—in a converted coat closet, large enough to hold only two people at a time. This allocation of laboratory space was recognition that both medical knowledge and the medical staff itself were becoming more sophisticated. By the 1890s, many of the staff members had received training in Europe that emphasized lab work to support bedside observations. Some staff members spent their free time as volunteers in the laboratory after completing their work on the wards and in their private practices.

Patient care, the stated goal of the Hospital, also changed in the three decades on Lexington Avenue, although the patient population continued to comprise predominantly Jews of the group known as the "worthy poor." The changes in care were basic and extensive. Once admitted, patients might have found themselves on one of the new specialty wards: the Pediatrics, Eye and Ear, Neurology, Genito-Urinary, and Dermatology Services were all created during this time. In 1896, a second dedicated operating room with attendant anesthesia and recovery space was created. After 1900, patients might even be x-rayed with new equipment that had just been received, and laboratory tests might be performed on their urine and blood.

Better patient care was also ensured by the creation of the House Staff and by the presence of the Training School for Nurses. At this time,

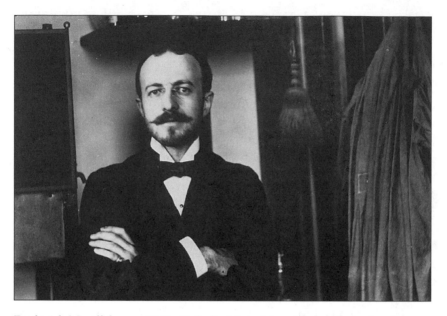

Frederick Mandlebaum, M.D., Pathologist, in laboratory at Lexington Avenue site, c. 1900.

the infamous competitive examinations were developed for applicants seeking a place on the Resident staff, a practice that lasted into the 1950s and the arrival of the National Resident Matching Program. Young doctors eagerly sought House Staff positions at Mount Sinai, because of its distinguished staff and the opportunity for learning, as well as the lack of available openings for young doctors of the Jewish faith at other institutions.

The nursing school brought an influx of student help to the wards, as well as one graduate, professional nurse to oversee and teach them, immensely improving and standardizing the quality of care given. Still, although the School was founded in 1881, it was not until 1885 that the female nursing students could appear on the male medical ward, and it was 1897 before they could work on the male surgical ward.[2,3]

Women also came to the new Mount Sinai as doctors. In 1872, Ann A. Angell was added to the House Staff (but apparently did not graduate), and Eliza Phelps was appointed Apothecary. Josephine Walter was said to be the first woman in the country to graduate from a formal house staff program when she received her Mount Sinai diploma in 1885. Mary Putnam Jacobi ran the Pediatric Division of the Dispensary, where most of the other women appointees could be found. (The Directors would not allow Jacobi's husband, Abraham, later known as the Father of American Pediatrics, to head both the inpatient and the outpatient divisions.) The female presence remained small, however, and women were banned from the House Staff entirely from 1911 to 1922.

Changes in medicine and society were combining to make hospitals in general a more acceptable place for all classes of people: the increased range of treatments available, especially in the surgical realm, with the growing use of aseptic and antiseptic technique; the lack of extended family networks to provide care as people moved to the City to find work in the growing industrial plants; and the improved, more sanitary

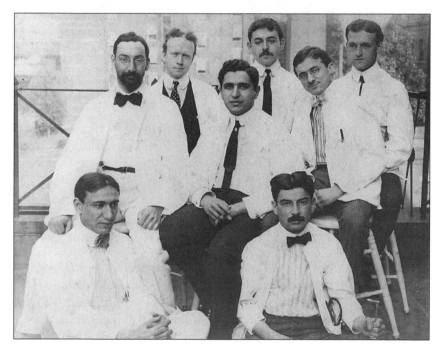

House Staff, January–June, 1902. Row 1: Drs. Meyer Stark, Major G. Seelig; Row 2: Drs. Alfred Fabian Hess, Edwin Beer, Eli Moschcowitz; Row 3: Drs. Fred H. McCarthy, D. Lee Hirschlet, S. S. Goldwater. Goldwater became the Superintendent of The Mount Sinai Hospital in 1903 and pioneered in the field of hospital administration.

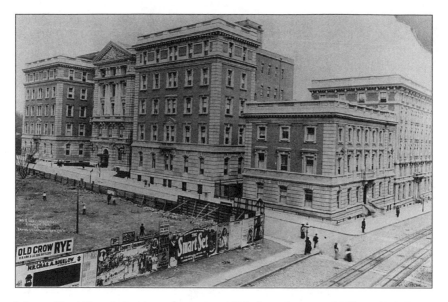

Mount Sinai Hospital at its current site, 100th Street between Fifth and Madison Avenues, 1904.

facilities that hospitals were providing. All of these factors and others convinced more and more people to spend periods of illness on the wards or in one of the private rooms found at the Hospital—a portent of things to come.

THE THIRD MOUNT SINAI HOSPITAL, 1904–

On March 15, 1904, the new home of The Mount Sinai Hospital, on Fifth Avenue at 100th Street, was dedicated. The expanded facilities—ten pavilions and 456 beds—provided the opportunity for increased patient care programs and research. The number of clinical departments grew as specialties received their own services: Otology (1909), Physical Therapy (1911), and Neurosurgery (1932). Other important divisions begun in these early years were Social Work (1906), the third such service in the country,[4] and Dietetics (1905); several clinics, including the Diabetes Clinic (1917), the Children's Health Class (1919), and a Mental Hygiene Clinic (1920), were opened. The Social Service Auxiliary, today's Auxiliary Board, also dates from this period. This organization was formed in 1916 to provide monetary and manpower support to social service–related activities at the Hospital, usually in conjunction with the Social Service Department. Its impact on the Hospital has been tremendous, and its record of success includes the founding of the Volunteer Department, the Patient Library, and the Hospital gift shops. Today the Auxiliary Board works tirelessly in supporting vital Hospital and community outreach projects.

The larger research facilities and an increased research program led to many important results that form the basis of this book. Beginning in 1899, the scientific environment led Mount Sinai itself to publish special reports noting various studies and summaries. In 1934, the *Journal of The Mount Sinai Hospital* was created as another venue for the publication of the scientific work emanating from the laboratories. The first Editor of the *Journal* was Joseph Globus, the well-known neuropathologist.

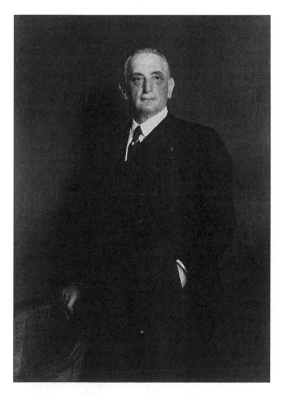

George Blumenthal, President of the Board of Trustees of The Mount Sinai Hospital, 1911–38.

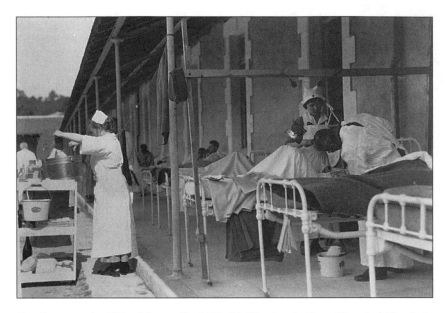

Outdoor ward of The Mount Sinai World War I unit, Base Hospital No. 3, in France, 1919.

In what has been a recurring theme in Mount Sinai's existence, six years after the move to 100th Street, the Hospital began renovations and additions to the existing buildings. In 1913, in the continuing search for adequate space, it announced plans to add seven more buildings. Four were completed by 1915, but World War I and the poor economy delayed until 1922 the opening of the Guggenheim Pavilion, the Einstein-Falk Pavilion for children, the Walter Children's Clinic, and the Blumenthal Auditorium.

The Great Depression deeply affected Mount Sinai. In 1928, the Hospital began planning another series of renovations, but these could not be completed until 1937 (the exception was the Semi-Private Pavilion, later known as the Stella S. Housman Pavilion, which opened in 1931. The Depression also lowered the patient census, particularly in the Private Pavilion, but also in the OPD. In 1931, salaries were cut. Two years later, the Social Service Department opened an occupational therapy workroom to provide rehabilitation and moral support for unemployed patients. The next year, private nurses were given the option of working either an eight-hour or the customary twelve-hour shift; the

Hospital believed that shortening the length of the shifts would make more jobs available.

The first half of the twentieth century brought the devastation of two world wars. Mount Sinai was active in both war efforts. In 1918, twenty physicians, two dentists, fifty nurses, and fifty-three enlisted men, many from the Mount Sinai staff, joined together to form Mount Sinai's unit, Base Hospital No. 3. This group was posted to an old monastery in Montpont, Dordogne, France, which they converted into a five hundred-bed hospital that ultimately housed 2,800 patients at a time.[5] On August 28, 1942, representatives of this unit passed their flag on to the leaders of the Third General Hospital, Sinai's World War II group. They served tirelessly in North Africa, Italy, and France before returning home in 1945. Mount Sinai had 802 staff members, professional and lay, in service to the country by the end of 1945, nine of whom died while serving.

It was in the area of teaching that Mount Sinai's program grew the most at the 100th Street site. In 1905, Mount Sinai held its first Clinical Pathological Conference; Sir William Osler was the speaker. These

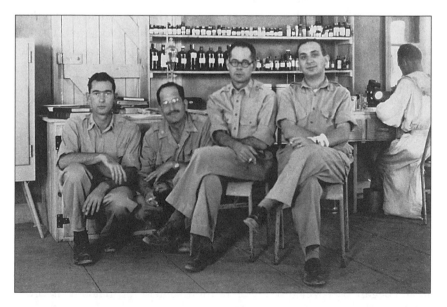

In the laboratory of the Third General Hospital, Mount Sinai's World War II unit. From left to right: Drs. Gerson Lesnick, Solomon Silver, Abou Pollack, Louis Wasserman.

conferences for the staff—later, outsiders were invited—expanded over the years and after World War I became a regular aspect of Mount Sinai's postgraduate teaching efforts. In 1923, the Hospital reached an agreement with Columbia University to provide formal postgraduate courses under Columbia's aegis. Undergraduate medical students from Columbia and from New York University also received instruction on Mount Sinai's wards.

In 1952, Mount Sinai celebrated its centennial in high fashion. A dinner was held at the Waldorf-Astoria Hotel, with the Mayor of New York City, The Honorable Vincent R. Impellitieri, the Governor of New York, His Excellency Thomas E. Dewey, and one of New York's Senators, The Honorable Herbert H. Lehman, in attendance, along with Dr. Arthur H. Compton, a Nobel Prize winner. To mark the occasion, the Hospital issued a book on its history,[6] and a maternity pavilion was opened—the first time Mount Sinai had an obstetrics service. Shortly after this, the Atran and Berg laboratory buildings were dedicated for the continued expansion of clinical and scientific laboratory work.

The post–World War II era was a turning point for Mount Sinai. The need for new clinical services—Obstetrics and Psychiatry, in particular—led to two campus expansions, as first the Klingenstein Pavilion (1952) and then the Klingenstein Clinical Center (1962) opened. The latter building allowed the Hospital to close the 1904 wards and remodel them into more modern accommodations, ending the period of large open wards at Mount Sinai. Unions came to the Hospital with a strike in 1959 that highlighted the change in hospital-employee relations from a patriarchal employer/caretaker relationship in which the staff accepted meals and accommodations in lieu of salary to a modern employer/employee relationship increasingly bound by regulations and contracts.

Other factors outside the institution had a profound influence on its functioning. One was the advent of Medicare and Medicaid in the mid-1960s, which changed the relationship between patients and hospitals, as well as between the government and hospitals. Hospitals were no longer charitable institutions giving away free care in exchange for government subsidies and tax exemption. Hospitals now were entitled to and began to expect and rely on reimbursement for that care. In order to obtain those funds, they had to comply with a raft of regulations, forms, and formalities and to implement organizational changes that would support these new programs. At Mount Sinai, this included opening a pioneering in-house Legal Department in 1972, perhaps the first such hospital department in the country.

Another societal change of major importance to Mount Sinai was the lessening of anti-Semitism in the medical profession. After World War II, federal money flowed to hospitals for the expansion of buildings and research programs. This allowed institutions around the country to expand their residency programs. The desire for the best candidates was stronger than the institutionalized anti-Semitism, and young Jewish physicians found many doors open to them that had previously been closed, including those at the new academic medical centers that had begun to form in the 1930s, where medical schools and hospitals were built in proximity to encourage the sort of translational research that is ubiquitous today.[7] Ironically, this diminution of prejudice adversely affected Mount Sinai; the Hospital lost residents to more academic settings and saw that, further down the line, it would lose young physician-scientists from its staff.

This change is related to another element that affected Mount Sinai—the transition of biomedical research from the clinically driven bedside-to-bench work in which the Hospital excelled to the basic science, laboratory-based molecular research that was not dependent on the presence of patients or physicians. In the 1960s, The Mount Sinai Hospital was ranked twenty-seventh in the country for receiving research funds from the federal government, a tremendous feat for a stand-alone hospital. But, as biomedical science continued to change, it was clear that Mount Sinai would lose ground.

Several department chairmen, including Hans Popper, of Pathology, Alexander B. Gutman, of Medicine, and Horace Hodes, of Pediatrics, suggested to the Trustees that if Mount Sinai was to maintain its high standards of patient care, it needed to recruit the best physicians and residents. For this to happen, Mount Sinai had to explore the concept of opening its own medical school. Despite the serious reservations of some, and the tremendous effort required to recruit and retain basic science faculty and to provide a building to house the research laboratories and teaching spaces necessary for the Medical School, the Trustees set about creating a school.

Joseph Klingenstein and then Gustave L. Levy headed the Boards of Trustees that during the 1960s led the efforts to create the School of Medicine. The provisional charter of The Mount Sinai Hospital School of Medicine was granted in 1963; the absolute charter was received in

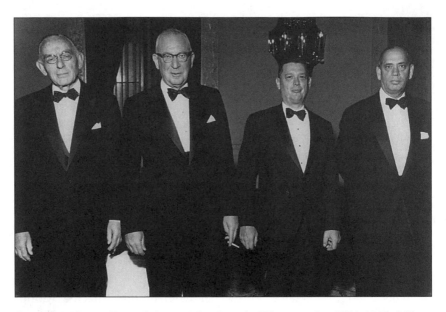

Four Presidents. From left to right: Joseph Klingenstein, 1956–1962; Milton Steinbach (MSSM), 1965–1968; George James, M.D., 1965–1972; Gustave L. Levy, 1962–1976.

1968, one year after the school affiliated with The City University of New York and the same year students first entered. Mount Sinai's clinical excellence was recognized when the new School was allowed to enroll both a first- and a third-year class in its first year of operation. To this day the School continues the postgraduate and house staff training programs originally created by the Hospital, as well as incorporating a Graduate School for Biological Sciences and M.D./Ph.D. programs.[8]

Throughout the 1960s and early 1970s, much of the fund- raising and building centered on creating the School, culminating in the dedication of the Annenberg Building in May 1974. The Hospital facilities might have weathered this benign neglect if the financial climate of the country had not turned so dark during the 1970s. Government support for health care and medical education shrank, and the Hospital posted a deficit for the first time in many years. The aging facilities, combined with town/gown issues between voluntary and full-time faculty, made matters worse. The President and Dean during these years, Thomas C.

Chalmers, worked with the Hospital Director, Samuel Davis, to begin a strategic planning effort aimed at making Mount Sinai one of the top ten academic medical centers in the country. Organizational changes were begun in the Hospital; departmental reviews were begun in the School. A new faculty practice plan began to function.

Matters improved slowly during the early 1980s, with the brightest note being the Trustees' commitment to rebuild the Hospital. In 1986, the Hospital began the demolition of the remaining 1904 buildings to make way for the new Guggenheim Pavilion, designed by the renowned architect I. M. Pei. This building opened in stages and was dedicated in 1992. Only three years later, a new research facility was opened on Madison Avenue to house patient care areas and additional Medical School laboratories to accommodate the growing research faculty.

In response to the more competitive, leaner times of the 1990s, The Mount Sinai Hospital, with John W. Rowe, M.D., serving as President, created a series of affiliations with area healthcare facilities. The Mount Sinai Health System at its largest included more than forty institutions. These loose connections were designed to bring Mount Sinai faculty

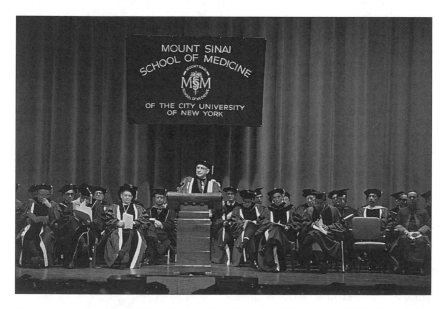

First commencement of the Mount Sinai School of Medicine, 1970. Hans Popper, M.D., Ph.D., at the podium.

and/or services to a wider area and to provide tertiary-care referrals to Mount Sinai. In 1996, development of the Health System was overshadowed by the announcement that The Mount Sinai Hospital was beginning merger talks with the New York University Medical Center. The goal of the merger was to promote cost efficiencies and to streamline back-office operations for the merged entities. The hospitals did not plan to merge clinical services but hoped that the merger would facilitate the adoption of "best practices" through a series of committees and task forces. However, in 2001, it was decided that the institutions would step back from further attempts to merge and would return to more campus-based governance and re-emphasize their historically distinct identities.

As The Mount Sinai Hospital celebrates its 150th anniversary, it is reaffirming its mission of excellence in patient care, education, and research. One factor that bodes well for the future is the continued active involvement and interest of the Trustees in the institution, to an extent not found at many modern hospitals. Over the years, it has been the Trustees who have charted the course, found the time, and found the money to make the dreams of the physicians and administrators happen. Leaders have always been found to take the Hospital through the difficult, changing times; this includes George Blumenthal, who raised the funds to build the buildings at Fifth Avenue and then, as President, expanded the programs and facilities in the early 1900s and Gustave L. Levy, who built the Medical School in the 1960s and 1970s.

In recent times, Alfred R. Stern presided over the early planning for the new hospital construction and oversaw the major administrative change in which a single President and Dean of the Medical Center was replaced by a Chief Executive Officer of the Center and a Dean of the Medical School. Under Frederick A. Klingenstein, the new Hospital building opened, and major academic expansion took place with the building of a new research building. And, under the stewardship of Stephen M. Peck, the Health System matured, the merger with New York University Medical Center in 1998 created Mount Sinai—NYU Health, and planning for expansion of research facilities was begun.

Medical staff, even "Giants," come and go. It has been the Trustees who have carried and maintained the vision of The Mount Sinai Hospital as "this House of noble deeds"[9] for 150 years.

PART I

THE FIRST DEPARTMENTS
Medicine and Surgery

THE DEPARTMENT OF MEDICINE

I

The Leadership of the Department of Medicine

OF ALL OF the "Giants" in Mount Sinai's past, few were bigger than the ones that ruled the medical wards at Mount Sinai. Names such as Libman, Brill, Baehr, and Oppenheimer would all find a place in a "Who's Who" of twentieth-century medicine. There were several factors that brought them to Mount Sinai during the first decades of the 1900s. The first was the stature of those who had come before: Abraham Jacobi, Edward G. Janeway, Alfred Loomis, and Alfred Meyer. There was the sense at Mount Sinai of being a member of an elite group of physicians, carefully selected and trained, nurtured with additional training abroad and then moved up the ranks. Also, there was the relentless anti-Semitism that kept some from pursuing residencies at other hospitals. It was clear that if one were a young Jewish physician with high ambitions, the wards of Mount Sinai were the place to be.

The groundwork for this environment was laid by the first physicians who staffed the Hospital at its opening in 1855. During the first fifty years of the Hospital's existence, it was not unusual for the physicians to be general practitioners in the broadest sense, seeing patients of all ages and performing deliveries and minor surgeries as needed. Abraham Jacobi, the "Father of American Pediatrics," was on Mount Sinai's staff for almost twenty years before he was given the title of Pediatrician. Prior to this he was a Consulting Physician. The "Consulting" title was accurate at the time. Mount Sinai's early staff usually consisted of four Consulting Physicians who visited the Hospital as needed or as they saw fit and as their active private practices allowed. The first staff of Consultant Physicians was Benjamin McCready, Chandler Gilman, William H. Maxwell, and William Detmold, an orthopedic surgeon in this prespecialty era. These men all had established reputations in the medical community, and their appointments augured great things for the young hospital.

The day-to-day medical affairs of the Jews' Hospital, as Mount Sinai was originally called, were run by the Resident and Attending

Physician, Mark Blumenthal, and then by his successor, Seligman Teller. Blumenthal was the official doctor for the Portuguese Congregation and had an active practice. As Resident Physician, he kept office hours to see patients who were applying for admission to the Hospital and was responsible for overseeing their care while they were in the Hospital. For these efforts, he was paid $250 the first year, a sum that later increased to $500. Teller, who served for twelve years, eventually received only $400 each year, but the Hospital found him an apartment nearby and helped pay the rent. He also maintained an active general practice on the side.

The Hospital had forty-five beds when it opened in 1855. The rules governing admission stated that all patients should be of the Jewish faith, with the exception of accident victims, and it was decided early on to exclude those with incurable, malignant, or contagious diseases. This rule was rather loosely interpreted, with the medical staff arguing persuasively that if typhoid cases could be segregated, the patients could be relieved of suffering while posing little danger to other patients. It was also a continuing source of dismay to the doctors and Directors that a number of chronic patients found their way to Mount Sinai's beds. The Directors urged the Jewish community leadership for many years to open a chronic care pavilion. This situation was alleviated by the creation of the Montefiore Home in 1884.

In 1872, the Hospital, cramped in its small quarters on 28th Street, moved to a larger space on Lexington Avenue, between 66th and 67th streets. The new Hospital had 120 beds when it opened and eventually grew to 200. The beds were divided solely by male and female; there was no separation of medical and surgical patients until five years later. The move to 67th Street precipitated two major changes for the medical staff. The first was the creation of a formal Medical Board to oversee "all matters appertaining to the Medical Management of the Hospital."[1] The second innovation was the creation of a house staff system. With the move to larger quarters, it was believed that two young physicians would be needed to live in and help the Resident Physician to oversee the 120 beds. Appointment to the House Staff would be by competitive examination, and the new Medical Board took it upon itself to test the applying physicians and to recommend appointments to the Directors for the House Staff positions.

This House Staff plan was changed in 1877 to conform to the newly divided Medical and Surgical services. After this time there were four positions: Resident Senior and Junior Physician and Resident Senior and Junior Surgeon. (The "Resident" was later changed to "House.") Again, those applying for these positions were vetted by the Consulting staff, initially through an oral exam and then through oral and written tests. These were "mixed" two-year internships; the doctors spent time on both services as Juniors and finished with a year as Senior on the selected service. They were years of intense learning; the resident oversaw all the patients, performed rudimentary tests, and aided accident victims. It was also a time when a tennis game on the court behind the Hospital could be interrupted by the sound of a steam whistle or (later) a gong announcing the arrival of an Attending. Since the tennis court could be accessed only from a window at the back of one of the wards, it could get exciting.

The Attendings on the medical service who served the Hospital on Lexington Avenue were a distinguished group. They included Alfred Loomis, Alfred Meyer, Edward G. Janeway, Julius Rudisch, and H. Newton Heineman. These men were important for their encouragement and support of the concepts that led Mount Sinai into the forefront of American medicine in the early twentieth century: the recognition of the role of the hospital as a teaching institution and of research as an important adjunct to hospital work. This included Meyer's creation of a library at the Hospital in 1883[2] and the efforts of many to convince the Directors of the value and need for a laboratory.

Several Mount Sinai physicians, especially the younger ones, traveled to Germany and studied the role of the laboratory, particularly pathology, in clinical medicine. Rudisch was trained in Germany and early on realized the potential of applying new laboratory techniques in chemistry and pathology to medicine. His interest was in diabetes, and he did later work in the medical applications of physics and electricity. He spent his retirement years studying chemistry.[3]

In 1893, the first rudimentary laboratory was established at Mount Sinai in a former cloak closet. H. Newton Heineman, M.D., paid for this laboratory. He also covered the salary of an assistant, making the fortuitous choice of Frederick Mandlebaum, who would lead the laboratories for the next quarter century. Heineman arranged and paid for Mandlebaum's training in Europe. In 1896, when Heineman retired to live abroad, Mandlebaum was made chief of the Pathology Laboratory.[4]

Another Attending of note was Edward Gameliel Janeway, "the greatest diagnostician of his day," according to Emanuel Libman.[5] A graduate of Columbia University's College of Physicians and Surgeons (P&S), Class of 1864, Janeway became a professor of Pathological Anatomy at Bellevue Medical College and later served as the school's Dean. He was a Health Commissioner of New York and took a special interest in tuberculosis. Heineman, Mandlebaum, and Janeway, among others, helped establish at Mount Sinai the value of a laboratory, not only to support the clinical work of the hospital but also to add to the base of scientific knowledge and to provide better training to young physicians.

The years on Lexington Avenue were a transitional time for Mount Sinai, as it was transformed from the care-taking facility of the mid-1800s into what is considered a modern hospital, with laboratories and specialized services. One of the components formed during these years was an Out-Patient Department (OPD). The work of the Hospital had always included taking care of accident victims, but the Hospital had long wanted to serve patients who required medical care but not hospitalization. This became increasingly important because the Hospital, no matter how many beds it contained, was never able to meet the demands on its services. By 1875, an Out-Patient Department was fully functioning, with an Internal (Medical) clinic. A separate staff ran the OPD at that time, with no oversight from the inpatient Attendings. In the 1920s, this changed, and one Chief of Service was put over both the inpatient and the outpatient staffs.

In 1893, the Hospital reorganized the medical staff to handle the ever-increasing volume of patients. A new category was created, the Assistant Attendings, later known as Adjuncts. On the Medical Service, the first two Assistants were Nathan Brill and Morris Manges.

Nathan Brill was born in 1860 and educated in New York, at City College. He interned at Bellevue Hospital, studied in France, and then worked on comparative anatomy and congenital defects of the nervous system. He learned his clinical medicine from E. G. Janeway. Brill was named Attending in 1898, serving until 1913. In his ward rounds he was quiet, serious, considerate, and unassuming. He was an authoritative master of diagnosis, renowned for scrupulous honesty and for defending truth. Brill's accomplishments were many. He defined endemic typhus (Brill's disease), coined the term Gaucher's disease (with Mandlebaum) and recognized it as a lipid storage disease, and described a form of lymphoma that became known as Brill-Symmer's disease.[6]

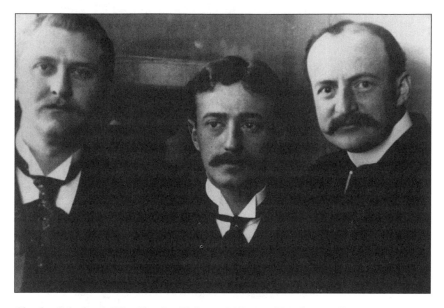

Charles Schultz, M.D., Charles Elsberg, M.D., and Nathan Brill, M.D.

Morris Manges became a full Attending in 1898. Manges was also a product of City College and received his M.D. from P&S. He studied in Berlin and Vienna and joined the Mount Sinai staff in 1892. A prominent consultant, Manges had appointments at various medical schools in New York City. Like other Mount Sinai physicians during these years, Manges had a wide range of interests and talents but was considered to be primarily a gastroenterologist.[7] He was an artist and a collector. He was a member of the American Climatological Association, the New York Pathological Society, the American Gastroenterological Association, and the Archeological Institute of America. He was also a fellow of The New York Academy of Medicine, to which he donated the first specimen of radium to be brought to the United States. A patient of his had acquired this specimen at his advice in 1902. The treatment failed, but the widow gave Manges the radium, who, in turn, gave it to the Academy.[8]

In 1904, Mount Sinai moved to its current home on 100th Street between Fifth and Madison Avenues. At the time, the Medical Service was in the hands of four men: Alfred Meyer, Julius Rudisch, Nathan Brill, and Morris Manges. With the much larger facilities at 100th Street, the House Staff was enlarged to four physicians in each year of the two-and-one-half-year program. By 1908, a separate Resident in Medicine was appointed to care for the Private Pavilion patients.

In 1905, a series of important meetings took place at Mount Sinai. One of the leaders in medicine, Sir William Osler, then at the Johns Hopkins University School of Medicine, was brought in to give a clinical conference at the Hospital. While he was visiting at Mount Sinai, the Trustees took the opportunity to speak with him about the role of medical education and research at a hospital such as Mount Sinai, laying the groundwork for the changes that would occur over the next decade. These included the expansion of the laboratories, the beginning of dedicated research and education funds to send young doctors abroad for training, the admission of medical students on the wards for clinical training, and the establishment of a formal postgraduate training program. Osler came to Mount Sinai in part because of his friendship with a Mount Sinai physician, Emanuel Libman.

Libman (1872–1946) interned at The Mount Sinai Hospital and studied in Vienna, Berlin, Munich, and Graz. He had plans to become a pediatrician but became excited by research while in Theodor von Escherich's laboratory in Graz, where he discovered the Libman Streptococcus.[9] Upon his return to Mount Sinai, he accepted an appointment as Assistant and then Associate Pathologist under Mandlebaum. His devotion to routine autopsies made him an unparalleled authority on clinical disease and helped give Mount Sinai a national and then international reputation. He started the bacteriology laboratory and pioneered in the early uses of blood cultures.[10] In 1903, Libman received an appointment in the Department of Medicine. His brilliance as a rapid diagnostician was modeled on Janeway's powerful memory and an "I have seen this before" attitude. Libman was a leader in the study of subacute bacterial endocarditis, including naming the entity on the basis of extensive casework. Noting that some lesions were bacteria-free, he described with Benjamin Sacks atypical verrucous endocarditis, which, with or without lupus erythmatosus skin lesions, now bears their joint eponym as Libman-Sacks endocarditis. In addition to these observations, his association of coronary artery thrombosis and its clinical presentations entitled him to be termed the founder of the "Mount Sinai School of Cardiology" by William Welch, another leader of American medicine at this time.[11]

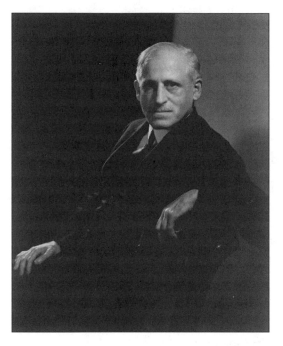

Emanuel Libman, M.D.,
Chief of a Medical Service,
1914–1925.

Libman was an early advocate of continuous medical education both at Mount Sinai and at The New York Academy of Medicine, and he gave or raised funds for several lectureships and traveling fellowships. He worked to save and find jobs for refugee doctors from Europe during the 1930s. He was an historian and rediscovered Thomas Hodgkin's grave in Jaffa; he also helped found the medical college at the Hebrew University in Jerusalem. Libman was in the first rank of both laboratory and clinical medicine, noted for his intellect and indefatigability. He was a loner with few social interactions but a distinct public persona. He was the only Mount Sinai physician to appear on the cover of *Time* magazine and to be profiled in both *The New Yorker* and *The Reader's Digest*, and his actions and interactions helped cement Mount Sinai's reputation at the highest rank.[12]

By the end of the 1920s, the Medical Services had assumed a more modern form. The inpatient and outpatient areas had been combined under one Chief, and the two staffs had begun to merge, although they never reached the level of integration desired. The Department had an active teaching program. The House Staff program continued to be very competitive and to provide excellent training to young doctors interested in both clinical and research work. Regular clinical-pathological conferences (CPCs) were held on Friday afternoons, filling the auditorium with both clinicians from the Hospital and members of the community. Undergraduate students from the New York University School of Medicine (NYU) and P&S received clinical training on the wards. In 1923, the Hospital began a postgraduate teaching program under the auspices of Columbia University. Several special lectures were also offered each year, including the William Welch Lecture and the E. G. Janeway Lecture (both endowed by Libman), which brought speakers from around the country and from around the world to lecture and to visit at Mount Sinai.

In 1920, the Hospital had three Attendings overseeing two Medical services, with five Associate Physicians and eight Adjuncts. There was the older Brill and Manges, along with the slightly younger Libman. (There was also a young Adjunct named Henry W. Berg, whose surgeon brother, A. A. Berg, would later endow a building at Mount Sinai in his honor.)[13] In 1922, Manges retired. Brill followed two years later, leaving Libman to run things alone until his own retirement in 1925. The Medical Services were without leadership in 1926–1927. In January 1928, a new generation of physicians was ready to take charge: Leo Kessel, Bernard S. Oppenheimer, and George Baehr. Two physicians oversaw the medical services, while the other was in charge of the Out-Patient Department every third year in succession.

Leo Kessel followed what had become the typical Mount Sinai pattern: born in New York in 1881, he attended P&S (1903) and obtained a House Staff position at Mount Sinai. He did clinical research on the thyroid, exophthalmic goiter (Graves Disease), pneumonia, and tuberculosis. He died in 1932 at the age of fifty-one.

Bernard Sutro Oppenheimer was, again, a native New Yorker and a product of P&S (1901), via Harvard University. He interned at Mount Sinai and then spent the typical year abroad studying pathology and physiology. He later went back to Europe to learn more about the budding field of cardiology and on his return helped establish Mount Sinai as an early leader in this field.[14] Well rounded and well traveled, Oppenheimer made another singular contribution to Mount Sinai: the establishment here of the tradition of the Gold-Headed Cane. This is modeled on a British ritual of giving a cane to a distinguished practitioner, which they pass on to a physician once they reach retirement age. The

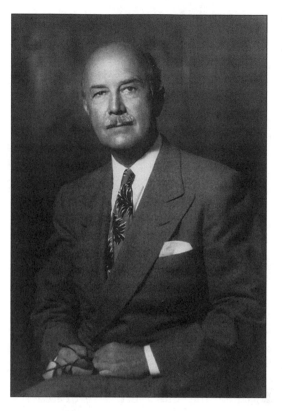

George Baehr, M.D., Chief
of the First Medical Ser-
vice, 1928–1950.

criteria at Mount Sinai is that the holder of the cane reflect the best values of a compassionate physician. This tradition has served to honor
many of Mount Sinai's most dedicated healers.[15]

But the man of this era who left the greatest mark on Mount Sinai
and on the world of medicine was George Baehr (1887–1978). He was
born and educated in New York, receiving his M.D. from P&S in 1908.
He then interned at Mount Sinai in surgery, because "he felt the discipline of surgical responsibilities would be good training."[16] He went
abroad to study pathology with Ludwig Aschoff in Freiburg and experimental pharmacology in Vienna. He was a member of the Sanitary
Commission that worked on typhus in the Balkans in 1915–1916 and
was captured during World War I. He was later part of a prisoner exchange and continued his research on the epidemic, eventually receiving decorations from both Serbia and Bulgaria. He returned to
Mount Sinai and in October 1918 was placed in command of the three

thousand-bed Mount Sinai Base Hospital No. 3 that served in France in 1918–1919. Upon his return to the States, he was appointed Associate Pathologist in charge of Morbid Anatomy and the Autopsy Lab. Baehr was named Chief of the First Medical Service in 1927. The weekly CPCs offered by Baehr and Paul Klemperer, the Chief of Pathology, became famous and were attended by hundreds of physicians from around the City. These lasted until Baehr's formal retirement from Mount Sinai in 1950. In his later years, Baehr was very active in helping Mount Sinai establish its school of medicine, using his contacts and his reputation to help smooth the way and to raise needed funds.

Baehr made seminal contributions to the world of medicine. He did early work in the laboratory and in the field on typhus and was the first to isolate *Rickettsia prowazeki* in the blood.[17] With many others at Mount Sinai during these years when Libman was ascendant, Baehr also did work on subacute bacterial endocarditis, publishing an important paper in 1912 that drew attention to the renal lesions in SBE.[18] Together with Klemperer and Abou Pollack, he enunciated the concept of collagen disease.[19] Also with Klemperer and Arthur Schifrin, Baehr published the first description of the vascular lesions in lupus.[20] In 1940, he was part of a team that made a major breakthrough in the treatment of syphilis that was announced at a press conference at The New York Academy of Medicine: a five-day intensive intravenous drip therapy using arsenicals, greatly shortening the time and cost of treatment.[21] The research was begun in 1932, and the researchers included Harold Hyman, Baehr, William Leifer, and Louis Chargin. This work was quickly eclipsed by the arrival of modern antibiotics and, although it constituted a breakthrough at the time, it is forgotten now.

Baehr was extremely interested in public health issues and healthcare delivery and received the Sedgewick Memorial Award in 1967 from the American Public Health Association. In 1931, he created the Consultation Service at Mount Sinai so that individuals of moderate means could take advantage of all of the diagnostic resources of Mount Sinai for a flat fee of $35. This was an important step for Mount Sinai and only the second such program in this country. The patients had to be referred by their private physicians, and, at the end of the workup, the test results were reported to the physician for his or her continued management. The Consultation Service continued until 1958, when changes in the healthcare system made it unnecessary. In 1947, Baehr helped establish the Health Insurance Plan (HIP) with his friend and patient New York City Mayor Fiorello LaGuardia, and over the years Baehr served as President and Medical Director of HIP, as well. In the Second World War, he was Chief Medical Officer for Civil Defense in the United States Public Health Service (USPHS).

Baehr's record of public service was exemplary. He served New York City (Board of Health and Board of Hospitals, for more than twenty-five years), New York State (the New York State Public Health Council, for thirty-five years), the nation (Health Council of the National Institutes of Health [NIH], the first scientific advisory board of NIH, the USPHS), and the international community (conferences on standardizing the nomenclature of causes of death). His administrative skills resulted in his election as President of Mount Sinai's Medical Board and of The New York Academy of Medicine. His remarkable career as pathologist, clinician, teacher, administrator, and public health proponent depended partly on his intellect and rapid decision making but also on his regal appearance, self-assurance, and love of power, which he used to further his ambitions for social justice.

After Kessel's death in 1932, Baehr and Oppenheimer assumed control of the two medical services. Baehr ran the First Medical Service wards and clinics, and Oppenheimer the Second Medical Service wards and clinics. Each service had a male and a female ward, with each housing between thirty-seven and forty beds. When Oppenheimer retired in 1940, Eli Moschcowitz took over the Second Medical Service.

Eli Moschcowitz (1879–1964) was born in Hungary and immigrated at age two to New York, where he was educated and received an M.D. from P&S in 1900. He interned at Mount Sinai and then spent a year in Ludwig Pick's pathological laboratory in Berlin. He came back to New York, to Beth Israel and then to Mount Sinai, as Attending Pathologist and Physician. Moschcowitz was the first to show that anaphylactic disease was accompanied by general eosinophilia.[22] His was the first description of thrombotic thrombocytopenic purpura, or Moschcowitz's disease.[23] He also was the first to describe pulmonary hypertension[24] and made significant contributions to the understanding of amyloidosis, colitis, glomerulonephritis, ileitis, and thyrotoxicosis. He was one of the first internists to emphasize the influence of the psyche in initiating and perpetuating diseases in individual patients, work that culminated in his book *Biology of Disease*.[25] An erudite diagnostician and teacher, he helped maximize and sustain the Hospital's Jacobi Library. Short and rotund in build, Moschcowitz had a delightful, wry sense of humor and

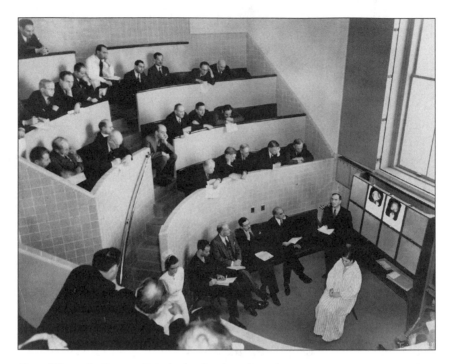

Grand Rounds, Dept. of Medicine. Reuben Ottenberg, M.D., is presenting. Next to him is B. S. Oppenheimer, M.D. David Beck, M.D., is two over from Oppenheimer.

was an accomplished sleight-of-hand magician who captivated his patients, young and old, with his expertise.

Throughout these years, the two medical services were housed to the east of the Administration (Metzger) Pavilion. Alvin Gordon, who began his internship in 1938, has described this arrangement:

> On the main floor of the medical building was the admitting and emergency wards (combined). Ward C was one flight up, Ward E one flight up from that, then H and K. C and K were assigned to the first medical service (Dr. Baehr) while H and E were the second medical service (Dr. Oppenheimer). Each floor had one huge room containing 27 beds, separated only by curtains. The beds were very close together. Ward C and E were for men, H and K for women. Behind each ward were about six small rooms, each with two beds. These rooms were used for

either dying patients or VIP's. . . . The only exception to this rule was Ward E, which had a six-bed room in the back. During my time on the house staff this room was used for a group of six patients who were undergoing an experimental program of a rapid (six-day) treatment of syphilis with continuous IV's of salvarsan.[26]

In a nod to the rise of specialties in medicine, the Department of Medicine was reorganized in 1939 to include six major areas of specialty along with the two general services: gastroenterology, metabolism-nutrition, hematology, allergy, thoracic diseases, and cardiology. The Chief and Assistant in each area were called Associates (or Assistants) in Medicine to differentiate them from the regular Associates and Assistants who were responsible for the routine work of the ward services. These specialists consulted throughout the Hospital, controlled their own specialty clinics, and participated in laboratory work either in their own laboratory, such as hematology, or with established laboratories, such as microbiology or pathology.

The advent of World War II both propelled and restrained changes in the Hospital. During the war years, there could be very few large-scale changes while the Trustees and staff struggled to get through the immediate crisis of the wartime shortages of staff, supplies, and money. All appointments made during these years were provisional, and the Hospital assured all physicians in military service that their positions would be waiting when they returned. The Trustees, the Association of the Junior Staff (now called the Association of the Attending Staff), and the Medical Board collaborated on a unique venture whereby the medical staff who were not in the military and who were continuing to practice placed a percentage of their earnings in a fund. The wife or other beneficiary of each medical staff member in the Armed Forces received a monthly stipend based on the number of dependents and the staff member's years out of medical school. This Fund lasted until six months after the war, and a total of $162,871 was paid out.[27]

But still, the world of medicine—and Mount Sinai—was changing quickly, with advances in therapeutics (penicillin in particular) as well as organizational changes in the Institution. In 1944, Mount Sinai appointed George Baehr Director of Clinical Research, and Isidore Snapper, the Chief of the Second Medical Service, became Director of Medical Education. These were geographic full-time positions, but this was a clear indication of where the future would lie. In 1948, Saul Jarcho was appointed the first full-time Associate Physician.

Isidore Snapper (1889–1973) took over the Second Medical Service at Moschcowitz's retirement in 1944. Snapper's career straddled three continents and many medical disciplines. He was born and educated in Amsterdam (M.D., 1911) and also studied in London and Groningen (Ph.D., 1913). He helped clarify the physiologic basis of red blood cell membrane permeability. Recognizing the difference between bilirubin crystallized from the serum of patients with hemolytic jaundice and that from patients with obstructive jaundice, he developed, with Albert van den Bergh, the "direct" and "indirect" bilirubin assays.[28] Later, he clarified glucuronic acid conjugation. He was appointed professor of medicine in Amsterdam at the age of thirty and was a European master of metabolic medicine. He was multilingual, and his frequent weekend voyages involved his lecturing Friday evenings, directing ward rounds on Saturday, and officiating at a soccer match on Sunday. As a Jew, he felt it wise to leave Holland in 1938 for an appointment at the Rockefeller Foundation in New York, and he was sent to their medical college in Beijing as professor of medicine. Imprisoned by the Japanese on December 7, 1941, he was exchanged in 1942 and served as adviser to the Secretary of Defense in Washington, D.C. In 1944, he was appointed Chief of the Second Medical Service at The Mount Sinai Hospital and full-time Director of Medical Education. Snapper wrote books and many articles on bedside medicine, bone disease, and multiple myeloma. After eight years, he left Mount Sinai and took a similar post at Cook County Hospital, Chicago. He returned to New York in 1953, first to Beth-El (Brookdale) Hospital and then to the Brooklyn Veteran's Administration Hospital. He was a brilliant diagnostician, a stimulating teacher, a creative thinker, and an entertaining showman. He was both imperious and approachable and brought increased international renown to Mount Sinai.

Snapper and Baehr got along like water and oil. There was intense rivalry between the two Medical Services and an overall choosing of sides, even among the Attendings. Snapper and Baehr shared a secretary and took turns firing successive job occupants over their perceived preferences for doing the other's work. There was turmoil, but great intellectual stimulation. Snapper's expertise in medical education helped the Hospital as it moved forward with the postwar expansion of the House Staff from thirty-four to sixty-two, the rise of the modern residency programs, which began in 1942, the rotation of the Residents in the Private and Semi-Private services through the ward service, and the training of veterans who returned from the war in need of updates and specialty training. Postgraduate training with Columbia University continued and grew. The CPCs, rounds, and special lectures again brought hundreds of physicians to Mount Sinai.

Research after the war continued to be a joint effort of the clinicians and the scientists in the various laboratories such as bacteriology or chemistry. Also, small departmental labs were created near the wards for more routine analyses. The work in the Department focused on studying the new antibiotics as they appeared, especially penicillin and streptomycin, and the different vitamins. The specialty groups continued to treat their patients and to run their own clinics and laboratories, overseen by Baehr and Snapper. In 1949, a program was begun to create groupings of doctors working on related research areas. Teams were created in cardiovascular disease, endocrinology, metabolism and nutrition, and radioactive isotopes. The goal was that "Such teams will meet regularly to discuss and program their work so that important planned procedures will replace small isolated projects and repetitious effort."[29] Laboratory space was tight, leading to the construction of the Atran and Henry W. Berg laboratory buildings in 1952–1953.

In 1949, Baehr announced that he would like to retire from Mount Sinai so that he could pursue the direction of the Health Insurance Plan (HIP) of New York. After his resignation from active service at Mount Sinai, he continued as a Consultant Physician and provided assistance as the Hospital moved to create the medical school in the 1960s. With the establishment of the School, Baehr was named a Distinguished Service Professor.

To replace Baehr as Chief of the First Medical Service and Director of Medical Research, Mount Sinai appointed Alexander B. Gutman, a Professor of Medicine at Columbia University and Director of the Columbia Research Service at Goldwater Memorial Hospital. He served with Snapper for one year, and, when Snapper left in 1952, became the first full-time Chief of Medicine, overseeing all of the medical services and activities.

Gutman (1902–1973) was born and educated in New York. He then took the unusual course of obtaining a Ph.D., studying the thyroid and amphibian metamorphosis. He spent 1925 and 1926 in the medical school of Halle, Germany, and received an M.D. in Vienna in 1928. He

Alexander Gutman, M.D.,
Professor and Chairman of
the Dept. of Medicine,
1950–1968.

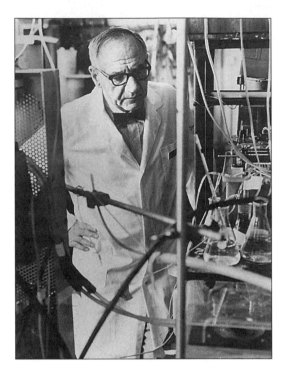

returned to New York to a career in metabolic medicine. At Columbia, he made the first analyses of thyroxin in the human thyroid, studied hyperthyroidism, the parathyroids, bone disease, serum alkaline phosphatase in liver disease, and serum acid phosphatase in metastatic carcinoma of the prostate. He identified Bence Jones protein in serum and introduced the term M protein in myeloma. In his last thirty years, he, along with his longtime colleague Tsai Fan Yu, elucidated the metabolic basis of hyperuricemia and gout and introduced the highly successful uricosuric treatment.[30] Gutman's approach to medicine focused on pathophysiology and clinical investigation; in addition, he was a superb bedside teacher. His lasting memorial is "the Green Journal" (*The American Journal of Medicine*), which he founded in 1946. For ten years, he edited the Cecil-Loeb textbook of medicine. He had a major influence on the sponsorship by the NIH of metabolic research. He was totally singleminded in his intellectual determination and industry, reticent, distant, and intolerant of errors.

Medical education was a primary concern during the Gutman years. When he took over the service, there were twenty Residents in Medicine, more than thirty rotating Interns, and twenty-two Research Assistants. Ten years later, the number of general medicine Residents had held steady, but the number of research positions had grown to almost thirty. (In 1963, the Medicine residency became three years in length.) In 1962, the Hospital began its affiliation with Greenpoint Hospital in Brooklyn, moving the next year to staffing the City Hospital Center at Elmhurst. This presented a challenge for the Department in terms of adequate attending and resident rotations and bringing the municipal hospital up to standard. In 1968, the Department began its affiliation with the Bronx Veterans Administration Hospital (VA).

In 1962, the medical ward service of 142 beds had an average length of stay of 24.5 days. This service was improved with the opening in December of the Klingenstein Clinical Center, which provided more modern facilities for the treatment of ward patients. That year there were

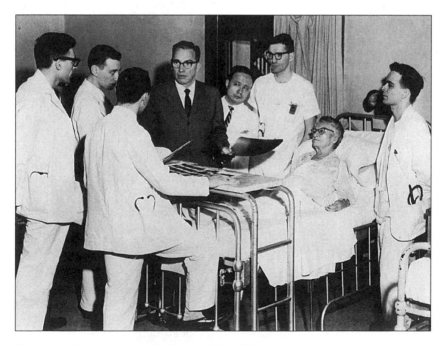

Ward rounds with Louis Siltzbach, M.D., 1950s.

also approximately 120 private and semi-private patients to care for each day, and the twenty-two medical and specialty outpatient clinics received 50,503 visits, representing about one-third of all outpatient activity. Medical care also became more technologically oriented during the 1960s. The first intensive care unit was created in 1962, and the Ames Coronary Care unit opened in 1968. In 1964, a six-bed Clinical Research Center (CRC) was established to allow physicians a place for the intensive study of patients. Sherman Kupfer was the first Director of the CRC.[31] This center was funded by a USPHS Grant and had expanded to twelve beds by 1966.

Gutman was a leading player in the drive to establish a medical school at Mount Sinai. In the late 1950s, he urged the Hospital to obtain an outside review of its research activities. This provided evidence of Mount Sinai's need for and its ability to establish a medical school. In 1966, Gutman became the first Chairman and Professor of Medicine in the new school. With the arrival of the students in 1968, the Department had to have ready a curriculum and clerkships for the students, a massive undertaking. The opening of the school also ended the many years of collaboration with Columbia University for undergraduate and postgraduate teaching.

When Alexander Gutman retired in 1967, both the Department of Medicine and the Hospital itself were much changed. To lead the Department in this new environment, Mount Sinai selected Solomon Berson, a clinician-scientist from the Bronx VA.

Berson (1918–1972) was born and educated in New York. He taught anatomy and physiology while a medical student and interned in Boston in 1945–1946. He came to the Bronx in 1948 for a medical residency and in 1950 became Internist to Rosalyn Yalow's Radioisotope Unit at the VA. In 1954, he was appointed Chief of the VA's first Radioisotope Service and in 1963 became a VA Senior Medical Investigator. The major contributions of this unit are described later in this chapter and are commemorated by the Solomon A. Berson Research Laboratory at the VA.

Berson was a biomedical scientist of Nobel laureate level, a first-rate professional mathematician, a virtuoso violinist and chess player, knowledgeable in history, archeology, literature, and art; there was no family TV. He was a revered role model for students and postgraduates for his teaching of medical science, his quiet yet decisive leadership, and his compassion for the frightened patient. His energy and curiosity

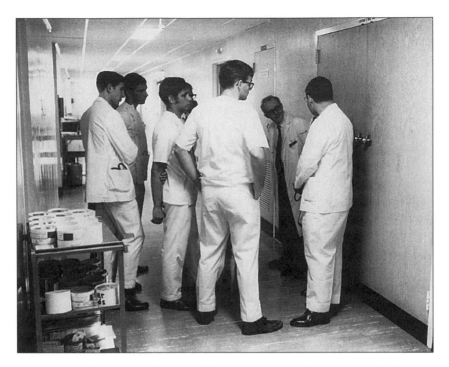

On rounds with Solomon Berson, M.D., Professor and Chairman of the Dept. of Medicine, 1968–1972.

were driven by a perpetual, selfless restlessness intolerant of complacency in both his staff and in himself. His one failing was in evaluating people, and Yalow's cooler head and superior insight were sometimes needed.

Berson was named Chairman at Mount Sinai in 1968, becoming the first Murray M. Rosenberg Professor of Medicine in 1969. This was a transitional time at Mount Sinai as the faculty tinkered with the curriculum of the School and tried to come to grips with town/gown issues between the voluntary clinical faculty and the growing full-time faculty. The advent of Medicare in 1966 also augured changes in medicine. In 1970, the Hospital underwent a clinical reorganization in which semi-private and semi-private division (ward) patients were combined into one group available for the treatment by and training of house staff. Many new divisions were formed in the Department during Berson's brief tenure, including Infectious Disease (1969), Oncology (1970), Rheumatology, and Liver Disease (both 1972.)

The end of the 1960s was also a time when the institution was focused on reaching out into the community more. One program that resulted from this orientation was the Narcotics Rehabilitation Center, which opened in 1970 and utilized methadone maintenance for the initial treatment of heroin dependency. Started by Barry Stimmel and Hillel Tobias, the Center was unique: it was the first such program in New York City to be located within an academic medical center; it was the first program in the City to initiate methadone maintenance therapy purely on an ambulatory basis; it was a pioneer in the use of a multidisciplinary approach to treatment that involved internists, psychiatrists, social workers, psychologists, nurses, vocational rehabilitation counselors, and former heroin users; and it served as the locus of many research projects related to heroin use and methadone treatment, including the first large-scale studies of the effectiveness of methadone maintenance.[32] The Center continues today to provide primary care to its current daily census of more than seven-hundred patients.

Berson never moved his research from the Bronx, and, after long days at Mount Sinai, he would make his way to the VA and his laboratory to continue his work with the radioisotope unit. One of Berson's first acts as Chairman was to secure an appointment to the faculty for Rosalyn Yalow. Yalow accepted the appointment, even though she had argued against Berson's accepting the chairmanship in the beginning. She was appointed a Research Professor in the Department of Medicine in 1968 and later became the Solomon Berson Distinguished Professor at Large.

Rosalyn Yalow (1921–) was born and educated in New York. She was the first physics major at Hunter College and later became the sole woman at the University of Illinois College of Engineering, receiving an M.A. in physics and then, in 1945, a Ph.D. in nuclear physics. She returned to Hunter College in 1945 to teach and perform research. She joined the Bronx VA Hospital radiotherapy service, part time in 1947 and full time from 1950 to 1980, serving as Senior Medical Investigator from 1972.

At the Bronx, Yalow developed a long-standing collaboration with Berson. Together, they first used radioisotopes to measure blood volume and the distribution of plasma proteins in body compartments, as well as to diagnose thyroid dysfunction. They postulated the presence of, and went on to demonstrate, insulin-binding antibodies in insulin-treated patients and then revolutionized medical science, especially endocrinology and metabolism, by developing the radioimmunoassay in 1957, first of insulin and later of growth hormone, ACTH, parathormone, and gastrin.[33]

In 1972, Berson died unexpectedly of a heart attack while away at a meeting. In 1977, Yalow received the Nobel Prize for their work. In her words of acceptance, she said:

> For the past thirty years I have been committed to the development and application of radioisotopic methodology to analyze the fine structure of biologic systems. From 1950 until his untimely death in 1972, Dr. Solomon Berson was joined with me in this scientific adventure and together we gave birth to and nurtured through its infancy, radioimmunoassay, a powerful tool for determination of virtually any substance of biologic interest. Would that he were here to share this moment.[34]

She continues as a Distinguished Service Professor at the Mount Sinai School of Medicine.

After Berson's death, Fenton Schaffner, an expert on liver disease, was appointed Acting Chairman of the Department.[35] It was a hard time for the Department. The Dean of the School, George James, and then its own chairman had died unexpectedly within months of each other. The physical facilities of the institution had suffered as all available money was spent to create the Medical School. The parameters of the faculty practice plan were being argued, and the voluntary faculty were unhappy. Federal funds for medical schools and research were drying up at the time the young school was trying to build an identity as an academic medical center.

In 1974, Richard Gorlin was appointed the new leader of the Department. Gorlin (1926–1997) was born in Jersey City and qualified at Harvard Medical School in 1948. He spent the next twenty-six years (apart from a year at St. Thomas' Hospital, London) at Brigham Hospital, rising to Chief of its cardiovascular division in 1969. His research fields were coronary artery disease, digitalis and vasodilators in heart failure, cardiac catheterization, ventricular enlargement, and thrombolysis in myocardial infarction.[36]

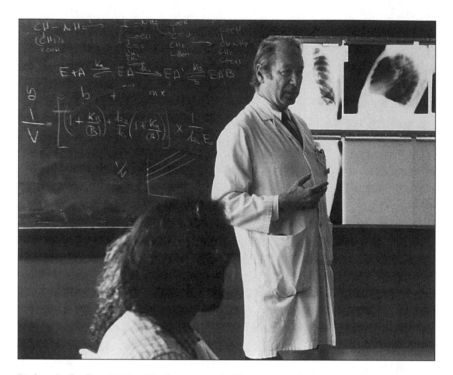

Richard Gorlin, M.D., Professor and Chairman of the Dept. of Medicine, 1974–1992.

Gorlin served as Chairman until 1992. In these eighteen years, he built seventeen successful subspecialty divisions, including molecular medicine, strengthened the Medical School in its early years, and helped plan the new patient care facility (the Guggenheim Pavilion), which was completed in 1992. In the early 1980s, he set up a humanistic medicine program to try to teach compassion to residents and medical students. Also in this era, he helped formulate the Department's response to the rise of AIDS.

Gorlin also spent a great deal of effort on ambulatory care. As reimbursement mechanisms changed, more medical care became ambulatory, and patients' length of stay became a constant concern. In 1982, he changed the General Medical Clinic into the Internal Medicine Associates, providing appointments for clinic patients and creating long-term patient-doctor relationships. As he stepped down from the chairmanship, he was appointed head of the Task Force on Ambulatory Care to help Mount Sinai chart its course in this area. In 1987, Gorlin became both President of the Medical Board and Dean for Clinical Affairs. From 1994, he was the Medical Director of the Mount Sinai Health System, helping to found one of the region's largest health networks. Gorlin died in 1997 and is commemorated today through the Richard Gorlin Heart Research Foundation Professorship of Cardiology and remembered for his compassion, warmth, and wisdom.

At Gorlin's retirement from the Chair in 1992, Ira Goldstein, a noted rheumatologist, was named the new Chairman. He had plans to expand the Department's research initiatives in molecular medicine and to bring these insights back to the patient. Sadly, Goldstein became ill on his first full day at Mount Sinai and died shortly thereafter. The divisional directors took over the day-to-day activity of the Department, and John Rowe, then President of Mount Sinai, became Acting Chairman. In September 1993, Barry Coller was appointed Chairman and Professor of Medicine.

Coller received his M.D. from NYU and spent the early years of his career at the State University of New York at Stony Brook, where he rose to be Professor of Medicine and Pathology and, ultimately, Distinguished Service Professor. A leading hematologist, Coller has done research on platelet physiology and pathology. He has developed a number of monoclonal antibodies and the technology for an automated assay to test the blood for platelet function. The holder of several patents, Coller represents the finest Mount Sinai tradition of translating research into better patient care. He was inducted into the Institute of Medicine of the National Academy of Sciences in 1999. A member of several professional organizations, he has served in many leadership roles, including as President of the American Society of Hematology. The author of numerous papers in his field, Coller is also the Editor of three editions of *Progress in Hemostasis and Thrombosis* and co-editor of *Williams Hematology*.[37]

Several important changes took place in the Department during the 1990s. One was the evolution of the care center model, in which patient beds are grouped by broad categories, including Cardiac, Perioperative Services, Oncology, and General Medicine. Transition to this model was completed throughout the Hospital in 1996. These units are staffed with teams of various specialists, nurses, and auxiliary staff. Another physical change was the erection of the Primary Care Building on Madison Avenue to house all internal medicine primary care, along with geriatric care. An important educational development was the work on the creation of the new curriculum of the Medical School, as well as the coordination of the residency program with all of the affiliates.

In August 2001, Coller resigned the Chairmanship to assume an important leadership role at Rockefeller University. He will be long remembered as a quintessential role model for future scientist clinicians and for his many innovative positive contributions to the Department of Medicine.

In November 2001, Paul Klotman was appointed the new Chairman of the Department. Klotman assumes the Chairmanship after a distingushed career serving as Chief of Nephrology since 1994.

While the future is unclear, what is certain is that Mount Sinai's Department of Medicine will continue to strive for excellence in all areas. With the past as prologue, there will be many more moments of greatness.

2

Division of Cardiology

AS IS TRUE for many of the great medical divisions at Mount Sinai, the history of cardiology begins in the basement. That's where, in 1909, Alfred E. Cohn first installed the electrocardiograph machine he had brought back with him from Europe, one of the first of its kind to be used in the United States. The electrocardiograph (EKG), developed by Willem Einthoven in 1901, allowed scientists to measure the heart's electrical impulses directly and in turn differentiated the newly emerging heart specialists who operated them from other practitioners.[1] Unfortunately, Cohn soon left Mount Sinai and took his apparatus with him. But, by 1914, Bernard S. Oppenheimer had procured another instrument that was similarly installed in a small, dark room in the subbasement of the laboratory. The Electrocardiographic Laboratory was officially opened in 1915 and placed under Oppenheimer's direction. Over the next eighty-five years, an extraordinary number of major contributions to the field of cardiology would grow out of these humble beginnings.

Oppenheimer had long been associated with Mount Sinai, having graduated from the House Staff in 1904. From early on, he was recognized as a physician of extraordinary skill. Howard Lilienthal recalled that Oppenheimer was one of only three candidates to examine a test case at the internship examination and arrive at the proper diagnosis.[2] Apart from his clinical contributions, Oppenheimer was also an active teacher. He was one of Mount Sinai's first instructors when the Hospital began postgraduate teaching, serving as chairman of the Medical Board's Committee on Medical Instruction from 1928 until 1939. Oppenheimer also established one of Mount Sinai's enduring traditions—the Gold-Headed Cane.[3] Oppenheimer was one of the first to use the electrocardiograph to study abnormalities of the wave form, and in 1917 he was awarded an American Medical Association gold medal for an exhibit on electrocardiographic changes associated with myocardial infarction.[4] Working in the laboratory with Oppenheimer during these early years was Marcus A. Rothschild, the Assistant Cardiographer, as well as Morris Kahn, Irving Roth, and Hubert Mann.

The most prominent figure associated with the founding of Cardiology at Mount Sinai was Emanuel Libman.[5] In the years prior to World War I, Libman was considered the country's outstanding authority on subacute bacterial endocarditis. He in fact named the disease.[6] He wrote and spoke profusely on the topic, and in 1923, with Benjamin Sacks, he also described atypical verrucous endocarditis, now known as Libman-Sacks endocarditis.[7] Libman also made some of the earliest correlations between coronary artery thrombosis and its symptoms.[8] It has been said that "so numerous, original, comprehensive and important have been the studies of the heart emanating from the wards and laboratories of Mount Sinai Hospital, that one may correctly speak of the Mount Sinai School of Cardiologists, of which Libman was the founder and guiding spirit."[9]

Following World War I, the pace of research and the number of EKG examinations performed in the Laboratory accelerated rapidly, thanks in part to a mobile EKG machine that was acquired in 1922. Research during the 1920s focused on the use of the EKG in the diagnosis and prognosis of myocardial disease and on new methods of analyzing the tracings.[10,11] Rothschild became head of the Electrocardiograph Laboratory in 1927 when Oppenheimer was appointed Physician to the Hospital. By that year, the Laboratory was performing two thousand EKG examinations annually and had catalogued a total of thirteen thousand since its inception. During Rothschild's tenure, his own research interests centered on the cardiac effects of anoxemia,[12] Arthur M. Master was performing clinical studies on rheumatic fever,[13] and Mann conducted important electrographic studies on bundle branch block.[14]

In 1934, William Hitzig[15] devised the first clinically applicable method for measuring circulation time to the right heart. By introducing ether into an antecubital vein, he was able to calculate "the ether time," a measurement of the circulation time from the antecubital vein to the capillaries of the lung.[16] This technique was used for a number of years to evaluate heart failure until more sophisticated methods were developed.

In that same year, Arthur M. Master was appointed head of the Cardiac Clinics and the Cardiographic Laboratory. Master had completed his internship at Mount Sinai in 1923 and, by the end of his more than fifty-year association with the Hospital, would leave an indelible mark

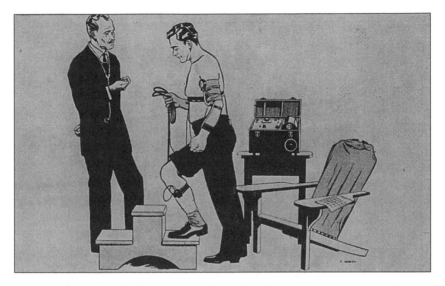

The Master 2-Step, the first successful standardized cardiac stress test. Illustration from the 1929 paper by Master and Enid Oppenheimer, "A Simple Exercise Tolerance Test for Circulatory Efficiency with Standard Tables for Normal Individuals." *Amer J Med Sci* 177 (1929): 233.

both on the division and on the field of cardiology. Master published one of his most important papers on the "two-step exercise test" in 1929. This was the first exercise test to be standardized for the weight, height, and sex of the patient and evaluated the function of the heart through blood pressure and pulse rate measurements taken before and after exercise. Although a wide variety of exercise tests were already in use prior to the publication of this paper, Master's was the first to "permit accurate measurement of the work performed, involve only an ordinary everyday muscular activity, and be simple enough for use in a hospital clinic or physician's office."[17]

Master's original contributions to cardiology were many. He was the first to report changes in the P-wave as a sign of acute myocardial infarction.[18] On the basis of his early seminal work on the relationship of obesity to heart disease,[19] Master was among the first to advocate a low-calorie diet for patients following coronary thrombosis; in collaboration with Harry R. Jaffe and Simon Dack, he observed that when those patients were placed on an eight hundred-calorie diet, basal metabolic rates, pulse rate, and blood pressure were all lowered, diminishing the work of the heart.[20] In 1936, Master and his colleagues reported on the treatment and progress of two hundred sixty-seven patients with coronary artery thrombosis. While previously reported mortality rates were between 38 percent and 53 percent, the mortality rate of these patients was only 16.5 percent; this difference was attributed, in part, to adherence to a low-calorie diet.[21]

In the years prior to World War II, other eminent New York physicians made important medical contributions that dramatically enhanced the practice of cardiology. These new techniques, used to visualize the heart and its vessels, were based on the work of Mount Sinai's Moses Swick, who developed intravenous urography.[22] In 1938, Robb and Steinberg at Bellevue Hospital introduced angiocardiography, which allowed cardiologists to visualize the ventricles and the aortic arch. The following year, Marcy Sussman performed the first angiocardiogram at Mount Sinai.[23] In 1947, six years after Cournand and Richards, also at Bellevue, introduced cardiac catheterization to the United States, Alvin Gordon performed the first cardiac catheterization at Mount Sinai.

Thus, Mount Sinai was able to keep up-to-date with the latest procedures, and the high level of research and scientific production that Master had encouraged in the 1930s continued. In 1940, the Department reported using fluoroscopy to evaluate the degree of myocardial involvement after recovery from acute myocardial infarction.[24] In 1942, Master added the results of an electrocardiogram to the standards he had previously developed for the diagnosis of coronary artery disease.[25] The "Master Two-Step Test" became the standard for assessing chest pain and for determining whether coronary artery disease was present. Many of these patients had a normal resting electrocardiogram, with characteristic abnormalities showing up only after exercise.

Many of Mount Sinai's cardiologists, including Master, Dack, and Jaffe, served in the Armed Forces during World War II. Nonetheless, research productivity continued.

After the war, it was decided that the research activities of the Hospital needed to be reorganized, and a number of clinical research units were established, including the Cardiovascular Research Group. The members of the group included staff from the Medical, Pediatric, and Thoracic Surgery services and from the Electrocardiography, Physics, and X-ray departments and was placed under the direction of Marcy Sussman, the Chief of Radiology. Responding to researchers' special interest in congenital heart disease, the Hospital established, in 1949, a single clinic for ambulatory cases of congenital heart diseases in children and adults. In that clinic, run initially by Frederick H. King and later by Sidney Blumenthal, a preliminary examination of all newly admitted patients with congenital heart disease was performed before the patients were sent on.[26] In 1950, the Research Group held a clinical conference on cardiovascular and congenital heart disease. The presentations detailed the work of the Group and the Clinic and were published in *The Journal of The Mount Sinai Hospital*.[27] One of the papers described the first successful subclavian artery to pulmonary artery anastomosis (Blalock procedure) performed at Mount Sinai.[28] By the end of the 1940s, in addition to the newly expanded cardiology programs, the Electrocardiography Laboratory had expanded to include three Adjuncts, one Research Associate, five Research Assistants, and nine "Residents." The lab had also attained a high level of international prestige, with members of the medical profession arriving from all over the world for a firsthand look at the work being done at Mount Sinai.

The concentration of leading cardiologists in New York City made it the logical site for the founding of the American College of Cardiology in 1949. Mount Sinai's own Simon Dack would later become President of the College in 1956, as well as the founder and Editor-in-Chief of the *American Journal of Cardiology* (it became the official journal of the College in 1988.) Dack served as Editor for thirty-five consecutive years, chronicling the rapid advances occurring in cardiology during this period.

In 1950, the Hospital's annual report stated that "in view of the increased life expectancy of the American population it has seemed desirable to establish new criteria of normal and abnormal blood pressure."[29] This gigantic task had been taken up a few years earlier by Master, who after a study in 1943 observed that more than 40 percent of the population over the age of forty would have been considered to be hypertensive according to the standards of the day.[30] To alleviate what he referred to as "an almost universal blood pressure phobia," Master collaborated with the American Medical Association and the Metropolitan Life Insurance Company to develop new ranges for normal blood pressure.[31] In 1954, simultaneous pressure tracings from the left atrium, left ventricle, and aorta were recorded for the first time in the exposed human heart at operation by members of the Cardiovascular Research Group.[32] For the first time, it became possible to measure precisely the difference in pressure across the valves, a great aid to the surgeon in evaluating the efficacy of a corrective procedure.

By the end of his tenure as head of the Cardiac Clinics and the Cardiographic Laboratory, Master had brought great renown and prestige to the Division of Cardiology at Mount Sinai, as evidenced by the fact that, in 1952, the American College of Physicians (ACP) invited the Hospital to conduct its annual cardiology course for graduate physicians. It was one of the first ACP courses to be based at a hospital without a university affiliation.

The year 1957 was an important year for Cardiology at Mount Sinai as it became an official Division of the Department of Medicine, and Charles K. Friedberg was appointed Division Chief. After having completed his internship at Mount Sinai in 1930, Friedberg had gone on to study physiology and pharmacology in Vienna and Rotterdam as a Libman Research Fellow. He then returned to Mount Sinai and worked with Louis Gross on rheumatic heart disease[33] and later with Libman on bacterial endocarditis.[34] His single-authored text, *Diseases of the Heart*, was seen as a monumental contribution to cardiac knowledge.[35] As Chief, Friedberg was highly involved in the activities of the Division, and he insisted on being present to hold the paddles during every defibrillation procedure. In addition, in 1957, a formal residency program was established, and the Department of Surgery performed its first open heart surgery.

Much of the work in the Division during the late 1950s and early 1960s focused on methods of recording sounds from the heart, including the use of intracardiac microphones. By recording the vibrations of the blood on either side of a valve, these microphones enabled physicians to localize heart murmurs more precisely than was possible from outside the chest wall.[36] In the late 1960s, research turned toward investigations of the causes and management of heart failure and cardiac arrhythmia. Important research was pursued during this period by Milton Mendlowitz, who was in charge of the Hypertension Clinic from 1950 to 1975. Also in charge of the circulatory physiology laboratory for many years, he published extensively on the digital circulation, heart failure, coronary occlusion and pulmonary embolism, arteriosclerosis and thrombosis, uterine and vascular physiology, and cloning of phospholipase C genes.[37] In collaboration with Stanley Gitlow, he also wrote extensively on hypersensitivity to norepinephrine in patients with essential hypertension.[38] Considerable research was performed in the Division in the 1950s, 60s and 70s, culminating in the awarding of competitive grants, international publications, and presentations. These included projects in heart failure (Richard Lasser), cardiogenic shock (Leslie Kuhn), computerized ECGs (Leon Pordy), heartblock (William Stein), vectorcardiography (Arthur Grishman), and hemodynamics (Howard Moscovitz and Alvin Gordon). During this time, Ephraim Donoso was recognized as an outstanding clinical teacher. Samuel Elster performed a number of important studies on the role of C-reactive protein in cardiac conditions and on acute rheumatic fever in adults. A superb clinician and teacher, he was one of the first to emphasize the importance of geriatrics and the aging population to the field of cardiology. Elster also served nine years as Dean of the Page and William Black Postgraduate School and as Dean for Continuous Education in the School of Medicine.

In February 1968, the Ames Coronary Care Unit was inaugurated; Leslie Kuhn was appointed the first director. At the time, it was one of the largest facilities in New York City designed exclusively for the medical care and treatment of heart attack victims. In 1970, the Division added two full-time faculty members to strengthen the Catheterization Laboratory. Arnold Katz subsequently became the first full-time Chief of Cardiology.

The Division was also strengthened with the arrival of Richard Gorlin as Chairman of the Department of Medicine in 1974. Gorlin was known for developing the formula used to measure the extent to which the heart valves of rheumatic heart disease patients were blocked.[39] Gorlin appointed Michael V. Herman Director of Cardiology, replacing Katz, and, in 1976, Louis E. Teichholz established Mount Sinai's first echocardiography laboratory.

In 1983, Valentin Fuster was recruited from the Mayo Clinic to serve as the Chief of Cardiology. Fuster was already well known for his research on the relationship between platelet function and atherosclerosis, which helped unify researchers in these areas.[40] Fuster had also conducted clinical trials that showed that platelet inhibitor drugs prevented occlusion of coronary bypass grafts. These trials had a profound and positive effect on the care of hundreds of thousands of patients who underwent coronary bypass graft surgery, which had become the most frequently performed major operation in the country. Antiplatelet therapy has since been adopted worldwide.[41]

Stimulated by Fuster's great energy and expertise, Mount Sinai's Division of Cardiology would make a number of important contributions to the field during the next fifteen years. Lina and Juan Jose Badimon developed a perfusion chamber to perform controlled evaluations of blood flow, platelet deposition, and thrombus formation under various experimental conditions.[42] These chambers became fundamental tools for future work on coronary artery thrombosis.

In 1984, Martin E. Goldman was the first to utilize intraoperative transesophageal color-flow Doppler echocardiography to guide the surgeon in the operating room, facilitating moment-to-moment decisions during heart valve repair and replacement.[43] In 1985, John A. Ambrose discovered the relationship between complex angiographic coronary lesion morphology and acute coronary events, dramatically altering the way patients were selected for angioplasty and bypass surgery.[44] In 1987, J. Anthony Gomes developed a noninvasive index of the risk of sudden death among heart attack survivors, based upon a combination of signal averaged electrocardiography, Holter monitoring, and left ventricular function.[45]

In 1988, Mount Sinai was one of only a few medical centers in the country that was investigating the use of lasers to remove plaques that block coronary arteries.[46] In collaboration with colleagues from the Mayo Clinic, Fuster and Badimon were among the first to demonstrate the ability of hirudin to prevent platelet deposition.[47] In 1990, the Molecular and Cellular Cardiology Laboratories were established, concentrating on investigation of cardiovascular diseases by utilizing the techniques of molecular and cellular biology. Fuster and Badimon were the first to report in vivo prospective evidence that infusion of high-density lipoproteins could reverse atherosclerotic lesions in animals.[48] In 1991, Mark B. Taubman and colleagues identified the proteins responsible for thrombosis and for inflammation in the blood vessel wall that contributes to the problem of restenosis following coronary angioplasty.[49]

In 1991, Fuster accepted a position at the Massachusetts General Hospital; he returned to Mount Sinai in 1994 to open the Cardiovascular Institute with the goal of bringing basic and clinical research to bear on clinical problems. Fuster assembled a team of investigators to create an internationally renowned research program. The Cardiovascular Research Program (CVRP,) a joint undertaking of the Zena and Michael A.

Wiener Cardiovascular Institute and the Samuel A. Bronfman Department of Medicine, has as its mission the establishment of a highly interactive and multidisciplinary basic research program to investigate diverse aspects of cardiovascular biology. The Cardiovascular Research Program under the direction of Juan Jose Badimon rapidly translates the results of basic investigation into improvements in disease diagnosis, treatment, and prevention. Jonathan Halperin, Associate Director of the Cardiovascular Institute, was the principal cardiologist responsible for the design and execution of the Stroke Prevention in Atrial Fibrillation Study to address the use of antithrombotic therapy for prevention of stroke in patients with nonvalvular atrial fibrillation.[50] The Section of Myocardial Biology, under the direction of Glenn Fishman, studies the molecular pathogenesis of myocardial diseases, focusing especially on various aspects of cardiac excitability and arrhythmogenesis, signal transduction, and cardiovascular development, growth, and failure. Under the leadership of Mark Taubman, the Section of Vascular Biology has existing research programs in atherosclerosis, thrombosis, lipoprotein biology, and angiogenesis. The Section of Lipoprotein Biology, directed by Edward Fisher, examines the biology and pathobiology of lipid disorders.

Zahi Fayad and Fuster have investigated the use of "black blood" magnetic resonance imaging (BB-MR) to image the human coronary arterial wall noninvasively. They and their colleagues were the first to produce detailed images of in vivo human plaque components using BB-MR[51] and the first to use the technique to characterize the atherosclerotic plaques in tortuous coronary arteries in intact swine.[52] Most important, they were the first to use BB-MR to image the human coronary artery lumen[53] and the first to produce in vivo microscopy images of the arterial wall of wild type and genetically engineered mice to identify and characterize atherosclerotic lesion burden without a priori knowledge of the lesion type or location.[54]

The success of the Cardiovascular Institute has helped to make the cardiology fellowship training program at Mount Sinai among the most sought-after in the nation, a success due in large part to Fuster. One of the country's most respected leaders in cardiovascular medicine, Fuster has received the Andreas Gruntzig Scientific Award of the European Society of Cardiology, the Distinguished Scientist Award of the American College of Cardiology, and the Lewis A. Connor Memorial Award of the American Heart Association, the first individual to earn cardiology's "triple crown" from the world's three major cardiological organizations. Under his leadership, with the support of the great pool of talent at Mount Sinai, which includes voluntary and full-time clinicians and basic and clinical researchers, the Cardiovascular Institute may very well reach its goal "to extinguish the spread of cardiovascular disease."[55]

3

Division of Clinical Immunology

THE DIVISION OF CLINICAL IMMUNOLOGY, created in 1978, is one of the younger divisions of the Department of Medicine. Established to develop a research program in immunology, it also was given responsibility for the clinical activities of the allergy clinics.

The understanding of the concept of allergy is recent, and Mount Sinai physicians have played prominent roles in its evolution. The term "allergy" was coined in 1906 by Clemens von Pirquet and Bela Schick to describe an altered response by the immune system to the effect of an external agent (an allergen). Von Pirquet also originated a skin test for tuberculosis. Schick, the creator of the Schick test for diphtheria, would later serve as Chief of Pediatrics at Mount Sinai.[1] When Schick arrived at Mount Sinai in the 1920s, the importance of allergy was still not thoroughly appreciated. In 1928, however, Gregory Shwartzman formulated the concept of hypersensitivity and described what has become known as the "Shwartzman Phenomenon."[2]

The Department of Medicine's early efforts in the study of allergic and immunologic disease were limited but valuable. These revolved initially around the work of Joseph Harkavy. Harkavy joined the House Staff at Mount Sinai in 1914 and after training was appointed to the coveted Admitting Physician position for a year. He served in World War I and then traveled to Europe in 1924 to study pathology and physiology. Upon his return to Mount Sinai, he was appointed Allergist to the Hospital.

In a 1930 study, Harkavy identified a chemical substance, not histamine, that was released in allergy.[3] Later work by others led to a fuller description of what is now known as slow-reacting substance of anaphylaxis (SRSA). Harkavy pioneered the study of the relationship between tobacco and allergy, specifically as they related to cardiovascular disease. In 1932, he demonstrated that it was not the nicotine in tobacco that directly causes disease but rather tobacco itself that can serve as an antigen, giving rise to an allergic state.[4] In 1941, there appeared a classic paper on the concept of vascular allergy, later to be termed the Harkavy Syndrome, a variant of Kussmaul-Maier disease relating to asthma.[5] He published a text on vascular allergy in 1963[6] and over the course of his career published more than sixty articles relating to tobacco allergy, hypersensitivity, cardiovascular disease, and asthma. A leader in his field, Harkavy held faculty positions at New York Medical College and Columbia University and was also Chief of the allergy section at Montefiore Hospital. He served as President of the New York Allergy Society and as Vice President of the American Academy of Allergy. He died in 1980 at the age of ninety-one.

In 1941, Harold A. Abramson was appointed an Assistant Attending in Allergy, rising to Associate in 1942. He continued as an Associate Physician (for Allergy) until 1959, becoming the Allergist to the Hospital when Harkavy reached Consultant status in 1949. With a major interest in asthma and pulmonary disease, Abramson was an early proponent of delivering aerosolized medication to the lungs and demonstrated the safety and efficacy of the technique.[7] In military service during World War II, he returned to Mount Sinai after the war and was the first ever to use aerosolized penicillin.[8] In his asthma studies on children, Abramson worked closely with M. Murray Peshkin, Mount Sinai's pediatric allergist.[9] Abramson developed an intense interest in psychoanalysis and in the psychosomatic aspects of allergy and asthma. He was involved in early studies of LSD and its medical application. He published extensively in the *Journal of Asthma Research*, a publication he founded with Peshkin, and was its editor until his death in 1980.

Abramson left Mount Sinai in 1959, at which time Sheppard Siegal was the sole Attending for Allergy, a position he held for many years. Siegal, an eminent consultant, is best remembered for his description of benign paroxysmal peritonitis, or Familial Mediterranean Fever.[10] He also did important work with members of the Dermatology Department outlining penicillin sensitivity.[11] Siegal served Mount Sinai for more than fifty years, and died in 1988 at the age of seventy-nine.

Studies of autoimmune phenomena have played a prominent role in Mount Sinai's history. None have been more illustrious than those of Kermit E. Osserman in the area of myasthenia gravis.[12] Trained in medicine, dermatology, obstetrics, and gynecology, Osserman had settled into a practice as a specialist in diabetes when, in 1950–1951, he saw one or two patients with myasthenia gravis and was both fascinated by the pathogenesis and challenged by the management of the disease. With the approval of Alexander Gutman, then Chief of Medicine, Osserman organized a Myasthenia Clinic in 1951 and, in true Mount Sinai fashion, scrounged laboratory space, personnel (including his wife and daughter), and financial support for research. It did not take long for the population living with myasthenia to learn that there was an individual who had genuine concerns for their plight, and they flocked to the Clinic. In twenty years, the Clinic registered more than 1,200 patients, all carefully studied and reported in meticulous detail by Osserman and his associate Gabriel Genkins.[13] Allyn Rule and Peter Kornfeld, working with Osserman, carefully documented the biologic aspects of the disease.[14] In 1952, Osserman and Lawrence Kaplan introduced the edrophonium test as an aid in diagnosis and later as an aid in management.[15] New drugs were subjected to rigorous clinical trials, and researchers, in collaboration with Allan Kark, Paul Kirschner, and Angelos Papatestas of the Department of Surgery, extensively studied the role of thymectomy as a treatment modality.[16] Osserman sensed the immunological implications of myasthenia long before the role of the thymus in immunologic disorders was appreciated. He and his colleagues made landmark observations, detecting circulating antibodies that, acting in concert with sensitized lymphocytes, led, in some way unknown at the time, to defective neuromuscular transmission.[17] The author or coauthor of more than one hundred publications, Osserman wrote *Myasthenia Gravis*, the first text on the subject.[18] A giant in the field, Osserman died prematurely in 1972, at age sixty-two, of a massive myocardial infarction, robbing Mount Sinai and the Department of Medicine of one of their brightest lights.

The study of allergy received little attention in the Department of Medicine for many years. During the 1970s, more Attendings were appointed, but fundamental research was a missing link. Finally, in July 1978, the Division of Clinical Immunology was created, and Frederick P. Siegal, the son of Sheppard Siegal, was appointed the Associate Attending in charge of this new Division. Siegal ran the service during the years that AIDS was being defined as a clinical entity. In an example typical of Mount Sinai's collaborative efforts, Siegal, along with members of the Division of Infectious Diseases, the Department of Microbiology, and faculty of other institutions, delineated many basic aspects of the disease.[19]

Frederick Siegal left Mount Sinai in 1984 and one year later was succeeded by Lloyd F. Mayer, a Mount Sinai School of Medicine graduate of the Class of 1976. Mayer, the first (1994) Dr. David and Dorothy Merksamer Professor in the Mount Sinai School of Medicine, is one of a handful of Mount Sinai–educated and trained physicians to occupy an endowed professorship at Mount Sinai. Trained in gastroenterology at Mount Sinai, Mayer returned after five years at the Rockefeller Institute and has established an internationally renowned laboratory, focused on the nature and functioning of the immune system. A specific area of concentration has been the role of T cells in immune deficiency. Mayer's group has long championed the concept that by failing to produce required cytokines or mediate appropriate cell:cell interactions, T cells and not B cells are the true culprits in primary immunodeficiency diseases. They were the first to show that T cells regulated immunoglobulin isotype (class) switching in humans and that there was a defect in these "switch" T cells in the hyper-IgM syndrome.[20] This model has been embraced by the scientific community and has led to new approaches in the treatment of these disorders. Mayer's laboratory was also the first to demonstrate that the epithelial lining cells of the intestine are active regulators of mucosal immune responses, responses that are distinct from those that regulate systemic immunity. These findings have had profound significance in the development of new anti-inflammatory drugs that have proven most effective in the management of inflammatory bowel disease.

Leading a discipline that crosses all borders, Mayer has assembled a superb faculty, almost all of whom have joint appointments and responsibilities in other divisions or departments. In 1986, Charlotte Cunningham-Rundles, M.D., Ph.D. was recruited from the Memorial Sloan-Kettering Cancer Center (MSKCC) where she worked on primary immunodeficiency disorders. Appointed Director of Mount Sinai's Immunodeficiency Clinic, she was the first to use interleukin-2 to treat primary immunodeficiency (common variable immunodeficiency or CVID),[21] work that emanated from her collaborations with Mayer at Rockefeller University and at MSKCC. This work was aided by the establishment of the Jeffrey Modell Foundation, a group founded by the parents of Jeffrey Modell after his death in 1986, at age fifteen, from a primary immunodeficiency.

Hugh Sampson, Mayer's counterpart in the Department of Pediatrics and also Director of Mount Sinai's General Clinical Research Center, has focused his efforts on the study of food-related allergic disorders, as have Scott Sicherer, Xiu-Min Li, and Anna Nowak-Wegrzyn. Sampson was the first to show that food allergy was the basis for a significant amount of atopic dermatitis in children, was involved in the identification of the specific allergens in peanuts, has developed formulas for food allergic infants, and has championed double-blind placebo-controlled food challenges as a true test for food allergy. The major interest of Scott Plevy's laboratory is the study of interleukin-12, an inflammatory cytokine that has a prominent role in the pathogenesis of intracellular infections and chronic inflammatory disorders. Karen Zier, Ph.D., also a member of the Institute of Gene Therapy, is investigating the immunology of T cells, specifically modifying tumor cell vaccines by means of genetic engineering to induce antitumor responses. Zier also directs the medical student research program, which over the years of its existence has encouraged and stimulated numerous students to engage in research, much of which has been enormously productive. Kirk Sperber, who remained on the faculty after completion of his fellowship, was the first to show that HIV infection alters the ability of monocytes to function as antigen presenting cells. He was also the first to generate human macrophage hybridomas, which have served as models for the study of intracellular infections in a number of disorders.

Mayer and his group have clearly upheld the legacy established by Schick and Shwartzman in exemplary fashion. The cutting edge science of the Division of Clinical Immunology will establish its own legacy for the next generation to aspire to.

4

Division of Endocrinology

LONG BEFORE THE SPECIALTY of endocrinology existed as an official division at Mount Sinai, there were physicians who were actively
involved in the field. Julius Rudisch was one of the Hospital's first
physicians interested in diabetes. Born in Russia, Rudisch studied medicine in Heidelberg before emigrating to the United States. Here he became friends with Abraham Jacobi, who enticed him to accept a position as house physician and surgeon at Mount Sinai in 1875. Four years
later he was appointed Attending Physician to replace Jacobi, who had
been named Pediatrician to the Hospital. Reticent with his colleagues
and quietly firm with his patients, Rudisch openly preferred the laboratory to the clinic. Among his most important accomplishments were
the methods he devised for detecting sugar in the urine.[1] He also reported on the statistics of cases of diabetes in the Mount Sinai Hospital
during the years 1890–1900. In this report, he concluded that "diabetes
is not altogether a disease of the race, but rather of the class."[2] Rudisch
retired and joined the consulting staff in 1913.

In 1917, "a special clinic for Diseases of Metabolism was established
in the Dispensary. The purpose of this clinic is to give intensive treatment along the most scientific lines to patients suffering from diabetes,
nephritis, and other chronic disorders."[3] This was the first such clinic in
the metropolitan area, and the second in the nation. Initially, the clinic
was organized and run by Arthur Bookman. During this period, without the availability of insulin, treatment for diabetes mainly involved
starvation diets. In 1924, George Baehr took over as Chief of the clinic,
followed by Herman Lande and then by Herbert Pollack.

In 1956, Henry Dolger was appointed to head the Diabetes Clinic.
A member of the Mount Sinai community since 1933, when he began his
internship, Dolger published a paper in 1946 that shocked the medical
community.[4] In it, he stated that, in using insulin, physicians were treating only the symptoms of diabetes, not the cause of the disease, and that
the incidence of retinopathy associated with diabetes was unrelated to

THE MOUNT SINAI HOSPITAL,

FIFTH AVENUE AND ONE HUNDREDTH STREET,

NEW YORK.

ANNOUNCEMENT

A special clinic for diseases of metabolism will be conducted in the Dispensary beginning Monday, January 15th, 1917, and will receive patients referred by other departments.

Chiefs of clinic are invited to refer patients with diabetes, nephritis and other conditions coming within its scope.

Patients will not be accepted beyond the capacity of the clinic to give them proper care. Those no longer requiring the special facilities of the clinic will be referred back to their original departments.

The clinic will be held Monday, Wednesday, and Friday morning from 9:30 to 10:30.

S. S. Goldwater, M.D.

Superintendent

Memorandum establishing the Diabetes Clinic, 1917.

the severity or control of disease but was clearly a function of disease duration. According to Joseph Barach, of the University of Pittsburgh, who attended the meeting where Dolger read his paper:

It is not too much to say that Dolger of New York actually startled us in the summer of 1946 at the Toronto Insulin Anniversary Celebration, when he reported that 80 to 90 percent of his diabetics have retinal lesions after 20 years of the disease, and that 100 percent have partial or complete blindness by the 25th year. When this bombshell was thrown into the arena many of us on our return home hurried to our records, to find out how true this was. So far, almost everyone who has discussed this topic seems to have corroborated Dolger's observations and faced the grim facts. Out of this there will finally come a revaluation of our knowledge on the subject and we will be better off for it.[5]

In 1948, Edwin Weinstein and Dolger analyzed the origin of common external ocular muscle palsies in diabetes. They demonstrated for the first time that the cause was tiny hemorrhages in the nucleus of cranial nerves III, IV, and VI, the innervators of the eye muscles. This led to a sharp reduction in the use of cerebral angiography in search of a non-existent tumor of the brain.[6] In 1952, when Mount Sinai opened its maternity pavilion and prenatal clinic, Dolger organized and headed the first diabetic prenatal clinic in New York City. Dolger was also one of the first to use oral drugs in the treatment of diabetes[7] and, with Stanley A. Mirsky and D. Diengott, demonstrated that oral sulfonylurea drugs acted via endogenous insulin only.[8] Like Dolger, Mirsky would spend his entire career at Mount Sinai and become one of its leading "diabetologists." In 1959, Dolger and Bernard Seeman published *How to Live with Diabetes,*[9] a text for the laity. It would be translated into many languages and go through four editions. Dolger was a founding father of the Juvenile Diabetes Foundation and served as President of the New York Diabetes Society.

Another prominent figure in the field of diabetes at Mount Sinai was Max Ellenberg. Early in his career, Ellenberg, in association with Kermit Osserman, had reviewed more than two hundred autopsies in diabetic patients, focusing on the cardiac complications. Noting that patients who had sustained myocardial infarctions with cardiogenic shock had a high incidence of liver damage, they went to the laboratory and, in an elegant study, were the first to recognize the role of shock in the genesis of central liver necrosis.[10] Widely recognized as an authority on the neurological complications of diabetes, Ellenberg, along with Harold Rifkin, authored the text *Diabetes Mellitus: Theory and Practice,* which has been regarded as the "diabetes bible."[11] In 1974, Ellenberg was elected President of the American Diabetes Association.

Throughout this period, members of the Department of Medicine were also involved in other areas of endocrinology outside the realm of diabetes, once again long before the formation of a formal division. Thyroid disease is a case in point. In 1879, Abraham Jacobi published a report on exophthalmic goiter in a child.[12] In the 1920s, Leo Kessel, an Attending in the Department of Medicine, also studied exophthalmic goiter. In the 1930s, when thyroidectomy was the therapy for uncontrollable hyperthyroidism, Solomon Silver, Richard Lewisohn, and Bernard S. Oppenheimer reviewed the operative mortality for hyperthyroidism (Grave's disease) at the Hospital.

Louis Soffer, who would later become the head of Endocrinology, first came to Mount Sinai in 1935. Soffer was a pioneer in the elucidation of adrenal disease and in the diagnosis and treatment of Addison's disease and Cushing's disease. His 1946 monograph, *Diseases of the Adrenals*,[13] was a significant contribution. Around this time, Soffer and J. Lester Gabrilove started an endocrine clinic; Joseph Gaines, the obstetrician/gynecologist, provided expertise in his area. In 1948, Soffer, Gabrilove, and their colleagues reported on the clinical use of adrenocorticotrophic hormone (ACTH) in a patient with myasthenia gravis and an associated thymic tumor.[14] Soffer would later comment that it "was the first demonstration of therapeutic effectiveness of this compound in disease. The observation of shrinkage of the thymic tumor which followed the administration of ACTH in this case laid the groundwork for the use of this agent in the treatment of lymphatic tumors."[15]

A Radioisotope Group was formed in 1948; in that same year, a publication by the group on the use of radioactive iodine in the diagnosis of thyroid disease established the foundation for the technique of scanning.[16] By 1959, the Physics Department had logged ten years of experience with radioactive isotopes and had reported on the largest group of patients to date treated with radioactive iodine for hyperthyroidism.[17] Solomon Silver, a renowned thyroidologist who first came to Mount Sinai as an intern in 1927, conducted pioneering research with radioactive isotopes in the diagnosis and treatment of thyroid disease. A member of the Department of Medicine and of the Radioisotope Group, he worked closely with Sergei Feitelberg, the Director of the Department of Physics. Many of the early papers of the Group helped establish the standards for the radioactive management of thyroid disease.[18] In association with Edith Quimby, of Columbia University, Silver and Feitelberg offered a course in the use of radioisotopes; the proceedings created the leading text on the subject.[19] Silver was also involved in planning and establishing the Mount Sinai School of Medicine. One of Mount Sinai's "Giants" by any criteria, Silver was a holder of the Gold-Headed Cane.[20]

J. Lester Gabrilove, currently the Division's senior practicing endocrinologist, first came to Mount Sinai as an intern in 1940. Involved in the early work on ACTH with Soffer, he was a co-author of *Diseases of the Endocrine Glands*.[21] During his long career, he has conducted extensive and important research on the feminizing and virilizing disorders of the adrenal and gonads, gynecomastia, Cushing's syndrome, thyroid toxicosis, and the medical treatment of prostatic hyperplasia with GnRH. Gabrilove received the Distinguished Endocrinologist Award of the American Association of Clinical Endocrinologists in 1995.

During the tenure of Alexander Gutman as Chief of the Department of Medicine in the 1950s, Endocrinology was made an official division, and Soffer was appointed the Chief. The "Soffer Years" were bright ones for the Division in both clinical and research areas. A fellowship was established; the first fellows were William Dorrance and Irwin Weiner. Cortisone had recently become available commercially and was tested extensively in the laboratory and at the bedside. As interest in the adrenal hormones accelerated, Milton Mendlowitz, Stanley Gitlow and their colleagues performed groundbreaking studies on the role of norepinephrine hypersensitivity in patients with essential hypertension.[22] Although they were basically cardiologists interested in hypertension, their interests came to include the functioning adrenal tumors. In 1959, the first of their many papers appeared on the use of measurements of norepinephrine catabolites to diagnose pheochromocytomas,[23] including the development of a simple method of measuring these catabolites by colormetric urinary analysis.[24] The group then went on to study the roles played by epinephrine and norepinephrine metabolism in the development of a number of clinical states.

With the appointment of Solomon Berson to replace Gutman, who had retired, as Chairman of the Department of Medicine in 1968, Mount Sinai was graced with a giant in the world of endocrinology. Unfortunately, Berson's sudden death in 1972 at fifty-four years of age cut short a brilliant career.[25]

Upon Soffer's retirement in 1972, Dorothy Krieger was appointed Director of the Division of Endocrinology. A member of the staff since her first day as an intern in 1949, her work focused on the role of neurotransmitters in the release of ACTH and then of other hormones. She studied the evolutionary origin of polypeptide hormones and their synthesis in the brain. She was the first to demonstrate that brain cells from the fetal preoptic area, where gonadotrophin releasing factor is synthesized, transplanted into genetically hypogonadal mice would reverse the deficiency and permit pregnancy to occur.[26] Tragically, Krieger's scientific career was cut short by a battle with breast cancer, which she lost in 1985.

The members of the Division of Endocrinology have been a remarkably productive group. Within the Division, there has been further subspecialization: Robert Segal and Steven Yohalem focused their efforts on thyroid disease, as have Edward Haber and Frank Ross. Ross has also been the Chief of Medicine at the Elmhurst Hospital Center affiliate for many years. Elliot Rayfield has had a major interest in pancreatic islet cell tumors; Charles Nechemias was in charge of the Diabetes Clinic for many years. In 1986, Walter Futterweit and Liane Deligdisch of the Department of Pathology were the first to define a direct role of androgens in inducing the morphologic changes of the Polycystic Ovary Syndrome in the ovary.[27] Alice Levine has made significant contributions to the understanding of male reproductive physiology. Jeffrey Mechanick has played an important role in the management of patients on total parenteral nutrition. All of the faculty have given freely of their time in teaching medical students, medical residents, and endocrinology fellows.

In 1986, Terry Davies was appointed Director of the Division of Endocrinology. Recruited to Mount Sinai in 1979, he had previously been at the National Institutes of Health and Newcastle-upon-Tyne in the United Kingdom. Davies has a distinguished record of groundbreaking contributions to the understanding of endocrine physiology and pathology since very early in his research career. Davies's laboratory is internationally recognized as one of the leading sites for innovation in our understanding of thyroid autoimmune pathology. A major focus of study at this time is the genetics of autoimmune thyroid disease. Davies is currently Editor of the journal *Thyroid*.[28]

During Davies's tenure, the Division has grown in stature and depth. There are now fifteen investigators in the Division, which is well funded from extramural grants. Davies has developed an extremely successful clinical training program and a postdoctoral research training program, each with eight fellows.

Since its inception, the Division has been at the cutting edge of clinical care and research in endocrine and metabolic disorders. Davies and his faculty will unquestionably exceed the contributions of their forebears in the years to come.

5

Division of Gastroenterology

PROGRESS THROUGH MULTIDISCIPLINARY collaboration has been a watchword of Mount Sinai throughout its existence. Nowhere is this in greater evidence than in the Division of Gastroenterology. J. Hugh Baron and Henry D. Janowitz have recently edited a very complete history of the Divisions of Gastroenterology and Liver Disease.[1] In three theme issues of *The Mount Sinai Journal of Medicine*, they and their co-authors reviewed in great detail the development and productivity of these groups. In almost every article, the authors stress the cooperation among the gastroenterologists, hepatologists, and the physicians of the Departments of Surgery, Radiology, Pathology, Urology, and other divisions of the Department of Medicine.

Medical specialization did not exist in the early years of the Hospital. Many practitioners performed their own surgery, and almost all surgeons had general practices, as well. Before the advent of aseptic surgery, abdominal surgery was nonexistent. As the first attending and resident physician in the 1850s, Mark Blumenthal cared for all medical and surgical patients. He certainly had his share of patients with abdominal and gastrointestinal disorders. Case No. 27, admitted on August 24, 1855, suffered from "quotidian fever" and jaundice. In one of the shortest lengths of stay recorded in the early casebooks, the patient was discharged as "cured" on the tenth hospital day.[2] Several patients with a similar illness were admitted during the first year of hospital operations. Patients who in retrospect almost certainly had appendicitis and/or gallstone disease were likewise admitted. On July 16, 1857, Patient No. 333 was admitted with symptoms classic of a peptic ulcer with posterior penetration and was treated empirically with bismuth and bicarbonate of soda by mouth and a plaster to the back. The patient improved and stated that she "had doctored for many, many years before entering the hospital, and nowhere did they ever do her any good except here."[3] This must surely have been one of the first testimonials given to the Hospital.

Edmund Aronson, in the early twentieth century, was the first physician at Mount Sinai to limit his practice to diseases of the gastrointestinal tract.[4] Morris Manges was, however, far better known for his expertise in gastroenterology. A founding member of the American Gastroenterological Society, Manges wrote extensively on many medical subjects but did not limit himself to diseases of the gastrointestinal tract. His translation of Ewald's two-volume *Diseases of the Stomach* from German to English introduced a major European text to America.[5]

In 1913, an outpatient Division of Gastroenterology was established, with Aronson as the Chief. In the Clinic, physiologic analyses on gastric and pancreatic secretions in health and disease were carried out, and therapeutic responses to available drugs were studied. One year later, in a reorganization of the Surgical Service, an intestinal service was created, with Albert A. Berg as the Chief. At Berg's urging, gastroenterologists, surgeons, physiologists, radiologists, and other specialists came together in the Clinic and on the wards to begin a collaboration that still continues and has led to many of Mount Sinai's major contributions over the intervening years.[6] When Aronson died in 1922, he was succeeded by Burrill B. Crohn.

When the words "gastroenterologists" and "Mount Sinai" are articulated, the name Burrill B. Crohn immediately comes to mind. A graduate of Columbia University's College of Physicians and Surgeons, Crohn began his internship in 1907 and was affiliated with Mount Sinai until his death in 1983 at the age of ninety-nine years. He published his first paper on Glanders[7] in 1908 but then entered the emerging field of gastroenterology. Following the completion of his training, he opened an office for practice and soon developed a substantial following of patients with gastrointestinal disorders. In 1925, Crohn and Herman Rosenberg, in a publication entitled "The Sigmoidoscopic Picture of Ulcerative Colitis,"[8] documented the first case of a carcinoma developing in a patient with ulcerative colitis. In this paper, they also described a case in which the colon and rectum were thickened and rigid and contained multiple discrete ulcers. Although unrecognized at the time, this was almost certainly a case of granulomatous colitis. In 1927, Crohn published the single-authored text *Affections of the Stomach.*[9]

When Crohn, Leon Ginzburg, and Gordon D. Oppenheimer published "Regional Ileitis" in the *Journal of the American Medical Association (JAMA)* in October 1932 and proposed "to describe, in pathologic and clinical details, a disease of the terminal ileum, affecting mainly

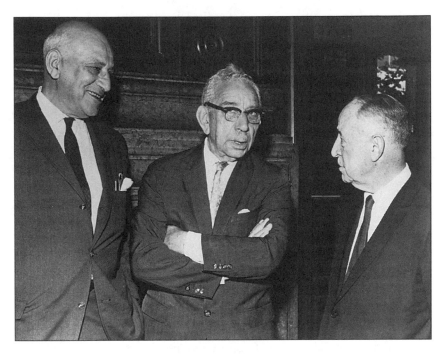

The three authors of the original paper on regional enteritis: Drs. Gordon D. Oppenheimer, Burrill B. Crohn, Leon Ginzburg.

young adults, characterized by subacute or chronic necrotizing and cicatrizing inflammation,"[10] they could have had no idea of the impact that this description would have on world medicine. It has been a source of continuing controversy that, in the spring of that year (prophetically, it was Friday, May 13), Crohn gave an oral presentation entitled "Terminal Ileitis" at the annual meeting of the American Medical Association and that he was listed in the program as the sole author, despite the undisputed role of Ginzburg and Oppenheimer in having done most of the groundwork. Two other extenuating facts, however, are less appreciated. One is that Crohn always contended that the single-author listing in the program was an error he had unsuccessfully sought to correct at the time. The second fact is that, also in May 1932, Ginzburg and Oppenheimer presented their own data on granulomatous ileitis and other lesions of the terminal ileum before the American Gastroenterological Association (AGA) with the pair listed as the only authors. When that paper was published in 1933, the authors made the following acknowledgment in a footnote on the first page: "The section on Localized Ileitis represents a joint study with Dr. Burrill B. Crohn."[11]

In any event, the pathway from Crohn's single-authored presentation to the subsequent jointly authored publication in *JAMA* was filled with turmoil. Indeed, the resolution was not reached without the convening of a formal committee of inquiry chaired by Mount Sinai's redoubtable Chief of Surgery, A. A. Berg. The ultimate outcome was an alphabetically listed authorship including Crohn, Ginzburg, and Oppenheimer. At Berg's insistence, his name was not included, although he had operated on all of the patients in the study. Can we conjecture that if he had put his name on the paper, and since the authors had agreed to an alphabetical listing, the disease would now be known as Berg's disease?

The fractious nature of this incident, however, never totally dissipated. In 1932, Crohn was already a well-established, successful gastroenterologist with a prestigious practice, while Ginzburg was a young surgeon and Berg's assistant in practice. Oppenheimer was an Assistant in the pathology laboratory. Crohn could readily sheathe his terrible swift sword of arrogance in a scabbard of smoothly polished charm; the brash young Ginzburg rarely bothered with such niceties. What the two men had in common, though, was that they were both intellectually curious, brilliant, proud, and opinionated. Their towering egos kept them in a state of smoldering animosity for the next fifty years, until Crohn's death in 1983 at the age of ninety-nine.

Nonetheless, as with so many other interdisciplinary efforts at Mount Sinai, Crohn and Ginzburg's collaboration was incredibly productive and stimulated an unparalleled flow of clinical and laboratory research on both of the principal chronic idiopathic inflammatory diseases: ulcerative colitis and what has become universally known as Crohn's disease.

Burrill B. Crohn lived a long and active life. He was able to be present at a major international symposium on Crohn's disease held at Mount Sinai in 1982, celebrating the fiftieth anniversary of the publication of the original paper. At that time he was ninety-eight years of age. His legacy lives on in the Burrill B. Crohn Research Foundation and in the Dr. Burrill B. Crohn Chair in Medicine, held by the Chief of the Division.

Crohn was succeeded by Asher Winkelstein as Chief of the Gastroenterology Clinic in 1922. In an almost forty-year career at Mount Sinai, Winkelstein made noteworthy contributions in the field of peptic disease, his major area of interest. He developed the continuous milk drip for the therapy of peptic ulcer and peptic esophagitis[12] and was the first to describe peptic esophagitis.[13] His studies of nocturnal acid secretion significantly advanced our understanding of the mechanism of acid secretion. A close collaborator of Ralph Colp, the surgeon, and bolstered by the work of the young surgeon Eugene Klein, Winkelstein was able to convince the former to perform anterior vagotomy when performing gastroenterostomy for ulcer disease. Blessed with a remarkably fertile and imaginative mind, Winkelstein was also an excellent violinist. In addition to the large body of work that he left behind, his son Charles, a psychiatrist, played a major role as Liaison Psychiatrist to the Department of Surgery for many years.

The past decade has seen the emergence of the term "translational research," modern terminology for the concept of bringing scientific research from the "bench to the bedside." At Mount Sinai, this is certainly not new. It has been going on for more than one hundred years, in fact, since the first laboratory opened in 1893. And nowhere was the concept more carefully honed than in the cooperation among gastroenterologists, surgeons, and the physiologist Franklin Hollander in using new findings from the laboratory to the benefit of the patient.

Already an established investigator in the field of gastric physiology by virtue of his studies in gastric secretion, Hollander was recruited to Mount Sinai in 1936 by the Surgical Service, but he soon became "Physiologist to the Hospital." In his thirty years as director of the Gastrointestinal Physiology Research Laboratory, Hollander contributed greatly to our understanding of the mechanisms of gastric secretion and the nature of the mucus barrier of the stomach. His studies on the vagal innervation of the stomach led to the development of the insulin test to determine the completeness of vagal interruption following surgery for peptic ulcer disease.[14]

Active on many editorial boards and a member of the most prestigious scientific societies, Hollander was honored by the AGA in 1965 with the receipt of the Julius Friedenwald Medal, given annually for outstanding achievement in gastroenterology. With peptic ulcer now considered to be primarily an infectious disease related to *Helicobactor pylori*, much of Hollander's work has lost some of its significance. What will never be lost was his role as an adviser, teacher, and mentor. Until his death in 1966 following a lengthy illness, Hollander helped nurture the investigative careers of numerous gastroenterologists and surgeons. With his death came the demise of his laboratory, which could not continue without him.

Even though a reorganization of the Department of Medicine in 1939 recognized gastroenterology as one of six major areas of specialization, gastroenterologists did not participate actively in medical ward teaching rounds in the Hospital. This did not change until 1958, when Alexander B. Gutman, the Chair of Medicine, created a separate Division of Gastroenterology and named Henry D. Janowitz as the Chief, a position the latter would hold for twenty-five years.

Janowitz interned at Mount Sinai and then served four and a half years in the Army Medical Corps during World War II as a gastroenterologist. Completing his residency after the war, Janowitz spent a number of years in full-time basic physiological research before embarking on a career that would be devoted to the combination of laboratory research and clinical practice. And what a career it would prove to be: fundamental contributions in gastrointestinal physiology related to gastric and pancreatic secretion (the latter in collaboration with David Dreiling of the Department of Surgery); the first clearcut evidence that an enzyme could inhibit acid secretion;[15] the development of an outstanding gastroenterology training program combining research and clinical training; leadership in American medicine; major clinical contributions to gastroenterology; and the support of a generation of clinical and physiological researchers in innumerable areas. Janowitz's trainees have become leaders throughout the world, and he has received numerous national and international honors, including the Julius Friedenwald Medal of the American Gastroenterological Society and Honorary Fellowship in the United Kingdom's Royal Society of Medicine.

When Janowitz became Chief of the Division in 1958, Mount Sinai had already been established as a GI medical and surgical referral center for half a century. Under his leadership, there was a dramatic increase in the number of patients with gastrointestinal disease, as well as an explosion in both laboratory and clinical research. With a personal clinical interest in inflammatory bowel disease (IBD), Janowitz played a major role in the establishment of the Foundation for Research in Ileitis, now known as the Crohn's and Colitis Foundation of America

(CCFA.) From its modest beginnings locally, the organization now has an annual budget of more than $21 million, more than sixty-thousand lay and physician members, and fifty-five chapters across the country with more than 350 support groups. With support of research as a prime goal, CCFA has provided the seed money for the majority of IBD investigators now funded by the National Institutes of Health.[16]

Henry Janowitz was a superb clinician; his judgment was impeccable. When he called a surgeon and said that he thought a patient needed an operation, the surgeon would be hard put to disagree. David Sachar has related a tale that speaks to Janowitz's prowess as a bedside teacher. In 1997, Janowitz sustained a hip fracture:

> During his hospitalization at Mount Sinai for corrective surgery and physical therapy, he was visited by a stream of attendings and colleagues. To each one of them, Henry delivered the most cogent, thorough, lucid, and precise summary of his medical condition, including the latest vital signs and functions, analgesic requirements and responses, and laboratory data and their interpretation. There was not a medical student, resident, fellow, or junior or senior faculty member who could not have benefited from the perfect model of bedside reporting provided by Henry's daily descriptions of his own clinical status![17]

It was during Janowitz's tenure as Chief that flexible endoscopy appeared on the scene, spurred and nurtured at Mount Sinai by Jerome Waye. As noted by the latter: "Changes in techniques and instrumentation progressed at a dizzying pace."[18] Early colonoscopy required fluoroscopy as an aid and led Waye to develop the nonfluoroscopic method of colonoscopic topography that has been universally adopted and has proven to be a landmark development in the use of this modality.[19] Waye became an international leader in endoscopy and eventually served as President of both the American College of Gastroenterology (ACG) and the American Society of Gastrointestinal Endoscopy.

Mount Sinai's reputation in gastroenterology and specifically in inflammatory bowel disease provided the institutional support and the patient base for its gastroenterologists of the past half-century to make noteworthy contributions to the art and science of the specialty. It has been noted that at least several dozen landmark papers on IBD have been published by the physicians of Mount Sinai.[20] These papers cover all aspects of IBD, including the natural history of the disease;[21] the first organized classification of the extraintestinal manifestations (the most often cited paper from the Division);[22] the measurement of clinical activity;[23] the relationships between cancer and IBD;[24] the risks of cancer in IBD;[25] and the first report of cancer developing in small-bowel Crohn's disease;[26] the radiological features of IBD;[27] the role of surgery;[28] the renal complications;[29] the association of amyloidosis and IBD;[30] the first demonstration of the use of colchicine to treat ulcerative colitis;[31] the first published trial on the use of fish oil in the management of ulcerative colitis;[32] the institution of novel and extraordinarily successful therapeutic modalities such as the use of immunosuppressive agents;[33] as well as the basic science and the role of immuno-modulators. The landmark studies of Daniel Present and Burton Korelitz in establishing immunosuppressive agents as first-line therapy in IBD have revolutionized the management of these illnesses. The entire body of work in inflammatory bowel disease emanating from Mount Sinai, spanning nearly seven decades, has been a prime example of multidisciplinary collaboration involving dozens of physicians and surgeons, from both voluntary and full-time faculty.

Like Crohn, the name Janowitz will be forever associated with Mount Sinai gastroenterology, as the Division has been named in his honor. Although he continued his practice, Janowitz stepped down as Chief in 1983 and was succeeded by David Sachar.

A graduate of Harvard Medical School and a fellow in Gastroenterology at Mount Sinai, David B. Sachar was appointed the first Dr. Burrill B. Crohn Professor of Medicine and the first full-time chief of the Division of Gastroenterology. Sachar had made his first significant contribution to world medicine while a research associate with the United States Public Health Service during his medical residency. Stationed in Bangladesh, he played a critical role in the development of oral rehydration therapy for cholera and other diarrheal diseases, an advance credited with saving millions of lives annually.[34]

A world-renowned specialist in inflammatory bowel disease, Sachar made important contributions to the field. He and his colleagues introduced modern life-table methodology for studies of postoperative recurrence of Crohn's disease;[35] identified risk factors for recurrence;[36] developed concepts of classifying clinical phenotypes by disease behavior;[37] and, as noted earlier, collaborated in the classification of the systemic manifestations of inflammatory bowel disease and the correlation of clinical findings with laboratory markers of activity. A founding director of the Burrill B. Crohn Research Foundation, Sachar was the first and so far the only American to be elected Chairman of the International Organization for the Study of Inflammatory Bowel Disease. An outstanding teacher, Sachar developed new resources and set new standards for clinical teaching nationwide as the first Chairman of the Clinical Teaching Project of the AGA. The recipient of numerous national and international awards, Sachar has been honored on many occasions at Mount Sinai with several faculty awards for excellence in teaching, the Alexander Richman Award for Humanism in Medicine,[38] the Jacobi Medallion, and the Gold-Headed Cane. Blessed with an ebullient personality and a great gift for speaking and writing, Sachar was able to attract a superlative group of young gastroenterologists to both the full-time and the voluntary faculties. One of them, Steven Itzkowitz, would succeed Sachar when he stepped down after sixteen years as Chief in 1999.

A graduate of the Mount Sinai School of Medicine, Steven H. Itzkowitz returned to Mount Sinai as Director of the Gastrointestinal Research Laboratory in 1988 after eight years at the University of California in San Francisco, where he received his gastroenterology training and served on the faculty. Nationally and internationally recognized for his research in mucin and molecular markers of colon cancer and inflammatory bowel disease,[39] Itzkowitz has taken the interests of the Division into new areas and will lead it to still greater heights.

6

Divisions of Hematology and Thrombosis Research

The Blood Bank

The diseases of the blood have occupied much attention.
—*Annual Report of The Mount Sinai Hospital*, 1924

BY 1924, this was already an understatement of the past and a prediction for the future. In 1908, Reuben Ottenberg had been appointed the George Blumenthal, Jr., Fellow in Pathology. He wrote his first paper as an intern at the German Hospital (later called Lenox Hill Hospital), and his 1908 publication, "Transfusion and Arterial Anastomosis," won the prize for the best paper of the year by a member of the house staff.[1] In this paper, Ottenberg describes a laboratory study of arterial anastomoses utilizing tiny silver wire rings rather than sutures to hold the blood vessels together during direct transfusion. He then describes the use of these rings in two patients being transfused and states that the blood was tested for compatibility prior to use, the first report anywhere of the clinical use of compatibility testing. Years later, Ottenberg was to note, "The subject is only brought in incidentally in a footnote. I was still an interne and did not realize how important the testing was to become. I should have made a separate article."[2]

Serving first in the Clinical Microscopy and Pathology laboratories and then in the clinics, Ottenberg was appointed to the inpatient Attending staff in 1920. While maintaining a busy practice and serving on the teaching service, Ottenberg continued to make fundamental contributions to medicine, especially in the evolving field of hematology, publishing almost one hundred papers. In notes accompanying his bibliography, Ottenberg writes that, in addition to the first use of blood

74

testing for transfusion compatibility, his most important investigative work was the first observation that patient antibodies against donor red cells could be harmful but not vice versa.[3] This report, coming shortly before World War I, helped establish the use of Group 0 individuals as universal donors.

In 1923, Ottenberg reported that jaundice and hemolytic anemia of the newborn might be due to blood incompatibility of mother and child.[4] The discovery of the Rh factor almost twenty years later by Karl Landsteiner and Alexander Wiener, and the description of erythroblastosis fetalis by Philip Levine, proved Ottenberg correct. He was also the first to suggest that human blood groups are inherited according to Mendel's law,[5] and, with Nathan Rosenthal, he described a new method of counting platelets using sodium citrate, a technique that remained in standard use for decades.[6] He observed that in septicemia, the largest number of bacteria are found at the time when the temperature is just beginning to rise, rather than at the height of the spike.[7]

Ottenberg also wrote a number of important clinical papers, including work on the diagnosis of painless jaundice, the toxic effect of sulfonamides, and septicemia following trauma. Suffering from stenosis of the internal carotid artery, Ottenberg reported his own case in 1955. In a matter-of-fact manner, he described his transient ischemic attacks, his episodes of amaurosis fugax, and the stroke from which he recovered four years before his death.[8] In 1954, Ottenberg received the Karl Landsteiner Award of the American Society of Blood Banks for his distinguished pioneering contributions to blood banking and hemotherapy.

Ottenberg was not alone at Mount Sinai in studying the diseases and the therapeutic uses of blood. Two vital contributions to the management of transfusion came from Mount Sinai in 1915. One spoke to the past, the second to the future. The first was Lester Unger's introduction of a new stopcock for direct donor-to-patient transfusion.[9] Connected to a syringe, the four-way valve allowed the operator to withdraw blood from the donor, mix it with either citrate solution or normal saline, and inject the mixture into the patient in one smooth operation. The second was Richard Lewisohn's description of the minimum amount of citrate required to prevent blood from clotting, making indirect transfusion possible and practical and allowing blood to be stored for later transfusion.[10] This was just the first of many contributions by Lewisohn to hematology.

Lewisohn was a prime example of the surgeon/scientist. Born in Germany in 1875, he graduated from the University of Freiburg in 1899, followed by postgraduate work in pathology and then surgery. He arrived in New York in 1906 and, once licensed, joined the staff of the First Surgical Service at The Mount Sinai Hospital. He advanced through the ranks, reaching Attending status in 1928 and retired from active status when he reached the mandatory retirement age in 1937. He then returned to the laboratory to work on cancer research. In 1954, a donor provided the funding to establish a Cell Research Laboratory, and, at the age of eighty, Lewisohn began his work anew. In 1955, one year after Ottenberg, he, too, was awarded the Karl Landsteiner Award and Medal of the American Association of Blood Banks. He died in 1961, secure in his legacy of the development of the citrate method of blood transfusion.

But, as Lewisohn himself said, "Any progressive step in medicine (or for that matter in many other branches of science) will usually be followed by an argument on priority."[11] The citrate method of transfusion was no exception. In 1944, Lewisohn described the events as follows:

> [Luis] Agote [Buenes Aires] should get proper credit. His paper appeared at exactly the same time as my original communication (January, 1915). He had the right percentage of sodium citrate (0.25 per cent). He reported 2 transfusions of 300cc. each. He did not answer the question of whether transfusions of average size (500 to 700 cc.) could be given with this method without causing toxic effects. Furthermore, he did not study the effect of anticoagulants on the coagulation time of the recipient. I have often said that when an idea is ripe it frequently occurs simultaneously to more than one person. Thus Agote and I, in different and far distant parts of this hemisphere, hit upon the right technique at the same time.[12]

Both direct donor-to-patient transfusion, using the Unger stopcock, and the use of citrated blood were used at Mount Sinai for many years until the value of sodium citrate was fully established. One reason for the hesitancy regarding the citrate method was the posttransfusion chills that often accompanied transfusions when citrate was added. In 1933, Lewisohn and Rosenthal demonstrated that the chills were caused by foreign proteins and that, with proper sterilization of the equipment, the reaction could for the most part be avoided.[13] This finding led to Mount Sinai's creation of the first Intravenous Therapy Department in the country in 1931 to ensure technical expertise in the proper handling of transfusions and intravenous lines. This work on the practical aspects of transfusion continued at Mount Sinai in the following decades, resulting in newer methods of blood typing and the automation of equipment and testing.

The early years of the twentieth century saw laboratory science make its appearance in hospitals. The venue was ideal for the study of hematological disease. In 1925, a separate hematology laboratory was authorized to coordinate the blood typing and tests needed for patient care, as well as to encourage research. Here, in 1925, Eli Moschcowitz described thrombotic thrombocytopenic purpura (Moschcowitz Disease),[14] and in the same year Nathan Brill, George Baehr, and Nathan Rosenthal elucidated giant lymph follicle hyperplasia, a form of lymphoma.[15] The latter became known as Brill-Symmers Disease, following a paper by Douglas Symmers in 1927.

In 1926, when there was a general reorganization of the laboratories, it was Nathan Rosenthal, an Associate in Medicine and a member of the laboratory Department of Hematology, who was appointed Hematologist to the Hospital. Born in New York City in 1890, Nathan Rosenthal graduated from Columbia University's College of Physicians and Surgeons (P&S) in 1913. He was an Intern, House Surgeon, and Research Fellow at The Mount Sinai Hospital and served in Mount Sinai's unit, Base Hospital No. 3, during World War I. On his return, Rosenthal received appointments as Assistant Clinical Pathologist and Assistant in Medicine. In 1925, when the laboratory was established, hematology was an emerging specialty, and Rosenthal was involved in many aspects of the field. Within a year of his appointment, Rosenthal established a Hematology Clinic for ambulatory care. He also organized a Hematology Service and Laboratory at the Harlem Hospital in 1927. Mount Sinai's laboratory and clinics attracted observers from around the world, and Rosenthal established a laboratory teaching program for fellows, as well as participating in Mount Sinai's postgraduate teaching of P&S students. This was one of the first centers for postgraduate training in hematology in this country.[16] Interested in cytology, lymphomas, leukemia, polycythemia, and hemorrhagic diseases and a keen observer, Rosenthal published extensively. In later years, his son, Robert, worked with him for a time, and, in 1953, in collaboration with O. Herman Dreskin, they described a new clotting factor, PTA

(Factor XI), the deficiency of which causes a bleeding diathesis.[17] In 1969, Stanley Lee, Fred Rosner, Robert Rosenthal, and the late Nathan Rosenthal published an article on one of the largest series of patients with reticulum or hairy cell leukemia.[18] In recognition of the elder Rosenthal's contributions to the understanding of this disease, his name was included.

In 1952, Rosenthal received the Order of Carlos Finlay from the Republic of Cuba and in 1953 was the first winner of the Harlow Brooks Medal of The New York Academy of Medicine. After his death in 1955, the monthly hematology seminars at Mount Sinai were renamed the Nathan Rosenthal Seminars in his honor. He had become known as the "dean of hematologists in the United States."[19]

During the 1930s and 1940s, many of Mount Sinai's brightest young house officers went into hematology. The staff during this period included Daniel Stats and Frank A. Bassen. Stats was a 1936 graduate of New York University Medical School (NYU). He began a surgical internship at Mount Sinai Hospital but had to switch to medicine when he developed dermatitis of the hands. He did fundamental work on the hemolytic anemias, especially those concerned with cold agglutination.[20] He also developed a new sedimentation test to determine red cell survival.[21] Under Rosenthal, he organized the teaching program in hematology. At Stat's untimely death in 1958 at the age of forty-six, the Department created a fund to establish the Daniel Stats Prize, to be awarded annually to the House Staff member who published the best original paper on the diseases of the blood.

Frank E. Bassen, a Canadian, received his M.D. degree from McGill University in 1928. He came to New York in 1932 and, after serving for a year as a Resident in Mount Sinai's Private Pavilion, went into practice and joined the staff as a Clinical Assistant in Medicine. In 1942, he was called to wartime service, rising to the rank of Major. He returned to Mount Sinai in 1946 and remained connected with the Hospital until his retirement in 1980. In 1950, Bassen and Abraham L. Kornzweig published the first description of what became known as familial abetalipoprotein deficiency, or the Bassen-Kornzweig Syndrome.[22]

In addition to an active and successful research program, a significant part of Nathan Rosenthal's legacy to Mount Sinai was the Blood Bank, only the second to be established in the United States, the first being at Cook County Hospital in Chicago. The addition of sodium citrate to blood had allowed for preservation, the use of proper steriliza-

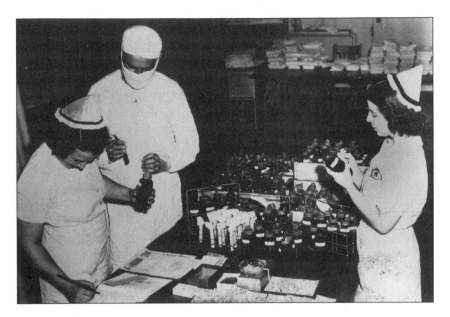

Blood Bank, c. 1945.

tion techniques had eliminated many major complications; attention was now turning to the use of stored blood. By 1937, Mount Sinai was administering more than one hundred transfusions each month. Blood was donated by patients, family, or friends, then collected and administered as fresh blood. Many times when patient and donor were not a good match, the blood was discarded, and the cost to the Hospital of providing fresh blood was high. Studies intensified on the use of stored blood versus fresh blood. By 1938, the Hospital decided to open a Blood Bank on an "experimental basis to determine its precise value in medicine."[23] Initially, the Blood Bank was open only three times a week at set hours. Rosenthal described the early program as follows:

> In order to concentrate all procedures in one unit, a special seven-bed ward with an icebox capable of storing 150 pints of blood at 2 to 4 degrees C was made available. Donors are registered, typed, and examined before phlebotomies are performed. The rapid slide method of typing (Coca) is used. High titre serum furnished by the Blood Transfusion Betterment Association is employed. Questionable groupings,

which occur rarely, are checked by the Schiff Modification of the Land-steiner tube method. . . . The phlebotomies are performed in the following manner: After surgical preparation of the arm with iodine and alcohol from axilla to wrist, and careful draping of the arm, a 13 to 15 gauge Luer needle with an 8 inch latex rubber tubing attachment is inserted into the vein through a procainized skin area. The blood is collected in a [quart-size] Mason jar to which has been added 50 cc. of 3.8 percent sodium citrate solution. . . .[24]

It was not long before the Blood Bank had the chance to prove its worth. In 1940, the Blood for Britain Project was established by the American Red Cross and the Blood Transfusion Association to provide blood plasma to England. Up to two hundred sixty donors weekly were handled by volunteer physicians, nurses, student nurses, and technicians. The Blood Bank was moved to larger quarters on the third floor of the Administration Building (Metzger) to accommodate the increased demand. With the United States' entrance into World War II, Hematology's research efforts intensified, focusing on how long red cells could survive for transfusion purposes and what conditions were required for airborne transportation. In 1943, Mount Sinai was the first hospital to complete its quota of blood plasma for the Civilian Defense Blood Bank.

The pace of the Department's work accelerated dramatically during and after the war years. Studies were carried out on the use of type O blood as the universal donor, on the role of the Rh factor in repeated transfusions, and on the entire gamut of hematologic diseases. In 1941, the number of clinic days increased from two to three; a weekly joint clinic with Radiotherapy was offered for the management of the leukemias, lymphomas, and lymphosarcomas. Educational efforts expanded, and the Hematology Journal Club opened its monthly meetings to practitioners from the area. In 1946, the Blood Bank performed 3,212 consultations, the Hematology Clinic saw 5,227 patients, and a Children's Hematology Clinic was established.

In 1939, the Department of Medicine had reorganized into six specialty "groups": gastroenterology, hematology, allergy, thoracic diseases, cardiovascular diseases, and metabolism and nutrition. Each group had an Associate in Medicine in charge, along with designated laboratory space and clinics. In 1950, Nathan Rosenthal reached retirement age, stepped down as Hematologist to the Hospital, and was succeeded by Louis R. Wasserman, who would head the program for twenty-two years. At this juncture, the Department had an active teaching program involving Residents in Pathology and Medicine, as well as Hematology Fellows. Successful postgraduate courses were offered through Columbia University and at The New York Academy of Medicine. The laboratory was performing all the hematological testing for the Hospital, in addition to providing a substantial research base.

Louis Robert Wasserman was only forty when he was named Chief of Hematology in 1950, but the reputation of his early work in iron metabolism and his prior years at Mount Sinai made him the perfect candidate for the position. Wasserman came to Mount Sinai as a Research Fellow in the Hematology Laboratory in 1937. He joined Mount Sinai's Third General Hospital during World War II and then was sent to the Donner Laboratory in Berkeley to work with John H. Lawrence from 1946 to 1949. He helped pioneer the use of radioactive isotopes for quantization of the circulation of red cell mass and in clinical studies of erythrokinetics. When he returned to Mount Sinai, he continued his laboratory research on iron metabolism and bone marrow physiology. But it would be in his lifelong clinical and laboratory studies of polycythemia vera that Wasserman would make his most lasting impact.

The group that Wasserman took over was on the cusp of change, some changes because of developments in the field, others because of the force of Wasserman's personality. Hematology had been a division of the Department of Medicine, as well as a separate laboratory division. In 1954, Hematology "was elevated to full departmental status, with the Blood Bank as one of its divisions."[25] There were two other divisions: the Hematology Laboratory and Clinical Microscopy. The Department had sixteen physicians on the inpatient and outpatient staff, a small group of Residents and two Research Fellows. Lester B. Hollander, the first Resident in Hematology, "graduated" in 1951. The teaching program included the Residents and Fellows in Hematology and other Departments, as well as students from NYU. Wasserman also worked out an agreement with the Brookhaven Laboratory Medical Group to rotate staff for teaching and to exchange data.

Hematology, in true Mount Sinai tradition, had long felt the need for more space. Wasserman quickly obtained enlarged quarters in the new research buildings that were being built, and early in 1955 Hematology moved into this larger space in the Atran-Berg buildings. It was hoped that the old Lewisohn Laboratory (a separate building) could be renovated for the Blood Bank, but this did not materialize. But, while the Blood Bank awaited new facilities, many changes took place there, as well.

One of Wasserman's first appointments was that of Peter Vogel as Director of the Blood Bank. Vogel trained in pediatrics at Mount Sinai, following his 1927 medical school graduation, and then worked in the tuberculosis clinics at The Mount Sinai and Harlem hospitals. He joined the Hematology Clinic in 1931 with a concomitant appointment in the Hematology Laboratory and was named Chief of Clinic in 1948, the same year that he helped the New York City Bureau of Laboratories set up its Rh typing laboratory. By 1951, the City's laboratory had become the busiest in the world. Vogel published on a variety of topics, including many relating to children. He did pioneering work with Philip Levine on erythroblastosis fetalis[26] and helped develop the first saline agglutinating anti-Rh serum. Vogel was a founder and the first medical director of the Blood Transfusion Association, a forerunner of the New York Blood Center, and was also very involved with the National Hemophilia Society. He reached Consultant status at Mount Sinai in 1961 but remained active for many years until his death in 1987.

One of the Blood Bank's innovations during Vogel's years was the development of the Walk-In Blood Bank, an attempt to get staff and employees to donate blood. Newer therapies, such as the early open heart surgery program and the use of the artificial kidney for renal dialysis, both of which required substantial amounts of blood, had put a strain on blood availability. Donors were initially paid fifteen dollars per unit and thirty dollars for a unit suitable for exchange transfusion for newborns. In 1951, a transfusion clinic and a laboratory were established. During these years, the Blood Bank also switched to collecting blood in plastic bags. The work of the Blood Bank and the laboratory increased dramatically. In 1955, they handled 4,516 donors, performed 42,134 specimen examinations and 180,893 blood tests, and provided 10,986 transfusions of stored blood.

The opening of Mount Sinai's first Obstetrical service in 1952 created opportunities and challenges, as the hematologists studied and treated the conditions relating to hematological disorders in pregnancy and in the newborn. The postwar period also saw the rise of the "War on Cancer," signaling increased efforts in the study of leukemia in the Department and the Institution. The Department received many research grants from the National Cancer Institute, as well as support from outside agencies to enhance training programs. In 1958, Mount Sinai joined the Cancer Chemotherapy Service Center of the National Institutes of Health to evaluate chemotherapeutic agents in the treatment of leukemia and allied disorders. In 1970, Hematology became a member of the National Cancer Institute Acute Leukemia Study Group.

Another area of activity that began during the 1950s and has continued to the present was in the innovative study and treatment of hemophilia. In 1953, with funds from the National Hemophilia Foundation, a weekly Hemophilia Clinic was established, with Martin C. Rosenthal in charge. A multidisciplinary team interested in the disease came together to manage the hemophilia patients; the Clinic was a success from the start. A most productive Coagulation Laboratory was also established in 1953. In 1963, the Blood Bank pioneered in the use of plasmapheresis therapy for hemophilia patients. In 1966, Solomon Estren, Julian Niemetz, and their colleagues made a landmark contribution to the emergency care of hemophiliacs with their use of animal antihemophilic globulin (AHG) concentrates in patients with circulating AHG inhibitor.[27]

As the Department's research efforts grew, basic scientists were added to broaden the scope of the research and fellowship training. By 1961, there were twenty-six Research Fellows, Clinical Fellows, Residents, and trainees in the Department, with a research budget close to $200,000. The Department had reorganized into seven different laboratories: coagulation, immunohematology, anemia, radioactivity, cytochemistry, special chemistry, and chemohematology. Researchers continued to study areas of long-term interest; including polycythemia vera, the hemolytic aspects of lupus erythematosis, the anemias, the role of vitamins, iron metabolism, and erythroblastosis fetalis. In 1958, Solomon Estren, Eugene A. Brody, and Wasserman published an important paper on the metabolism of vitamin B12 in pernicious anemia and the megaloblastic anemias.[28] Wasserman lobbied the administration to add a virologist to his staff, but the founding of the Medical School in 1963 changed the way staff needs were evaluated and prioritized. Eventually, Charlotte Friend, a young virologist, was added at Wasserman's urging, but she was named a full Professor in the new Center for Experimental Cell Biology, not in Hematology. Friend discovered and worked with an animal leukemia virus that became known as the "Friend leukemia virus."[29]

In 1957, Richard Rosenfield was named the Director of the Blood Bank, a position he would hold for almost thirty years with great distinction. Graduating from medical school in 1940, Rosenfield spent six years in the U.S. Army Medical Corps as an internist and laboratory officer. He joined the staff of the Hematology Clinic and the Hematology Laboratory at Mount Sinai in 1948 and also took a part-time position as Hematologist in the Rh Laboratory of the New York City Department of Health, an appointment he maintained for twenty years. In 1967, he accepted the added challenge of becoming the Editor-in-Chief of the journal *Transfusion* and subsequently served on the editorial boards of numerous hematology journals. Rosenfield's research interests were expressed in more than two-hundred publications and spanned the field from the practical development of tests and equipment[30] to the classification of the blood groups[31] to the basic science of blood and blood typing.[32] He was also well known for his efforts in the study of ABO disease.[33] He later collaborated with Sheldon Cherry, an obstetrician, and others in the study of erythroblastosis fetalis.[34] In 1967, Rosenfield participated in the care of an extremely rare type Rh Null obstetrical patient, aiding in the delivery and treatment of her newborn son, whose life was in danger because the infant had not inherited his mother's rare blood type.[35] Rosenfield's many contributions to hematology and blood banking were recognized when he received the Karl Landsteiner Memorial Award for Medical Research in 1972, making him the third Mount Sinai physician so honored, and the Philip Levine Award from the American Society of Clinical Pathologists in 1975. He also received the Humanitarian Award from the National Foundation in 1981.

The Blood Bank moved to larger, more modern quarters in the basement of the Klingenstein Clinical Center in 1963. Changes in the operation of the Blood Bank included many innovations developed in the Department. Mount Sinai became a member of the New York Blood Center in 1967. Four years later, routine hepatitis screening of blood was instituted. Rosenfield created a full-time, two-year training program for blood bank directors; its graduates would take leadership positions around the world. In 1974, a Nurse Intravenous Team was created to assist in patient care and to provide specialized training for the nursing and ancillary staff.

By 1964, the Department of Hematology was noted as being "the largest and most active of its kind in the New York metropolitan area."[36] At mid-decade there were sixteen full-time hematologists, three full-time Ph.D.s, fifteen part-time hematologists, one part-time Ph.D., and fifteen Residents and Fellows. The training program included the Mount Sinai affiliates, the City Hospital Center at Elmhurst, and the Bronx Veterans Administration Hospital. The Department, now responsible for all testing, performed more than 500,000 procedures for the first time in 1967. There were six clinics each week and an extensive teaching program. The Nathan Rosenthal Hematology Seminars drew speakers from around the world and were well attended by area physicians interested in hematology. When the first medical students arrived at the Mount Sinai School of Medicine in 1968, the Department accepted responsibility for teaching courses in laboratory procedures and clinical hematology and offered a number of electives.

Like other great leaders, Wasserman surrounded himself with unique and productive individuals. Victor Herbert's research vastly improved understanding of the nutritional anemias. He also assisted in the administration of the Department during this period, prior to his move to the Bronx VA. In 1966, Wasserman invited William Dameshek, the world-renowned hematologist and founder and Editor-in-Chief of the journal *Blood*, to join the Department. An inspiring teacher and colleague, he was at Mount Sinai for only three years when he died unexpectedly in 1969 of a ruptured thoracic aneurysm.

Also recruited in 1966 was Louis Aledort, who was appointed Director of the Coagulation Laboratory and Chief of the Hemophilia Clinic. Aledort's early research focused on platelet mechanisms and function, including the first description of the mechanisms controlling platelet contractile proteins.[37] Later papers dealt with hemophilia, the delivery of patient care, and AIDS. While in charge of the Hemophilia Clinic, Aledort designed a comprehensive care model to deal with all aspects of hemophilia, emphasizing patient education, to allow the patient to optimize his own life. In 1972, Mount Sinai was named an International Hemophilia Training Center and became a federally funded diagnostic and treatment center.

Aledort published almost two hundred papers and served on national and international associations in hemophilia. He was Medical Co-Director of the National Hemophilia Society for many years and during that time played a controversial role in defining a policy for the hemophilia group to follow in the early years of the AIDS epidemic. The impact of AIDS on the hemophiliac community was a medical, scientific, and social tragedy. The cautious strategies of Aledort and the

National Hemophilia Society were viewed by some, in retrospect, as misleading and harmful.[38] For many years, Aledort was Vice-Chairman of the Department of Medicine and an Associate Dean in the Medical School. In 1993, he was invested as the Mary Weinfeld Professor of Clinical Research in Hemophilia.

Wasserman's own clinical and laboratory research interests continued to focus on polycythemia vera. A centerpiece of this effort was the formation of the Polycythemia Vera Study Group in 1967.[39] This group, composed of physicians and investigators from around the world, met to try to reach agreement on some of the basic questions in polycythemia vera, questions about the natural history of the disease and the optimum therapy that would lead to the longest, uncomplicated survival. Sponsored by the National Cancer Institute and under Wasserman's leadership, the group established the first reliable set of diagnostic criteria for polycythemia and evaluated many different therapies. The value of the Study Group for this disease, in addition to serving as a model for other conditions, cannot be overstated.

Wasserman was a driving force to be reckoned with. Not only did he acquire departmental status for the Hematology Division, but he also influenced Mount Sinai policy in many ways while serving on important committees. He demanded excellence and was, above all, a superb teacher and mentor whose many trainees went on to serve hematology well. Wasserman was involved in professional associations around the world, including serving as the President of the American Society of Hematology (ASH). He was particularly interested in the education of hematologists; in 1979, the ASH established the Wasserman-Ham Lecture in recognition of his service to that group's educational efforts.

Upon Wasserman's retirement as Chief in 1972, Hematology was reorganized, with the clinical activities placed again under the aegis of the Department of Medicine. The changes occurred during a difficult period for the Department of Medicine. The Chairman, Solomon Berson, had died unexpectedly; Fenton Schaffner was designated the Acting Chairman. Ralph Zalusky was appointed Acting Director of the Division of Hematology and was also responsible for the Clinical Microscopy Laboratory. Rosenfield was placed in charge of a new Hospital Department of the Blood Bank and Clinical Microscopy; Shaul Kochwa was placed in charge of the Immunohematology Laboratory.

In 1974, Richard Gorlin began his tenure as the new Chairman of Medicine and over the ensuing years absorbed the various components of Hematology into Medicine. Paul Berk was named Chief of the Division of Hematology in 1977. A graduate of P&S, Berk trained under Nathaniel Berlin at the National Institutes of Health and was subsequently appointed head of the Liver Disease section of the National Institute of Arthritis and Metabolic Disease. His work on the life cycle of the red blood cell led to research on bilirubin metabolism and in turn on the liver itself. Berk and his colleagues discovered the fatty acid binding protein[40] and made other seminal contributions to the study of liver disease. In 1980, Berk became the second Albert and Vera List Professor of Medicine (Wasserman was the first). He served as the Co-Chairman of the National Polycythemia Study Group with Wasserman and was President of the New York Society for the Study of the Blood. A Hemoglobinopathy Clinic was established in 1980 to coordinate research programs and patient care for inherited diseases of hemoglobin structure or production.

Another outstanding recruit in 1977 was Yale Nemerson, who became the Philip J. and Harriet L. Goodhart Professor of Medicine and established a new Thrombosis Division to coordinate blood coagulation research within the Department of Medicine. Working to define the mechanisms that initiate the blood coagulation process, Nemerson studied human tissue factor and its relationship to various coagulation factors, particularly Factor X and Factor VII.[41] Internationally recognized for his research, Nemerson was awarded the Dameshek Prize by the American Society of Hematology in 1981. In 1987, in collaboration with scientists at Yale, Nemerson isolated and cloned the complete structural gene for human tissue factor.[42]

The early 1980s witnessed many changes for the Division of Hematology, one of the most important being Rosenfield's elevation to emeritus status in 1985. Looking back on Rosenfield's career, Maxwell Wintrobe noted that Rosenfield "is unique in that he is the only person who has done research with all three of the protagonists in the blood group debates—Levine, Wiener, and Race—though separately of course."[43] Charles G. Zaroulis, James Louie, and Michael Greenberg each then directed the Blood Bank for a short period until 1989, when the appointment of Morton Spivack provided stability for twelve years until the latter's retirement. A defining event in hematology during Berk's tenure in the 1980s was, of course, the beginning of the AIDS era. Fortunately, virus testing became available in 1984–1985 so that the blood supply could be more adequately screened.

Berk was responsible for the institution of Mount Sinai's bone marrow transplantation program. A certificate of need was granted by the New York State Health Department in 1990. Stephen Fruchtman was appointed Director of the Stem Cell Transplantation Service, and the program rapidly expanded its activities.[44] In collaboration with the New York Blood Center and its Director, Pablo Rubenstein, Fruchtman established a hematopoietic stem-cell bank that utilized placental blood drained from the umbilical cord after delivery, performed HLA typing of the blood, and then stored it for future use. A recent report by Fruchtman and his colleagues documents the first use of an autologous cord blood infusion given to a twenty-month-old baby who developed severe aplastic anemia following a liver transplant.[45]

In 1990, Peter Harpel was named Chief of the Division of Hematology, succeeding Paul Berk, who became Chief of the Division of Liver Diseases. The former Director of the Coagulation Laboratory at the New York Hospital, Harpel performed research focused on the action of blood proteins in the process of clot formation and dissolution.

The appointment of Barry Coller, a renowned hematologist, as Chairman of the Department of Medicine in 1993 added a luminary in the field to the roster of the Division. Coller continued his groundbreaking platelet studies and proved to be an outstanding mentor, despite the restrictions on his time created by his administrative responsibilities.

The death of Louis Wasserman in June 1999, after more than a sixty-year affiliation with Mount Sinai, marked the end of an era. Harpel retired in the same year as Chief of the Division and was succeeded by George Atweh, who had been at Mount Sinai since 1992. An eminent scientist and a recognized authority in the molecular biology of hemoglobin and its disorders, Atweh served as the Associate Program Director for the General Clinical Research Center, as well as the Director of the Sickle Cell Program. In 1999, Atweh and other Mount Sinai researchers announced a new pharmacologic treatment modality for sickle cell disease.[46]

Atweh was fortunate in recruiting Carolyn Whitsett as Director of the Blood Bank in 2000 after Spivack's retirement. A distinguished "blood banker," Whitsett trained at the New York Blood Center and has been involved in setting national policy and priorities through her role on the Advisory Council of the National Heart, Lung, and Blood Institute.

As the new century dawns, Hematology at Mount Sinai is poised to continue its pioneering traditions of the past. The fellowship program is now a combined effort of the Divisions of Hematology and Oncology. The Division of Hematology remains one of the largest such groups in the world. In the Division's own words, "the principles that we espouse are ones in which basic and clinical research are conducted by an inter-active group of physicians and scientists who work together to bring advances in basic research to the clinic in an expeditious manner."[47]

7

Division of Infectious Diseases

MORE THAN A century before the creation of the Division of Infectious Diseases in 1968, the physicians of the Hospital were contributing to the diagnosis and management of the entire spectrum of infectious disease. Major epidemics of typhus and cholera devastated New York in the 1840s; an epidemic of Asiatic cholera in 1849 killed thousands. These diseases, plus typhoid and tuberculosis, were affecting large numbers of the rapidly increasing Jewish population of the city, a population that the Jews' Hospital, opening in 1855, was meant to serve. Nevertheless, before the Hospital's opening, the Directors (later called Trustees) resolved that patients with typhoid could not be admitted. It would be more than six months before the medical staff could convince the Trustees that the disease was not contagious when patients were hospitalized and housed under sanitary conditions. The same was true of typhus. However, patients with tuberculosis were not barred and accounted for a number of the early admissions. The medical staff was not immune from infectious disease: Ernst Krakowiczer, the surgeon, died of typhoid in 1875.

Just as today, laboratory investigation was vital to the Hospital in managing infectious disease and led to important discoveries. In 1897, Charles Elsberg, Mount Sinai's Assistant Pathologist, published on studies he had performed utilizing the Widal test (a test of blood serum that utilizes agglutination of blood cells) to diagnose typhoid. Shortly thereafter, the use of the test would be crucial in determining the source of an outbreak of typhoid among the nursing staff; a carrier was identified. Later, Nathan Brill identified a group of patients who seemed to have typhoid but who had negative Widal reactions. His definitive study in 1910 established endemic typhus (Brill's disease) as a distinct entity. In the first decade of the twentieth century, Emanuel Libman, who had discovered *Streptococcus enteritis* while studying in Europe in the late 1890s, continued his bacteriological studies, reported on the use of blood cultures in diagnosing the causative agents of infection, and published his landmark studies on bacterial endo-carditis.[1]

Although improving sanitary conditions in New York diminished the incidence of typhus and typhoid, the advent of World War I once again brought Mount Sinai physicians to the fore in the battle against typhus. In 1916, George Baehr and Harry Plotz were sent to Serbia as members of the Strong Commission to study an outbreak of typhus. Baehr and Plotz were captured and for a time were prisoners of war. After their return to the United States, Plotz and Peter Olitzky, with a group partly sponsored by the Hospital, went to Mexico for study of another outbreak of typhus. Olitzky contracted typhus while there but recovered. In 1921, Leo Loewe, an internist working in the bacteriology laboratory of the Hospital, reported the first cultivation of Rickettsia-like bodies from the blood of patients with typhus fever and from the blood and multiple organs of guinea pigs infected with the blood of typhus fever patients.[2]

The influenza epidemic of 1918 put Mount Sinai to the test in two geographically disparate areas. Base Hospital No. 3, the Mount Sinai unit, cared for hundreds of influenza patients while stationed in France. At home, eighty-five nurses contracted influenza, eighteen developed pneumonia, and five died, as did a member of the House Staff. The surgeon, Alexis Moschcowitz, while in the military, was appointed a member of the Empyema Commission established to deal with the ravages of empyema, which too often followed postinfluenzal pneumonia. The recommendations of the group reduced the mortality rate from more than 50 percent to less than 5 percent.[3]

In the years between the two world wars, infectious disease continued to account for a substantial number of admissions. For example, in 1983, a letter was sent to the Hospital: "Gentlemen: I, Mary . . . , known on your records as Mary . . . (or Typhoid Mary #2) . . . was in your hospital from October 1938 to February 1939 with typhoid fever, later removing my gallbladder so I would not be a carrier. Since that time, I have enjoyed perfect health."[4] Bacterial infection of the lung remained a major problem; patients with putrid lung abscesses and empyema occupied a large number of beds on the surgical service. The one-stage procedure for drainage of a lung abscess was developed by Mount Sinai's thoracic surgeons.[5]

Patients with syphilis had been admitted to the Hospital from its earliest days and treated in large numbers in the Dispensary as outpatient services expanded. The synthesis of arsphenamine in 1909 allowed for an effective treatment for the first time. In 1940, Louis Chargin, the Chief of Dermatology, and his colleagues, in collaboration with George Baehr, Chief of the First Medical Service, reported on a novel intensive five-day course of arsphenamine treatment that produced striking results.[6] Although the treatment was revolutionary in concept, the availability of penicillin at the end of World War II soon relegated the group's contribution to obscurity.

The increasing use of penicillin and the rapid development of new antibiotics dramatically altered the management of infection and infectious diseases. Diseases that had been responsible for so many deaths in the past were now curable. But, over time, a new phenomenon appeared—antibiotic resistance. Stanley Schneierson, the Hospital's microbiologist, developed antibiotic sensitivity testing to a fine degree.[7] Many physicians were engaged in clinical testing to determine the proper dosage of the new antibiotics. Gradually, a new specialty evolved—physicians expert in the management of infection, in the utilization of appropriate antibiotics, used either singly or in combination, and in understanding the complex interplay between antibiotics and other drugs.

With the opening of the new Mount Sinai School of Medicine in 1968, a Division of Infectious Diseases was established by Solomon Berson, the Chairman of Medicine. Molecular biology was moving to the fore, and Shalom Z. Hirschman, then a Senior Investigator in the Molecular Virology Division of the National Cancer Institute, was recruited to head the Division.

Hirschman instituted a fellowship, obtained a training grant from the National Institutes of Health (NIH), and began recruiting additional faculty. His first new full-time faculty members were Burt Meyers and Gerald Keusch. Hirschman established hospital-wide programs in Infection Control and Antibiotic Control, both of which have made major contributions to medicine and the Hospital. With the advent of the era of human immunodeficiency virus (HIV) and the Acquired Immunodeficiency Syndrome (AIDS), Hirschman helped establish the AIDS program at Mount Sinai and was instrumental in obtaining early grants for the study of AIDS. He served as Vice Chairman of the Department of Medicine for four years following the death of Solomon Berson.

In addition to his patient care, teaching, and administrative duties, Hirschman continued to conduct active basic scientific research. With interest centered on hepatitis B, Hirschman and his colleagues were the first to describe the DNA polymerase of the virus.[8] Subsequent studies touched on many aspects of viral replication, including the ability to replicate the hepatitis B virus through transfection of cells with viral DNA in culture.[9] Extensive clinical research was also carried out on new antimicrobial agents. In 1996, Hirschman described the "switch-type" immunomodulatory properties of a new chemical entity, a peptide-nucleic acid.[10] These immunomodulators have opened a new and exciting area of medical research, offering new tools for the study of immune functions and, moreover, opened new approaches to the therapy of HIV infection and AIDS. Hirschman stepped down as Chief of the Division in 1996. Now working in industry, he remains a member of the faculty and Consultant in infectious diseases.

Other Mount Sinai investigators have made important contributions to our knowledge of AIDS and its causative agent, the Human Immunodeficiency Virus (HIV). Almost all of the work has been a collaborative effort among the Divisions of Infectious Diseases and Clinical Immunology, the Department of Community and Preventive Medicine, and other departments of the Medical Center. One of the first descriptions of the clinical syndrome was reported by Frederick Siegal and colleagues in 1981.[11] Much of what we have learned about HIV and AIDS comes from large-scale multicenter studies, and Mount Sinai has been a site for several landmark studies. The Transfusion Safety Study, directed by Thomas C. Chalmers, Henry Sacks, and Louis Aledort at Mount Sinai, was the first to show that the HIV antibody test could reliably detect infectious units of blood or blood products and helped to greatly reduce the risk of HIV infection from transfusion.[12] Mount Sinai's Unit of the AIDS Clinical Trials Group (ACTG), led by Henry Sacks and Jeffrey Jacobson, a large nationwide collaboration of medical centers studying new treatments for HIV and AIDS, has enrolled nearly two thousand subjects in dozens of different treatment trials.[13] Rhoda Sperling, of the Department of Obstetrics and Gynecology, was the principal investigator on a milestone study known as ACTG 076, which established for the first time that treatment with zidovudine (AZT) for pregnant women and their infants drastically reduced the transmission of HIV from mother to child and led to a dramatic reduction in the number of babies born with HIV.[14]

Meryl H. Mendelson, one of Hirschman's Fellows and Mount Sinai's Director of Infection Control, played a vital role as a member of national study groups in assessing the incidence and potential risks to healthcare workers of needlestick injuries and also the possible hazards of skin, mucous membrane, and blood contacts with HIV-infected patients.[15] Her work led to changes in hospital procedures, including the use of blunt needles for high-risk procedures in infected patients and the development of safer access systems for intravenous use.[16]

In another area of infectious disease, the studies of Burt Meyers have had a significant impact on antibiotic usage. Just prior to coming to Mount Sinai, he and his colleagues were the first to report on the treatment of bacterial endocarditis with cephalothin.[17] In collaboration with the oral surgeons and members of the Division, Meyers was the first to recognize that biopsy was necessary to diagnose invasive mucormycosis premortem.[18] Major advances have been made in the understanding of the pharmacokinetics of antibiotics in the elderly.[19] Meyers, Director of Transplantation Infectious Diseases at Mount Sinai since 1995 and a charter member of the New York State Transplant Council, has devised novel therapies to deal with infection, especially tuberculosis, in this highly immunosuppressed population.[20] Glenn Hammer, Eric Neibart, and Jeffrey Gumprecht, superb clinicians and teachers all, have also provided outstanding consultative services throughout the Hospital, especially to the surgical services, in the antibiotic management of complex infections, whether they be the primary cause of admission or postoperative in nature.

Mary E. Klotman was named Chief of the Division of Infectious Diseases in 1996 to succeed Hirschman. Originally recruited to Mount Sinai in 1994 from the National Institutes of Health, where she had been a senior investigator in the laboratory of Robert Gallo, her research has focused on the molecular pathogenesis of chronic viral infections, especially HIV, and the development of novel therapeutic and preventive strategies. Recent important observations include the demonstration that HIV resides in kidney cells[21] and that antiviral therapy can relieve some of the clinical manifestations of the renal component of the disease, but the virus persists. Understanding how to deal with this reservoir for the virus will be an important step in the goal of eradicating the virus from infected individuals. A great teacher and mentor of younger faculty, Klotman holds the Irene and Dr. Arthur M. Fishberg Chair in Medicine, as well as joint appointments in the Department of Microbiology and in Mount Sinai's Institute of Gene Therapy and Molecular Medicine.

While, for the first time since the start of the AIDS epidemic, the death rate from HIV infection has declined in New York, new challenges exist. Laboratory-based research efforts in the Division continue on the identification of a unique natural factor released by normal human immune cells (CD8+ cells) that has potent inhibitory activity against HIV. A new sensitive assay to monitor the course of infection in patients responding to therapy is being jointly developed by laboratory and clinical investigators. Complementary clinical investigations in AIDS continues through the NIH-funded Mount Sinai clinical trials program, the study of HIV in women (WIS study), and the evaluation of new agents through pharmaceutical-sponsored trials. In a further study of the beneficial effects of thalidomide, Jacobson and his colleagues have shown that this drug enhances the healing of painful esophageal ulcers in HIV-infected individuals. Clinical trials of potential HIV vaccines as well as immunological approaches to therapy have been initiated. An exciting new initiative between members of the pediatric and adult divisions of infectious diseases has been the development of agents that might be used topically to block the transmission of sexual diseases, including HIV and herpes simplex. Mount Sinai investigators have received a new NIH program project grant to bring these much needed agents to the clinic.

In collaboration with the Division of Nephrology, NIH-funded laboratory-based efforts are focused on the development of viruses, stripped of their potential pathogenic genes, as vectors to deliver therapeutic genes to patients. These efforts complement the recent institutional commitment to advance the basic and clinical science of gene therapy.

The hospital epidemiology research program continues to evaluate strategies to improve the safety of the hospital setting for both staff and patients. Recent efforts focused on programs geared to limiting the spread of antimicrobial-resistant organisms in the hospital.

Now in the fourth decade of its existence, the Division of Infectious Diseases continues to make valuable contributions to the patient care, teaching, and research missions of the Medical Center. The Division has recently been awarded a new NIH training grant to mentor new physician scientists in the study of viral infections. With strong leadership and a dedicated faculty of both full-time and voluntary physicians, the Division has amply justified Solomon Berson's vision.

8

Division of Liver Diseases

WITHIN THE FIRST six months of the June 5, 1855, opening of the Jews' Hospital, two patients with "intermittent bilious fever" were admitted. The first (Case No. 48) had an enlarged tender spleen and was treated with quinine and "sulphas" and an ointment applied to the splenic area; she improved. The second (Case No. 50) almost certainly had gallstones, with a stone in the bile duct. She had an attack of acute right upper-quadrant pain associated with jaundice, fever, and a tender liver and spleen. A similar attack had occurred one year earlier. She improved and was discharged as "cured."[1]

In a recent review of the history of liver disease at the Mount Sinai Hospital,[2] Fenton Schaffner notes that there were also cases of liver abscess, echinococcus cyst, and acute yellow atrophy of the liver diagnosed and reported in the Mount Sinai Hospital Reports for the years 1899, 1901, and 1903. These cases were able to be studied because of the opening of the Hospital's first laboratory in 1893. As a result of religious proscriptions and the absence of a pathology laboratory, autopsies were rarely performed in the early days of the Hospital; those that were performed were limited in scope. Chemical determinations of liver function did not exist; indeed, the first chemistry laboratory was not opened until 1902, a time when the planning was already under way for the move to the Hospital's current site. It was not until 1890 that a biliary tract operation (cholecystostomy) was performed. As a consequence, the liver was rarely, if ever, visualized in the early years. Schaffner's review traces the growth of the study of the liver at Mount Sinai and also cites eighty of the most important publications about the liver that emanated from the clinics and laboratories of the institution during the twentieth century.

The move of the Hospital to 100th Street and Fifth Avenue in 1904 provided more beds and allowed for an increase in staff. The laboratories were expanded and housed in a separate building. New tests were added to the armamentarium of the chemistry laboratory, and members of the laboratory and clinical staff engaged in a number of research projects. Study of the liver, however, lagged behind. Whatever progress might have been made in the study of liver disease was, like all research, stymied by the advent of World War I and its aftermath.

Paul Klemperer, appointed Director of Pathology in 1926, was the catalyst in stimulating interest in liver disease research. One of his first publications from Mount Sinai was a study of the pathology of catarrhal jaundice.[3] He later described sclerosing cholangitis.[4] Klemperer welcomed the clinicians to the laboratory, paving the way for a spate of publications on liver tumors, the hepatic manifestations of other diseases, and the effect of drugs on the liver.[5] Experimental studies were undertaken to investigate the consequences of drug toxicity. A detailed description of chemically induced jaundice by Reuben Ottenberg and Rose Spiegel served as the standard reference on the subject for many years.[6]

The appointment of Harry Sobotka as Director of the Chemistry Laboratory in 1928 proved to be another stimulus to the investigation of liver disease. A student of bile metabolism himself, Sobotka encouraged chemical studies of hepatic illness. In 1937, Sobotka published *Physiological Chemistry of the Bile*,[7] based on his original investigations of bilirubin and bile salt metabolism. As new tests of liver function were developed, they were evaluated in various disease states. Progress was being made, but, once again, war (this time, World War II) intervened. Those members of the Mount Sinai staff who served with the Third General Hospital in the African and Italian campaigns, ending the war in France, gained experience in liver disease, caring for large numbers of soldiers with hepatitis.

In 1944, Isidore Snapper and George Baehr were appointed full-time Attendings and Chiefs of the two medical services. The former was also appointed Director of Graduate Medical Education; Baehr was appointed Director of Medical Research. Snapper, interested in liver disease, studied benzoyl glucuronate formation in the liver and devised a quantitative measurement to detect its presence.[8] Solomon Lichtman who, before the war had studied the "hepatorenal syndrome" with Arthur Sohval,[9] in 1953 published the two-volume *Diseases of the Liver, Gallbladder and Bile Ducts*,[10] which became the definitive text on the subject for many years and went through three editions. A liver clinic was established; Alexander Richman, the gastroenterologist, was its Chief. Richman served Mount Sinai for almost forty years. A gentleman, scholar, ethicist, and humanist, he was honored by his family, which created the Alexander Richman Award for Humanism in Medicine, given annually to a deserving member of the faculty.

A meteoric rise of interest in liver disease took place in 1957 with the appointment of Hans Popper as Chairman of the Department of Pathology. A founding member of the American Association for the Study of Liver Disease (AASLD) and the International Association for the Study of the Liver, Popper was already a giant in the field of hepatology. Just prior to his move to Mount Sinai, he and his colleague Fenton Schaffner published *Liver: Structure and Function*,[11] a unique text that correlated histology and pathology with function. In 1958, Popper was joined at Mount Sinai by Schaffner, who would lead the clinical efforts of the newly formed liver group. Together they would create an internationally recognized center of excellence in the study of liver disease. Collaborative projects were developed between basic scientists and clinicians leading to the acquisition of numerous grants and new clinical programs. Schaffner noted that "the Popper years saw an explosion in description and discovery, and in the number of papers published, which amounted to more than 1000 in a period of thirty years. The main topics were hepatic fibrosis, cholestasis with special emphasis on morphology and bile salt metabolism, toxic liver injury, metabolic transformations, and carcinogenesis."[12]

In 1965, eight years after Popper's arrival, Alexander Gutman, Chairman of Medicine, created an independent Division of Liver Disease, splitting hepatology from gastroenterology, and named Schaffner as Chief. A native of Chicago, Schaffner was trained in medicine and pathology, becoming expert in the field of electron microscopy, a technique that was invaluable to the group in its early days. The author of more than four hundred publications, he co-edited the classic series *Progress in Liver Diseases*, over a twenty-nine-year period and was one of the first Associate Editors of *Seminars in Liver Disease*. Like Popper a founding member of the AASLD, Schaffner served as its President in 1976. He was also instrumental in the founding of the American Liver Foundation.

Schaffner served as the acting Chairman of the Department of Medicine from 1972 to 1974, following the death of Solomon Berson. As a clinician, Schaffner had no peer. His judgment and compassionate care were impeccable, and he was revered by his patients and the many physicians who consulted with him. He played a vital role in the devel-

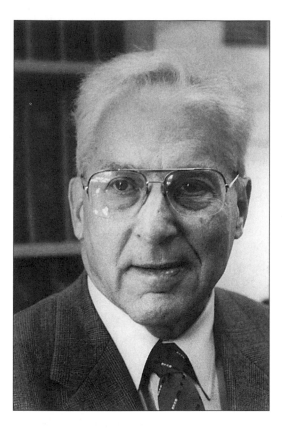

Fenton Schaffner, M.D.,
Chief of Division of Liver
Disease, 1965–1989.

opment of Mount Sinai's liver transplant program, which performed its first transplant in September 1988, and in the program's early days he referred a lion's share of the patients. A master teacher, Schaffner left a legacy that lives on in the many clinician/scientist hepatologists he trained who now occupy leadership positions around the world. Schaffner retired as Chief of the Division in 1989 but remained active for several more years. He died in 2000.

Another most important member of the Division throughout its existence is Charles Lieber. A world-renowned clinician/scientist, Lieber is based at the Bronx Veteran's Administration Medical Center and has made fundamental contributions to the understanding of the pathogenesis of alcoholic liver disease. His more than six hundred publications have covered every clinical and research aspect of the effects of alcohol on the liver.[13]

One of Schaffner's first fellows, Franklin A. Klion, has also been a notable member of the Division since its inception. Taking over the Liver Clinic upon Richman's retirement, Klion was an early member of the liver transplant team. In 1992, Klion along with Thomas L. Fabry, a gastroenterologist and also a member of the transplant team, published the highly successful *Guide to Liver Transplantation*.[14] In the book's foreword, Paul D. Berk points out the truly collaborative nature of Mount Sinai's transplant program, another prime example of the spirit of cooperation that has characterized Mount Sinai's clinical successes throughout its history.[15]

In 1989, Berk succeeded Schaffner as Chief of the Division of Liver Disease. Originally recruited to Mount Sinai in 1977 to be the Chief of the Division of Hematology, Berk had previously served as Chief of the Section on Diseases of the Liver in the Digestive Diseases Branch of the National Institute of Arthritis, Metabolism and Digestive Diseases of the National Institutes of Health (NIH). His parallel careers in hematology and hepatology stem from the major focus of his research in bilirubin metabolism. He and his colleagues have made valuable contributions in this area, including the identification of the fatty acid binding protein.[16] An established authority on jaundice and the hereditary hyperbilirubinemias, Berk also has clinical and research interests in primary biliary cirrhosis, hemochromatosis, the porphyrias, and hepatitis C. Berk was instrumental in organizing the fundamental medical support aspects of Mount Sinai's liver transplant program and has been a staunch advocate ever since. Berk served as President of AASLD and Editor-in-Chief of *Hepatology*. A founding Editor of *Seminars in Liver Disease*, he has continued in that role for twenty years. In 2000, Berk was elected to a two-year term as Chairman of the Board of Directors of the American Liver Foundation. On that occasion, Barry Coller, Chairman of the Department of Medicine, commented, "With his tremendous ability and breadth of experience, he is an ideal leader."[17] Truer words were never spoken.

Other members of the Division have played major roles in the management of the large number of patients with liver disease who have been attracted to Mount Sinai. Nancy Bach, a fellow when the transplant program began, "was the one who set the tone for the cooperation of the Division with the transplant team."[18] She was joined by Leona Kim-Schluger when the latter completed her fellowship.

A major recruitment to the enterprise was Henry Bodenheimer, Associate Professor of Medicine at Brown University, who returned to Mount Sinai in 1991, twelve years after completing the liver fellowship. Currently the Director of the Liver Diseases Fellowship Program and Deputy Director for Medical Services in the Recanati/Miller Transplantation Institute, Bodenheimer was the first to observe immune abnormalities in primary sclerosing cholangitis.[19] He is a leader in multicenter trials of therapy for both hepatitis B and C.[20]

Scott Friedman was another "returnee" to Mount Sinai in 1997, recruited by Berk to be Director of Liver Research. A graduate of the Mount Sinai School of Medicine (1979), Friedman then forged a highly successful career at the University of California, San Francisco. He is recognized as a world leader in understanding the molecular mechanisms involved in the development of hepatic fibrosis. Friedman was the first to isolate and characterize the hepatic stellate cell, which is now known to be the key cell type responsible for scar production in the liver.[21] This research has expanded into a comprehensive program exploring the cellular and molecular basis of liver fibrosis and opens new pathways for the understanding and treatment of chronic liver disease, whether due to viruses, alcohol, or metabolic disorders.[22] Clinical trials have been designed to test the role of antifibrotic agents, another prime example of translational or bench-to-bedside research.

In 2001, Berk stepped down after a total of twenty-four years as a Division Chief. During his tenure as Chief of the Division of Liver Diseases, the faculty grew to sixteen members, and its annual clinical practice activity increased more than tenfold. Both basic and clinical research have expanded in a similar fashion, the former supported by NIH grants and foundations. Multiple clinical trials have been sponsored by the pharmaceutical industry. A goal of the Division is to have virtually every patient participating in one of its multifaceted clinical research programs.

Berk was succeeded by Friedman, who is only the third Chief in thirty-five years to lead the Division of Liver Diseases, a division that has had an illustrious past and will certainly have a brilliant future.

Adapted from an article by Fenton Schaffner, M. D. in *The Mount Sinai Journal of Medicine* 67 (2000): 76–83.

9

Department and Division
of Neoplastic Diseases

THE STUDY AND treatment of cancer at Mount Sinai transcends any one Department or Division, encompassing the efforts not only of oncologists but also of chemists, microbiologists, cell biologists, pathologists, radiologists, radiotherapists, environmental scientists, and surgeons, among others. As a result, the story of milestones in cancer treatment at Mount Sinai is disbursed throughout the pages of this book, as each Department mounted its own research efforts to advance physicians' knowledge of neoplastic diseases. This chapter touches on efforts in the Department of Medicine, as well as in the Department of Neoplastic Diseases, which existed from 1973 to 1993.

Historically, cancer was treated with external remedies as well as attempts to regulate the humors within the body. As time progressed, surgery was added to the armament against tumors, but only in areas easily accessible to the surgeon's knife. With the discovery of x-rays at the end of the nineteenth century, radiation therapy was added when it was shown to shrink tumors. There then followed a period of experimentation to discover the minimum dosage necessary for the maximum effect. During the second half of the twentieth century, there began a chemical assault on cancer using new medicines developed in the burgeoning laboratories of research institutions and pharmaceutical companies.

Mount Sinai's efforts have spanned many eras of cancer care and many departmental boundaries. One of the early pioneers was the surgeon Richard Lewisohn. When he reached official retirement age in 1937, he "retired" to a newly established cancer research laboratory that he created within the Department of Pathology. At this time, cancer researchers were seeking chemotherapeutic agents that could slow or stop the growth of tumors, with many laboratories and pharmaceutical companies joining forces to isolate and to test such compounds. Early on, Lewisohn collaborated with Lederle Laboratories in the testing of its products. His early efforts focused on using splenic extracts to arrest tumor growth in mice, with enough success to merit mention in *Time* magazine.[1] Subsequent studies assayed the ability of yeast extract, pantothenic acid, riboflavin, and then other grain extracts to halt breast cancer growth in mice. In 1944, Lewisohn and his colleagues Cecele Leuchtenberger, Daniel Laszlo, and Rudolph Leuchtenberger published two papers establishing folic acid and then xanthopterin as tumor inhibitors.[2] Laszlo and Cecele Leuchtenberger also devised a rapid test for tumor growth inhibitors.[3] An important paper followed in 1945, entitled "The Influence of 'Folic Acid' on Spontaneous Breast Cancer in Mice."[4] This study identified the active component as teropterin, a folic acid analog, which had been obtained from Lederle Laboratories.[5] As efforts proceeded to develop what eventually became pure aminopterin, Lewisohn used his imperfect supplies of teropterin experimentally to treat George Herman "Babe" Ruth, who was suffering from nasopharyngeal cancer. Treatments started late in June 1947 with daily injections of teropterin. Dramatic improvement was observed, and Lewisohn presented the case at the International Research Cancer Congress in September. Unfortunately, relapse occurred, and Ruth was admitted to Memorial Hospital in June 1948. Although, by then, the drug had been purified and had been used by others with success, Memorial Hospital treated Ruth with radiation therapy alone, and he died August 16, 1948.

By this time, Lewisohn wanted to retire once more,[6] and the Cancer Research Laboratory did not survive in its then current form. Cancer research at Mount Sinai was not ended, however. Isidore Snapper, Chief of the Second Medical Service, had an interest in myeloma and was studying the therapeutic properties of stilbamidine. He involved a young Resident named Ezra Greenspan in the work, thereby initiating a lifelong career in cancer investigation and treatment.

Following his residency, Greenspan served in the United States Public Health Service and became the Acting Chief of its Clinical Research Unit in Baltimore. There he was able to pursue his new interest in the chemotherapeutic management of malignancy. It was a perfect example of being in the right place at the right time. Cancer was becoming a major topic of interest during these years, with the relentless fear and hopelessness associated with the disease giving way to hope as new chemotherapeutic agents were being identified. Large amounts of federal and private money were being made available for cancer research. Adding to this impetus was the National Cancer Institute Act of 1937 and the evolution of the American Cancer Society from the American Association for the Control of Cancer in 1944.

Greenspan's contribution to cancer care, and to Mount Sinai, was in showing that there was no one magic bullet but that, by using combinations of drugs, clinicians could make significant gains in the treatment of cancer. This work, which began in Baltimore, continued upon his return to the Department of Medicine at Mount Sinai in 1952, when he became an Attending and assumed the direction of the Cancer Detection Clinic. The premise of using combinations of potentially toxic chemicals to treat cancer was not greeted enthusiastically by the medical community either at Mount Sinai or elsewhere. Also, many at Mount Sinai, a hospital with few basic scientists on staff, did not understand the complex interactions of the cancer drugs. But Greenspan persisted, ultimately publishing landmark papers on the treatment of ovarian and breast cancer by combination chemotherapy in *The Mount Sinai Journal of Medicine*.[7] As Greenspan has noted, traditional cancer journals would not accept his work in the early 1960s; he also commented that he was fortunate in that the administration in the Department of Medicine and the Research Committee at Mount Sinai allowed him to continue in his efforts, even though, early on, few understood the value of his work or the science behind it.[8]

Combination chemotherapy was extended to other malignancies and included new drugs as they were developed. Greenspan, in collaboration with Howard Bruckner and others of the Department of Neoplastic Diseases and members of the Department of Obstetrics, Gynecology, and Reproductive Science, reported the first use of platinum in the United States for the treatment of ovarian cancer.[9] Greenspan established the Chemotherapy Foundation in 1968 to stimulate cancer research and to provide education to oncologists and patients. The Foundation now supports research through grants at seven major medical centers in the New York metropolitan area and conducts an annual international symposium for professionals. Over the years, the Foundation has also provided significant support to clinical and laboratory research programs at Mount Sinai. In 1997, the Ezra M. Greenspan, M.D. Professorship in Clinical Cancer Therapeutics in the Department of Medicine was created. The author of almost two hundred papers and several monographs, Greenspan has been honored by Mount Sinai and his colleagues for his leadership in cancer chemotherapy for half a century.

Although the advent of the Medical School in the late 1960s led to a marked increase in full-time staff and faculty, Greenspan, a member of the voluntary staff for his entire career, was named Chief when a formal Division of Oncology was created within the Department of Medicine in 1970. Greenspan's efforts to create new laboratories and to initiate a training program were crucial to the selection of Mount Sinai in 1973 by the National Cancer Institute as one of seven medical centers to train physicians in the latest diagnostic and treatment techniques in cancer. The impetus for this effort was led by Louis Wasserman, Director Emeritus of Hematology, whose Division was well known for its research in the leukemias and lymphomas.[10] With an eye toward further enhancement of Mount Sinai's cancer program, the Hospital decided to create a separate Department of Neoplastic Diseases to house a core of clinicians and scientists to coordinate multidisciplinary approaches to cancer care and research. A new cancer treatment center was also proposed.

After the establishment of the new Department, there still remained the Division of Oncology in the Department of Medicine. It served as the base for Greenspan and for most of the medical oncologists on the voluntary staff, all of whom contributed greatly to the institutional cancer programs. Seymour Cohen, Nathaniel Wisch, Lynn Ratner, and their associates and colleagues all participated in the many cancer protocols and were active in the teaching of residents and students. The efforts of the Division of Oncology continued to focus on a clinical and research program devoted to combination chemotherapy and immunotherapy, often in collaboration with the Department of Neoplastic Diseases. Research on cancer cell differentiation, based on a discovery by Charlotte Friend, in the Center for Experimental Biology at Mount Sinai, was spearheaded by Samuel Waxman, a member of the voluntary staff of the Division of Oncology. In 1971, Friend and her colleagues noted that dimethyl sulfoxide (DMSO) could induce cancer cells to progress or differentiate to a normal pattern of development, opening the way to new, less toxic forms of cancer therapy.[11] Waxman's work on differentiation therapy has been recognized around the world, and in 1985 he organized the first international conference on differentiation therapy in cancer.

The new Department of Neoplastic Diseases became operational in July 1973, with James F. Holland as its first full-time Chairman. Holland came to Mount Sinai from the Roswell Park Memorial Institute, where he was Chief of Medicine and Director of the Cancer Clinical Research Center. As befits the 1972 winner of the Albert A. Lasker Award, Holland had already made landmark contributions to cancer chemotherapy. He and his colleagues had pioneered multi-institutional trials that proved the value of aggressive combination chemotherapy in many solid tumors, as well as in the lymphomas and leukemias. Indeed, Holland's most important accomplishment was in proving that acute childhood leukemia was curable, work that was done while he was Chairman of the Cancer and Leukemia Group B (CALGB), an NIH-funded international cooperative program that evaluates new treatment protocols in leukemia. CALGB remains active to this day, with significant expansion of its activities.

Holland had to create the Department. He coordinated the construction of the nineteen-bed Clinical Center for Neoplastic Diseases on the sixth floor of the Klingenstein Clinical Center, designed to include laminar air-flow beds to provide a sterile environment for patients. The facility opened in 1974, staffed by nurses specially trained to deal with the particular needs of cancer patients receiving chemotherapy and immunotherapy for advanced cancer. The unit expanded over the years and by 1988 had grown to thirty-five beds, when it was dedicated as the Derald H. Ruttenberg Cancer Center, named for a Mount Sinai Trustee who provided substantial support for the Department. The next year, the Center moved to the new Guggenheim Pavilion and expanded to fifty-three beds, with more than one hundred twenty-five physicians and scientists contributing to the multidisciplinary research and patient care efforts.

From its inception in 1973, the Department's clinical research effort was the search for the ideal protocol to cure advanced cancers. Shortly after the introduction of daunorubicin (Adriamycin), the group published, in 1973, the first paper on its use in the treatment of acute myelocytic leukemia. In the same year, a second paper established the superior benefit of using the drug in combination with cytosine arabinoside, a protocol that remains the "gold standard" in 2001.[12] The use of cisplatin was extended to other gynecological malignancies besides the ovary and then to testicular tumors, where the drug has provided the most effective adjuvant chemotherapy available, with more than 90 percent of patients now being cured of their disease. Continuing study on the treatment of breast cancer demonstrated that five-drug therapy is superior to three-drug therapy as an adjuvant regimen.[13] By the late 1980s, immunotherapy research was centered on the value of interleukin-2. There were also collaborative efforts on pancreatic cancer, mesothelioma, brain tumors, and gastrointestinal cancer. Along with and resulting from all of this work was Holland's textbook, written with Emil Frei III, called *Cancer Medicine*, first published in 1973 and now in its fifth edition.[14]

Recent exciting research has found a new family of highly active anticancer compounds.[15] There has also been breast cancer research on envelope gene sequences and possible viral causes of breast cancer, leading to a report on the entire structure of the provirus, 9.8 kilobases long, 95 percent homologous to the mouse mammary tumor virus.[16] Pursuant to this, researchers are now working on environmental sources for breast cancer.

The Department of Neoplastic Diseases was a vibrant, active organization centered on Holland and his clinical colleagues, such as Takao Ohnuma (who was also Chief of the Department's laboratory efforts in chemotherapy), Vincent Hollander, Howard Bruckner, Larry Norton, Janet Cuttner, and Paolo Paciucci. John Roboz and George Bekesi were the mainstays of the laboratory efforts for decades. Many Researchers, Residents, and Fellows received their training in the Department. In 1982, Holland was installed as the Jane B. and Jack R. Aron Professor of Neoplastic Diseases, and the Department attracted several generous supporters over the years, including the T. J. Martell Foundation and the Ruttenberg Family. Physical facilities for the Department improved near the end of the 1980s with the opening of the Chemotherapy Day Unit to treat ambulatory patients who receive chemotherapy infusions. As noted earlier, the Ruttenberg Cancer Center moved to the new Guggenheim Pavilion, providing modern space for inpatient treatment. In 1989, the Department revitalized the Tumor Registry (now known as the Cancer Registry), a listing of cancer patients that notes the diagnosis, stage, and treatment provided over the lifetime of each patient. This registry is important for clinical investigation, as well as medical education and basic science research.

In 1993, when Holland reached official retirement age for a Chairman, the decision was made to dissolve the Department of Neoplastic Diseases and to once again coordinate cancer activities within the Department of Medicine. This new beginning was stimulated by the arrival of a new Chairman of Medicine, Barry Coller. Holland, now a

Distinguished Service Professor, remains active, with more than five hundred publications to his credit. The tremendous contributions he has made over the course of his career have been recognized in many ways, including the establishment of the James F. Holland, M.D. Professorship in Neoplastic Diseases and a symposium and issue of *The Mount Sinai Journal of Medicine* devoted to Holland on his sixty-fifth birthday.[17] On that occasion, Ohnuma noted that Holland had coined the term "precurable" in 1983 to identify those tumors that for the moment were incurable but would some day be conquered by new therapies.[18] Holland's "unrelenting pursuit of cancer cures"[19] has continued into the twenty-first century.

In 1993, Stuart Aaronson was appointed Director of the Derald H. Ruttenberg Cancer Center and the second Aron Professor of Medicine. Before coming to Mount Sinai, Aaronson was Chief of the Laboratory of Cellular and Molecular Biology at the National Cancer Institute and was widely known for his studies of normal growth regulation and of genetic aberrations that underlie cancer's abnormal growth pattern. Two years after Aaronson's arrival, the inpatient unit of the Division was transformed into the Oncology Care Center, and a multidisciplinary staff was created to more efficiently meet the needs of the patients. Aaronson and the staff of the Division of Neoplastic Diseases continued and expanded the research efforts of previous years. And, in 1997, the new Ruttenberg Cancer Center laboratories in the East Building were dedicated, comprising forty-thousand square feet of space and devoted to further understanding and combating cancer.

Another milestone in the cancer story at Mount Sinai was reached in 1998 when Janice Gabrilove was appointed the first James F. Holland Professor in Neoplastic Diseases and the Chief of the Division of Neoplastic Diseases within the Department of Medicine. A 1977 graduate of the Mount Sinai School of Medicine, Gabrilove returned to Mount Sinai with several research triumphs already behind her. She was a pioneer in research on hematopoietic cytokines and with her colleagues at Memorial Sloan-Kettering Cancer Center was the first to purify and clone the human granulocyte colony stimulating factor (GCSF), known today as Neupogen.

With Gabrilove's arrival, the Annual Report for 1998 states the mission of the reorganized, and renamed, Division of Medical Oncology, goals that have led the Division into the twenty-first century:

The Division of Medical Oncology is focused on the development of rationally based, hypothesis driven translational research, taking advantage of fundamental observations derived from basic research endeavors and directed toward an understanding of the molecular mechanisms that underlie the pathogenesis of malignant disease. In addition, the division is committed to a mission embracing education, basic and clinical research and outstanding patient care in a multidisciplinary, disease oriented manner.[20]

The Division today is actively participating in the New York Cancer Project, a twenty-year cooperative effort that will attempt to discover the causes of cancer. Also, a new patient care area is being readied for ambulatory patients on the lobby level of the Guggenheim Pavilion, further enhancing the Division's ability to meet its ambitious goals for the twenty-first century.

10

Division of Nephrology

HOMER SMITH, the renowned nephrologist, once said, "We are what we are because we have the kind of kidneys we have."[1] In like manner, Mount Sinai's Division of Nephrology is what it is because of the kind of physicians who were interested in diseases of the kidney. Many of them were active in the field long before it became a formal division. In 1917, Albert A. Epstein, who had come to Mount Sinai in 1911 as an Associate Attending Physician and Associate Physiological Chemist, described the causation and therapy of edema in chronic parenchymatous nephritis, Epstein's Disease.[2] Epstein's article was reprinted as a landmark article in 1952 in an issue of *The American Journal of Medicine* celebrating Mount Sinai's one hundredth anniversary. The annotation by Alexander B. Gutman, Editor-in-Chief of *The Journal* (and also Chief of Medicine at Mount Sinai), stated:

> This was the first explicit application of Starling's principle, stating the role of the plasma proteins in the distribution of body water, to the problem of edema formation in what is now known as the nephrotic syndrome. It has since been made clear that other factors also are important in this connection but even these are hinted at in Epstein's insistence upon the essentially extrarenal nature of "chronic parenchymatous nephritis," a position far in advance of his time.[3]

One of the early leaders of the renal group was Marvin F. Levitt, who first came to Mount Sinai as an Intern in 1944. Three years later, Wilhelm Kolff, who had devised what has been referred to as the first practical artificial kidney machine, came from Holland (along with his machine) to Mount Sinai. Kolff stayed for less than a year, however, and dialysis was not pursued earnestly by the group. Nonetheless, in 1947, Mount Sinai won an American Medical Association award for its exhibit on the artificial kidney at the Association's annual meeting in Atlantic City. According to a report by the staff, "At first we were reluctant to expose our patients to a new form of treatment with which we were relatively unfamiliar."[4] In fact, the first series of patients treated with the machine were critically ill and dying of uremia; all other conservative methods of treatment had been tried and had failed. According to Irving Kroop, a Resident at the time and a coauthor of the report, the machine was used only in the evenings when the operating room was empty. As the newest technology of the day, the procedure attracted many visitors to the operating room galleries.

Another pioneer in renal care was the surgeon Stephan S. Rosenak. Born in Hungary in 1901, Rosenak studied medicine in Germany and interned in Budapest, where he developed the first peritoneal catheter in 1926.[5] He received appointments at Mount Sinai in 1941 in the Outpatient Department and in the Chemistry laboratory. Eventually, he received an appointment in Surgery and then in Urology. In collaboration with Gordon Oppenheimer, the urologist, he developed an improved peritoneal dialysis drain.[6] In the laboratory, Rosenak worked with Bernard S. Oppenheimer, the cardiologist, to study the effects of nephrectomy on renal hypertension.[7]

The year 1951 brought a new Chief of the Department of Medicine who stimulated research in the area of renal medicine. Alexander Gutman had done previous work on hyperthyroidism, but in the late 1940s his interest turned to gout. Working with Tsai- Fan Yu, he made important contributions in elucidating the metabolic defects of gout and in advancing clinical management of the disease. Among other accomplishments, they were the first to establish the usefulness of long-term uricosuric therapy in preventing tophaceous deformities and disabilities[8] and were also the first to suggest the bidirectional transport of uric acid.[9]

During this period, other members of the staff continued to pursue the use of the artificial kidney. As the technology began to improve, the employment of dialysis expanded, and, in 1957, "a proper facility was made available, using modern equipment (some of new design engineered at this Hospital) and operated under competent supervision. This unit will provide the services of an artificial kidney."[10] This, the first artificial kidney center in New York, was organized and directed by Sherman Kupfer. Kupfer joined Mount Sinai as an Intern in 1948, later completed his residency at the Hospital, and has served the Medical Center continuously ever since in a variety of roles. With Rosenak, Kupfer designed a new hemodialysis machine that utilized parallel tubes for more efficient use of the membrane surface area for dialyzing.[11] However, the apparatus was still replete with problems. Primarily, it was large and cumbersome. For every new procedure, it had to be transported to the operating room, assembled, and then sterilized. Before dialysis could begin, a surgeon had to gain vascular access to insert catheters into an artery and a vein. The machine frequently broke down. Nevertheless, patients from all over the area were brought to Mount Sinai for treatment with the artificial kidney. A mobile dialysis unit was also introduced. If patients at local hospitals were too sick to be moved, the staff would load the machine onto the back of a fire truck and drive to the other hospital. The majority of the patients treated at this time had acute renal failure, due to either poisoning or other catastrophic causes.

In addition to designing the new artificial kidney machine, Kupfer developed a new catheter for peritoneal dialysis.[12] Early in his career, Kupfer was also involved in physiological studies on experimental shock and coronary artery occlusion and on the hemodynamic effects of extracorporeal circulation. The work, accomplished in conjunction with Leslie Kuhn, of the Division of Cardiology, demonstrated that intra-arterial blood transfusions were of no value in increasing aortic pressure and that the sought-after rise in pressure could be induced instead by increasing vascular resistance through balloon obstruction of the lower abdominal aorta.[13] Later, with Peter Stritzke of the Division of Nuclear Medicine, and Lewis Burrows, of the Department of Surgery, Kupfer originated and patented the noninvasive technique known as functional imaging, using radioactive tracers to measure kidney blood flow and function.[14] Kupfer has also had a significant impact on the Hospital and the School. He served as Senior Vice President for Research and Education from 1974 to 1985; as Deputy Dean from 1981 to 1985; and as the first Chairman of the Research Committee and Institutional Review Board of the School and was the first Director of the Clinical Research Center from 1962 to 1985. Kupfer currently serves as Editor-in-Chief of *The Mount Sinai Journal of Medicine.*

When the Department of Medicine was reorganized in 1939, renal disease had not been named as an area of specialization. In 1959–1960, however, a formal Division of Nephrology was created, and Levitt was appointed its first Chief. A scintillating teacher, blessed with a marvelous sense of humor, and totally devoted to Mount Sinai, Levitt would serve the institution for more than half a century. Throughout his career, Levitt did research on the homeostatic mechanisms by which salt and water balance and extracellular volume are preserved in kidney function. In 1959, Levitt instituted a fellowship program in renal medicine. A. Daniel Hauser became the first renal fellow; the second was Marvin Goldstein. In 1959, Hauser and Lawrence Berger established an outpatient kidney clinic. Hauser's research interests were in renal function, sickle cell disease, the effects of calcium on the kidney, and mechanisms of urine concentration. Goldstein studied the mechanisms of diuretic actions, renal concentrating and diluting functions, and renovascular hypertension. He and Jacob Churg, the pathologist, also investigated the hemolytic-uremic syndrome.

Richard Stein, another fellowship graduate, began his association with Mount Sinai in 1961. He was one of the first investigators to characterize the effects of changes in salt and potassium balance, hormonal stimuli, alterations in blood flow, and chronic diseases of the kidney on renal tubular function; many of his publications have had great impact.[15] Stein is a past President of the New York Society of Nephrology and has been honored by the National Kidney Foundation. Also honored on a number of occasions by the students of the Mount Sinai School of Medicine for his teaching abilities, Stein has served as Vice Chairman of the Department of Medicine for more than two decades.

The creation of an independent division with its own clinic proved salutary. Levitt built a very strong team of nephrologists, many from the fellowship program, others recruited from elsewhere. The research program flourished, and, as the use of dialysis increased, patients with chronic renal disease were attracted to the Hospital. The expanding dialysis program was instrumental in helping to establish Mount Sinai's kidney transplant program; the first kidney transplant was performed in 1967. The two programs have complemented each other ever since. The development of the end-stage renal disease program and its coverage by Medicare in 1973 paved the way for a period of exponential growth in the management of chronic renal failure. Dialysis services continued to grow under the direction of Juan Bosch, Beat Von Albertini, and Sheldon Glabman.

Glabman directed the dialysis unit from 1969 to 1986. In 1977, the Robert Wood Johnson Jr. Renal Treatment Center was opened. A cooperative effort of the Departments of Medicine and Surgery, the unit provided facilities for hemodialysis, transplant patients, and other kidney disorders. Glabman, along with Allan Lauer and other colleagues, began studies on the use of continuous arterio-venous hemofiltration; its first clinical use in the United States was at Mount Sinai.[16] More recently, Glabman has played an important role in the Department of Medicine's efforts to reduce length of stay.

The current Director of the dialysis unit is Jonathan A. Winston, also a graduate of Levitt's training program. In recent years, Winston and colleagues from the Divisions of Nephrology and Infectious Disease have made seminal observations on clinical aspects of HIV-associated nephropathy.[17]

In 1963, Ruth Abramson came to Mount Sinai as a renal fellow. The work of Gutman and Yu on uric acid piqued her interest, and she initiated studies in uric acid transport. Abramson then performed micropuncture studies in the rat kidney to measure uric acid in the nephron. During the 1970s and 1980s, in collaboration with Michael Lipkowitz, she was able to isolate and clone the recombinant protein in the rat kidney responsible for urate transport in plasma membranes.[18] Subsequent studies identified the human homolog of the rat urate transporter and mapped it to chromosome seventeen.[19] Abramson and her colleagues are currently investigating the expression of the uric acid transport protein during different stages of fetal development. Abramson has also played a major role in the School of Medicine as Associate Dean for Research and as Chairperson of the Institutional Review Board for fifteen years.

Upon Levitt's retirement, Stein served as Director of the Division from 1989 until 1994, when he was succeeded by Paul Klotman. Klotman joined Mount Sinai from the National Institutes of Health, where he was Chief of Viral Pathogenesis in the National Institute of Dental Research. His laboratory is internationally known for its work in understanding the molecular basis of HIV pathogenesis, particularly that of HIV-associated nephropathy, and in the development of novel molecular approaches to therapy. Researchers in the laboratory were the first to identify and characterize a gated channel that conducts nucleic acid into cells.[20] Using transgenic technology, they were also the first to prove that HIV can directly infect human kidney cells.[21] Under Klotman's direction, the lab is currently developing appropriate vectors to target renal and lymphoid tissue, using adeno-associated viruses, liposomes, and a novel toxin-based strategy for DNA transduction, as well as appropriate animal models to assess in vivo efficacy and toxicity.[22] In the fall of 2001, Paul Klotman was named the new Chairman of the Department of Medicine.

From the observations of the early clinicians interested in kidney disease to the preeminence of the Division's current cutting edge science, nephrologists have played a compelling role in Mount Sinai's never-ending quest for excellence. The Division is well positioned to continue that pursuit well into the future.

11

Division of Pulmonary Medicine

FROM THE DAYS of Alfred Meyer, Mount Sinai's first pulmonologist, the Division of Pulmonary Medicine has continuously excelled in its clinical and research endeavors. Meyer first came to Mount Sinai as an Intern in 1878; he was appointed Attending Physician six years later. Shortly thereafter, he established the medical library. According to Meyer, "I did this partly from a sense of gratitude (I was not quite 29 years of age), and partly because I had recognized the need of one when I was an interne only five years before."[1] It would be only the first of Meyer's many contributions. Chairman of the Library Committee for fifteen years, Meyer was also Secretary of the Medical Board for seven years and Chairman of the Training School for Nurses Committee from 1894 to 1899. The latter position entailed providing medical care for sick nurses, which during Meyer's tenure included an outbreak of typhoid.

Meyer is best remembered for his indefatigable efforts on behalf of tuberculosis patients. In 1899, he was appointed Attending Physician at Montefiore Hospital's tuberculosis sanatorium in Bedford, New York. While there, he introduced work therapy, encouraging the patients to tend to garden plots. In 1904, he was integral in establishing the sanatorium at Ray Brook on Saranac Lake, making New York the second state in the country to provide a sanatorium for the poor. He subsequently organized meetings at The New York Academy of Medicine that resulted in the installation of a municipal sanatorium in Otisville. He traveled to Europe to stimulate interest in the International Congress on Tuberculosis, held in Washington in 1908. At the conference, he collected $30,000 to bring a tuberculosis exhibit to the New York Museum of Natural History. In 1917, he created the tuberculosis division at Mount Sinai; two years later, he was one of the incorporators and first Directors of the New York Tuberculosis Association. Another of Meyer's far-reaching accomplishments occurred early in his career, namely the introduction of the oxygen tank for use in the Hospital. In 1923, Benjamin Eliasoph introduced an oxygen tent of his own design.

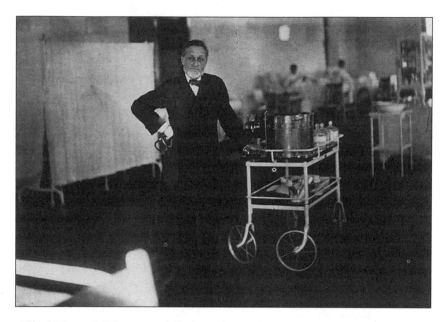

Alfred Meyer, M.D., on a medical ward, c. 1910.

When Meyer wasn't busy promoting the care of tuberculosis patients, he played the piano, was an active member in New York society alongside his wife, and enjoyed backpacking in the Adirondacks. Meyer's work did not go unnoticed. At the laying of the corner stone of the third Mount Sinai Hospital, in 1901, Mayor Seth Low is said to have exclaimed that "if the Hospital had been responsible for nothing else but the development of Dr. Meyer it would have justified its existence."[2] Meyer retired from active service and was appointed Consulting Physician in 1920.

When compared to the efforts of subsequent Mount Sinai pulmonary disease specialists, Meyer's concentration on tuberculosis was unique. Unlike the chest physicians at other hospitals who were, for the most part, phthisiologists, the Mount Sinai group of pulmonologists were primarily (though not exclusively) interested in lung abscess, empyema, and other nontuberculous lung infections. The first leader of this group was Harry Wessler. Appointed to the House Staff in 1908, Wessler also worked as a volunteer in the pathology and x-ray departments. This training greatly influenced Wessler's subsequent career, and he maintained appointments in both the Department of Medicine and the Department of Radiology throughout his tenure at Mount Sinai. Not a prolific writer, Wessler preferred to discuss his findings with colleagues, rather than publish them. Nevertheless, in collaboration with Coleman B. (Kelly) Rabin, he wrote a description of adenoma of the bronchus that was classic,[3] and Wessler and Leopold Jaches's book, *Clinical Roentgenology of Diseases of the Chest,*[4] became the standard text on the subject for decades. After witnessing an "epidemic" of lung abscess following tonsillectomies at the Hospital, Wessler propounded the concept that putrid lung abscess resulted from the aspiration of putrid material from the mouth or throat.[5] Wessler also played an important role as a catalyst, stimulating other members of the medical staff in their clinical and research pursuits. It was Wessler who encouraged Amiel Glass, the surgeon, to study the anatomy of the bronchial tree. The result was Glass's landmark description of the bronchopulmonary segments.[6] All of this aforementioned clinical research was integral to the development by Neuhof and Touroff of the one-stage operation for draining putrid lung abscess.[7] Another highly respected member of the pulmonary group was Herman Hennell, who, in addition to conducting clinical research on suppurative lung disease, did have a significant interest in tuberculosis.

Wessler continued to work closely with Rabin. Rabin had come to Mount Sinai as an Intern in 1922, when he began a seventy-year association with the Hospital, which was interrupted only by a pathology fellowship in Berlin. In 1935, Wessler left Mount Sinai to become Chief at Montefiore Hospital, and Rabin was appointed Associate in Medicine. His knowledge and training were so broad that during his tenure he also held appointments in the Departments of Radiology, Radiotherapy, and Pathology. Making use of this vast knowledge, and using x-ray and fluoroscopy, Rabin was able to localize lung abscesses with great accuracy, enabling the use of the one-stage drainage procedure. But the technique required Rabin to be present for almost every operative procedure to help locate the abscess. In his own words, "After spending days and nights over a period of years, in the operating room, since we had so many cases, I felt I had to evolve some way by which I'd be released from this chore."[8] What he devised was the method of "spot localization." By injecting lipiodol and methylene blue into the intercostal space just over the abscess and then making a film, he could determine the relationship of the lipiodol to the abscess and tell the surgeon before the operation where the latter would find the abscess in relation to the methylene blue spot.[9,10] In 1939, when the Department of Medicine was reorganized to formally include six divisions, Rabin became the first official Chief of the Division of Thoracic Diseases.

Rabin's meticulous elucidation of the pathology and therapy of inflammatory and neoplastic lung diseases in great measure helped to expand the scope of the new broad field of pulmonary medicine. His laboratories were the morgue, the operating room, the X-ray facility, and the patient's bedside. In addition to his groundbreaking work on lung abscess, his landmark descriptions of pleural tumors,[11] bronchial adenomas,[12] and the topographical classification of primary lung cancers[13] all evolved from rigid adherence to scholarship in these laboratories. His texts on radiology of the chest were read worldwide.[14,15] Rabin was also involved in founding the American College of Chest Physicians and served as its President in 1969. He retired as Chief of the Division in 1960 but remained a Consulting Physician and continued as Associate Attending Radiologist. An innovative researcher, a scholar, a doctor's doctor, and a dedicated teacher, Rabin was also a man of wit and good will, beloved by those who knew and worked with him.

Following Rabin as Director of the Division was Louis Siltzbach. Siltzbach had come to Mount Sinai in 1942 as an Adjunct Physician in Chest Diseases. In 1946, he founded and became Chief of the Sarcoidosis Clinic; he would soon become a world authority on the disease. He was one of the first to demonstrate the efficacy of adrenal corticosteroids in suppressing granuloma formation in the treatment of sarcoidosis.[16] He went on to establish definitively the specific diagnostic role of the Kveim test in 1954, which subsequently became known as the Kveim-Siltzbach test.[17] His description of three radiographic stages of sarcoidosis brought a chronological order to what had previously appeared to be seemingly unrelated clinical syndromes.[18] As an organizer, speaker, Chairman, and Executive Secretary for the International Conferences on Sarcoidosis, Siltzbach set the standards to be met by satisfactory Kveim-Siltzbach test suspensions.[19] Moreover, he pioneered the universal application of the test and proved that sarcoidosis was a distinct worldwide clinical entity.[20] With more than fourteen thousand patients enrolled in the world's largest sarcoidosis clinic since the program began, Mount Sinai has honored Siltzach's legacy; the clinic remains the only location in the United States that performs the Kveim-Siltzbach test.

Another of Mount Sinai's pulmonary giants was Irving Selikoff. Selikoff joined Mount Sinai in 1941 as a Volunteer Assistant in Morbid Anatomy, then went to Sea View Hospital, where along with Edward Robitzek he published the first successful clinical trial of isoniazide in the treatment of tuberculosis.[21] Upon returning to Mount Sinai to join the Thoracic Diseases Division, Selikoff made a second important discovery. He noted the unusually high occurrence of lung disease among patients in his practice who worked at the United Asbestos and Rubber Company. Recognizing asbestos as the cause of pulmonary fibrosis, lung and digestive tract cancers, and mesotheliomas that occurred two decades or more after exposure, Selikoff conducted the epidemiological studies necessary to persuade physicians of a causal relationship.[22] This work laid the foundation for the establishment of strict asbestos exposure limits and encouraged concern over the potential hazards of other materials. Later, Selikoff reported that asbestos exposure increased the risk of lung cancer for smokers.[23] Often credited with the development of the field of environmental medicine, Selikoff was Director of Mount Sinai's Environmental Sciences Laboratory, Director of the Division of Environmental Medicine, and Professor of Community Medicine. Among his many honors, he received the prized Lasker Award. Selikoff is considered to have saved thousands of lives through his work in removing asbestos from the construction industry. Upon his death in 1992, Mount Sinai inaugurated the Irving J. Selikoff Occupational Health Clinical Center and the Irving J. Selikoff Asbestos Archives and Research Center. The archives hold his research documents, the largest and most detailed collection in the world of health records of asbestos-exposed persons.

Following Siltzbach's retirement, Alvin S. Teirstein was appointed Chief in 1974. Teirstein first came to Mount Sinai as a rotating Intern in 1953, then completed a medical residency and cardiopulmonary laboratory fellowship. During his first two years as Chief, Teirstein reorganized the Division into a full-time structure and initiated the medical and respiratory Intensive Care Units. His own research has involved studies on sarcoidosis, environmental lung disease, lung cancer, and mesothelioma. Teirstein developed a fiberoptic bronchoscopy program, utilized for both diagnosis and treatment, especially in sarcoidosis and interstitial lung disease.[24,25] In the 1980s, Mount Sinai physicians were one of the first groups to use the bronchoscope to make the diagnosis of lung diseases in patients with AIDS[26] and to intensively investigate the pulmonary manifestations of that disease. After twenty-seven years as a Division Chief, Teirstein, a charismatic teacher, mentor, and role model, with a legendary sense of humor, stepped down in 2001 and was named Director of the newly established Vivien Richenthal Institute for Pulmonary and Critical Care Research and the George Baehr Professor of Medicine.

David Nierman, a long-time member of the Division, Director of the Medical Intensive Care Unit, and a national leader in chronic critical care, succeeded Teirstein. Nierman's research interests have focused on designing prediction models of survival in various groups of critically ill patients and metabolic responses to chronic critical illness. All of the members of the Division have continued the tradition of their forebears in advancing pulmonary and critical care medicine. Neil Schachter has made many significant contributions to occupational lung disease both here and abroad; Judith Nelson has introduced the concept of palliative care to the Intensive Care Unit; Maria Padilla has become renowned for her studies of lung transplantation in patients with interstitial lung disease. The Richenthal Institute has begun extensive studies on the pathogenesis of lung cancer in women.

Were Alfred Meyer alive today, he could take great pride in what his successors have accomplished over the past century. He would also be fascinated to see the multiple areas of productive research going on in the Division and the magnitude of the clinical problems that are now being dealt with.

12

Division of Rheumatology

THE TERM "RHEUMA," which literally means "flowing," was used by Hippocrates to describe an excess of watery humor thought to flow from the brain. Ancient Greek physicians used "rheuma" interchangeably with "catarrhos" to describe a variety of illnesses, including joint problems. In 1642, Guillaume de Baillou (Ballonius), a French physician, coined the word "rheumatism" to distinguish noxious humors that affected joints from those that caused catarrh (hay fever, colds, and the like): "The whole body becomes painful, the face in some becomes red, the pain rages especially about the joints, so that indeed neither the foot nor the hand, nor the finger can be moved . . . without pain and outcry. . . . Although the arthritis is in a certain part, this rheumatism itself is in the entire body."[1] Today, rheumatic disease covers a wide gamut of illness, the common denominator being pain and inflammation involving muscles and joints.

The specialty of rheumatology did not exist in the early years of the twentieth century. There was little knowledge or interest in diseases of the muscles and joints on the part of the general medical community. At Mount Sinai, however, musculoskeletal problems (i.e., arthritis) were treated on the Medical Service; trauma, bone tumors, and infections were within the province of the surgeons. When Mount Sinai's first orthopaedic outpatient clinic was established in 1909, Philip Nathan, known for his work with arthritic patients, was placed in charge. He would become the first Chief of the orthopaedic inpatient service one year later.[2] Arthritis was the poor relation of medical research. The situation began to change in the 1920s, first in Europe; in 1934, the American Rheumatism Association was established and held its first formal meeting. Several years later, at Mount Sinai, Maurice Wolf, a European refugee physician, was placed in charge of an outpatient arthritis clinic. In the past fifty years, the field has burgeoned, spurred on by the Omnibus Medical Research Act of 1950, which established the National Institute of Arthritis and Metabolic Diseases (NIAMD) in the Public Health Service.

All of this notwithstanding, Mount Sinai's physicians were making seminal contributions to the understanding of the illnesses that constitute the field of rheumatology long before the term became fashionable. As a consequence, the current Division of Rheumatology is heir to an illustrious history in the subspecialty. In 1924, Emanuel Libman and Benjamin Sacks provided the first description of the characteristic heart lesions that can occur in patients with lupus erythematosus.[3] A decade later, George Baehr recognized the exacerbating effects of sun exposure and "wire loop" kidney lesions in patients with lupus.[4] Gregory Shwartzman devoted his career at Mount Sinai to the study of the pathogenesis of tissue lesions induced by endotoxin and immune complexes.[5] In 1942, the term "diffuse collagen disease" was introduced by Paul Klemperer, Mount Sinai's Chief of Pathology, as a critical unifying element in scleroderma, lupus, and related disorders.[6] The pathologists Jacob Churg and Lotte Strauss provided the first description of allergic granulomatosis, now generally known as the Churg-Strauss syndrome.[7]

Also in the early 1950s, one of the first gout clinics in the United States was established at The Mount Sinai Hospital by Alexander B. Gutman, then Chief of Medicine, and his long-time associate Tsai-Fan Yu, Emeritus Professor. The clinical effectiveness of probenecid in lowering the serum urate and diminishing the size of gouty tophi was established at Mount Sinai.[8] The effectiveness of colchicine taken daily as prophylaxis against recurrent attacks of acute gout was documented by Yu and Gutman in a landmark report in 1961,[9] and this finding was subsequently corroborated by Yu in follow-up studies that extended for more than thirty subsequent years.

A defining moment for the specialty occurred in 1956 when Charles Plotz and Jacques Singer, working in the serology laboratory, developed and standardized the latex fixation test for the diagnosis of rheumatoid arthritis.[10] Plotz, who had been on the faculty of Columbia University's College of Physicians and Surgeons, followed Gutman to Mount Sinai when Gutman was recruited as the Chief of Medicine. Plotz was named head of a section of rheumatology and was working in the laboratory on tests for rheumatoid factor. Singer came from Israel to become a fellow in the laboratory. The original papers on the technique became *Citation Classics*; the ease and applicability of the latex technique advanced studies in immunology to a profound degree.

Harry Spiera became Plotz's first clinical fellow and then joined the latter in practice. In 1966, Spiera, Plotz, and Selvan Davison published the first description of polymyalgia rheumatica in the United States and helped define the condition as a distinct entity.[11] When Plotz left Mount Sinai to become Chief of Rheumatology at Downstate Medical Center, Spiera succeeded him. With the advent of the Medical School, Spiera and Solomon Berson, then the Chairman of the Department of Medicine, created a formal Division of Rheumatology; major support for a fellowship was obtained from the Arthritis Foundation.

Spiera went on to develop the Rheumatology training program; more than forty fellows were trained, a significant percentage of whom opted for academic careers. Laboratory and clinical research flourished during Spiera's tenure. Numerous studies were carried out on rheumatoid factor with Irwin Oreskes and his colleagues; the presence of the factor was found to be nonspecific. Charles Steinman developed a system to map anti-DNA antibodies.[12] Spiera and his colleagues provided the first reports of early coronary artery disease in young patients with lupus[13] and on the first use of sulfamethoxazole-trimethoprim in the management of Wegener's granulomatosis.[14] Under Spiera's direction, Mount Sinai has become a major referral center for disorders such as giant cell arteritis, scleroderma, and Sjogren's syndrome, dedicated to providing excellent care and furthering basic knowledge pertinent to rheumatologic diseases. Leslie Dubin Kerr remained on the full-time faculty after completing her fellowship and has focused her research activities on the complications of the rheumatic diseases.

In 1997, Peter Gorevic was appointed the first full-time Chief of the Division of Rheumatology. Gorevic had spent a year at Mount Sinai during the 1960s doing graduate work, so he is, in a manner of speaking, another "returnee." Internationally recognized for his basic research in amyloidosis and cryoglobulinemia, Gorevic has served on advisory panels for the National Institutes of Health, the Arthritis Foundation, and the Lupus Foundation. With a major interest in the clinical care of the rheumatologic problems of the elderly, Gorevic has created a focus for the Division in the area of geriatric rheumatology and has developed interdisciplinary training programs with the Department of Geriatrics and Adult Development.

Although chronologically young in age as a Division of the Department of Medicine, the Division of Rheumatology has a sustained record of outstanding leadership and contributions to the field. It is now well positioned to propel itself to a still higher level of excellence.

Department of Surgery

THE HISTORY OF SURGERY at the Jews' Hospital begins June 8, 1855, when patient No. 1 in the case books of the Hospital was admitted three days after the opening of the Hospital doors. L. S., a forty-two-year-old male with a fistula-in-ano, was successfully operated on by Israel Moses and was discharged in good condition five days after surgery.[1] Where this procedure was performed is unclear, since there were no operating rooms in the original Hospital building. It was probably performed in the patient's bed.

The initial surgical staff consisted of five men. There were three Consulting Surgeons: Valentine Mott, Willard Parker, and Thomas Markoe, all of whom had volunteered their services well in advance of the opening of the Hospital. The other Attending Surgeon in addition to Moses was Alexander Mott, the son of Valentine.

The consultants were already well known in the field. The elder Mott was "the most distinguished surgeon of the first half of the nineteenth century here in America"[2] and world renowned for his surgical prowess. Willard Parker, the first to successfully drain an appendiceal abscess in the United States (1843), made significant contributions to the development of Mount Sinai. It was he who led the establishment of the Medical Board in 1872, holding the first meeting in his home and becoming its first Chairman. A fine clinical teacher, Parker remained on the staff until his death in 1884. The third Consultant, Thomas M. Markoe, was a leading orthopedist; his text on diseases of bone was a standard for many years.

Although the Consultants did see patients, the operative procedures were performed by Moses and Alexander Mott. Yet, the importance of these Consultants cannot be underestimated; their willingness to serve and their presence within the Institution helped establish the Jews' Hospital's reputation as a house of excellence from the outset, providing it with legitimacy and enhancing the Hospital's ability to raise needed funds.

Israel Moses, a member of a prominent Jewish family, had served in the United States Army prior to joining the Jews' Hospital. With the outbreak of the Civil War, Moses resigned to go back into the military. There he served with great distinction in the capacity of both military surgeon and military hospital director. Mustered out of the army in 1865, he did not return to the Hospital but lived out his life in Philadelphia, where he focused his attention on the need for sanitary reform and was involved in the formation of the American Public Health Association. Moses died in 1870 at the age of forty-seven. In 1944, the Trustees commissioned a portrait of Moses, which was painted from a photograph housed in the American Jewish Historical Museum. That portrait now hangs in the Department of Surgery, one of the few portraits of the active physicians from those early days known to exist.

In the first seven months of the Hospital's existence, five operative procedures were performed. A number of the early cases were orthopedic in nature, including the first child (Patient No. 9) to be admitted to the new Hospital.[3] Strict rules were established for the conduct of the Attending Surgeons. They were required to visit the Hospital at least every second day and to sign an attendance book. An absence of six consecutive days was considered a resignation. They were also required to attend in all cases of emergency or accident when called for by the Resident Physician and Surgeon. These rules for the mandatory notification of Attendings and their required presence for almost every case persists to this day. In great measure, these regulations helped establish the excellence of the surgical service.

The surgeons of the Jews' Hospital became increasingly busy, and there were numerous additions to and resignations from the staff. The revolutions in Europe in 1848 had forced a number of well-trained individuals to flee to the United States, many of whom settled in New York. One such individual was Ernst Krakowiczer,[4] well trained in pathology and surgery, who was appointed an Attending Surgeon in 1859. Krakowiczer would serve the Hospital steadfastly until his death from typhoid in 1875 during one of the many epidemics of that disease to affect New York City in the latter part of the nineteenth century.

The Civil War years and the Draft Riots of 1863 saw a marked increase in the number of cases of trauma admitted to the Hospital. Of the 364 admissions in 1864, fifty-three were soldiers. In that year, 115 operations were performed, of which eleven were "capital." There were eleven orthopedic procedures, including two above-knee amputations and resections of the knee joint and elbow joint.

The Orangemen Riots of 1871 brought another influx of seriously wounded (civilians this time) into the already overcrowded Hospital, but by then the new building on Lexington Avenue between 66th and 67th streets was well on its way to completion, and the physicians and surgeons were anticipating the move to new and more spacious quarters. However, there still were no operating rooms in this new structure. In the last year of occupancy of the original building, there were 650 admissions, eight births, and 276 operative procedures, including thirty-three major cases. Only four could be classified as general surgery: a resection of a breast cancer, two rectal procedures, and an attempted repair of an imperforate anus. The majority of the remaining procedures involved the drainage of abscesses and suturing of lacerations.

The move to the new site in 1872 coincided with the formation of the Medical Board. One of the first acts of that body was to recommend the creation of a House Staff. Even at this early stage of development of the Institution, excellence was paramount, and appointment to the House Staff would be by competitive examination. Krakowiczer became the surgical member of the Examination Committee. The Outdoor Dispensary was established, including a Surgical Division. Staff members were appointed to the Dispensary, but this was their only responsibility; it would be many years before this staff would be allowed inpatient responsibilities.

Surgical volume continued to grow, and, finally, in 1876, "the long felt need for the surgeons has been supplied by taking a part of the synagogue, which was larger than required, and erecting a partition. . . . This room . . . has been supplied with hot and cold water. . . . An operating table has been furnished and a platform raised and arranged for witnessing the operations; a case for preserving surgical instruments has also been supplied."[5] In this one room, all cases, whether clean or dirty, were operated on. In an era before the understanding of antisepsis and asepsis, and in the face of almost prohibitive mortality rates, surgery remained limited to operations for infection, amputations, and the occasional removal of a breast. Orthopedic procedures still appeared to dominate the surgical reports. In the year following the construction of the operating room, a modest percentage of the procedures performed would be considered major by today's criteria, but there were no intra-abdominal procedures recorded.

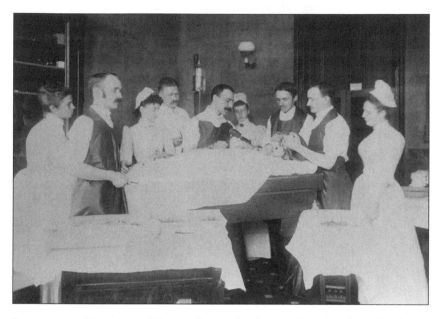

Surgery, possibly a mastoid operation, at Lexington Ave. site. Anna L. Alston, the Director of the Mount Sinai Hospital Training School for Nurses, is on the far left. Note the wooden tables in the front and the IV in the back center.

In 1877, the medical services and staff were divided into formal Medical and Surgical Services. The House Staff was also separated into Medical and Surgical Divisions; each Division had a Senior and a Junior Resident who were required to live in. Appointments to the House Staff were for two-year terms. Newly appointed house officers could choose their service. They would spend their first six months on the service of their choice and the next six months on the other. The entire second year would be spent as either the House Physician or the House Surgeon. A diploma was conferred at the completion of the training period.

With the ever-increasing patient volume, three new Attending Surgeons were appointed in 1877. Daniel Stimson, a military surgeon with the Seventh Regiment and the son-in-law of Willard Parker, is the best remembered. Arpad Gerster would later comment, "I have seen few men operate with greater elegance than Stimson."[6]

The introduction of asepsis and antisepsis by Lord Joseph Lister in 1867 was one of the greatest contributions made to the development of surgery, helping to establish it as a specialty independent of general medicine. Unfortunately, Lister's concepts were generally treated with disdain in America until the late 1880s. Without a doubt, the man responsible for making this country's surgeons aware of the value of Lister's work was Arpad Gerster.

Arpad Gerster, a giant in surgery, was appointed to the staff in 1880. Born in Hungary in 1848, Gerster emigrated to the United States in 1873. At a time when there were really no specialists, Gerster was the first in New York to limit his professional activities to surgery.[7] An early appointment to the German Hospital (now the Lenox Hill Hospital) was followed by his appointment to Mount Sinai. In 1888, Gerster published *The Rules of Aseptic and Antiseptic Surgery*,[8] one of the earliest and unquestionably most important American books on the subject. Illustrated with half-tone photographs taken by Gerster himself from the operating rooms of both the German Hospital and Mount Sinai, the book went through a second and third edition in two years. In the preface to the first edition, Gerster stated, "It can not now be successfully denied that *the surgeon's acts determine the fate of a fresh wound, and that its infection and suppuration are due to his technical faults of omission or commission.*"[9] With Gerster, there was no such thing as passing the buck. Publication of the book preceded the use of sterile gloves in the operating room. Rubber gloves were not used at Mount Sinai until introduced by George Brewer in 1899. The other symbol of sterility and cleanliness, the pristine white coat, was introduced in 1890 by Southgate Leigh, then a House Surgeon.

Not only had Gerster's "practice of asepsis opened the cavities of the body for operative procedure—chiefly the abdominal"[10] but also, to some physicians, such as William J. Mayo, who became a particular friend, Gerster was "the man who I believe did more for American surgery as a whole than any other man of his time"[11]—high praise from one of the most celebrated physicians in the Western Hemisphere. Gerster's surgical experience was vast. Among his more than eighty publications, he was the first to suggest that cancer might be disseminated by a surgical procedure.[12] In collaboration with Bernard Sachs, he published on the surgical management of epilepsy. Gerster also published on a wide range of topics in orthopedics, urology, and plastic surgery and spearheaded major advances in abdominal surgery, especially in surgical approaches to cancer of the rectum and in appendicitis in pregnancy.

The first Mount Sinai surgeon to be elected to the prestigious American Surgical Association, Gerster was an active participant in the meet-

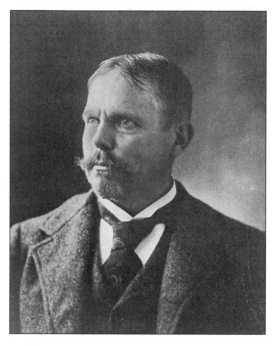

Arpad Gerster, M.D., Chief of Surgery, 1882–1914.

ings as both a speaker and a discussant.[13] He served as the group's Vice President in 1909 and President in 1912. Gerster, in his day, had few peers as an operator or as a teacher. He was, in addition, a skillful artist and musician and a master of language. His autobiography, *Recollections of a New York Surgeon*,[14] published in 1917, vividly portrays the development of surgery at the time and is a striking testimonial to this remarkable man. For many years, Gerster spent his vacations in the Adirondack Mountains. It is there that he was buried after his death on March 11, 1923. Gerster's legacy was the outstanding group of surgeons trained by him who furthered the level of surgical excellence on the Surgical Service for the ensuing half-century. The list includes Howard Lilienthal, Albert A. Berg, Edwin Beer, Charles Elsberg, and Alexis Moschcowitz.

Mount Sinai would become "home" to others besides those who emigrated from Europe or who had trained at the Hospital. John A. Wyeth, a native southerner, was appointed to the staff in 1882. Remembered by his peers for his gentle southern accent and for his calm and easy demeanor, he would have a major impact on graduate medical education in New York. In 1883, Wyeth established the New York Poly-clinic, an institution devoted exclusively to postgraduate medical edu-cation. He enlisted a number of Mount Sinai physicians to ensure the success of his new venture.

Wyeth's surgical technique was widely praised. He was also a pro-lific scientific writer, publishing on fecal fistula after appendicitis, la-parotomy and intestinal suture, surgery for urethral-rectal fistula, and amputations through the hip joint. In addition, he published several surgical texts, as well as his autobiography, *With Sabre and Scalpel: The Autobiography of a Soldier and Surgeon*.[15]

With the separation of the House Staff into Medical and Surgical Di-visions and the growth of the Surgical Service, it was inevitable that a House Staff appointee would eventually choose surgery as his primary service. And so it was that, in 1887, Howard Lilienthal became the first individual to do so.

And what a choice it was! Although he would eventually become one of the founding fathers of thoracic surgery, Lilienthal was the epit-ome of the general surgeon.[16] He became Gerster's assistant at a time when much of their surgery was still being done in patients' homes. While the surgeons would bring their own instruments and other equipment, it was the patient's responsibility to provide an appropriate table. The latter, being frequently inadequate, led to the development of one of Lilienthal's many inventions: a portable operating table, the first of its kind. Its design would become the precursor of the field operating tables used in World War I.

Lilienthal devised a number of widely used instruments. These in-cluded a self-retaining trocar and cannula for the aseptic evacuation of fluid from distended viscera, the first usable metal detector for surgery, a rib spreader, a guillotine for cutting the first rib, removable plates for fracture fixation, and silver wire for use as suture material in the pres-ence of infection.

Lilienthal's paper on the repair of tendons and nerves in the wrist in 1892 was the first of his more than three hundred publications. In an era when most excisions of the gallbladder were performed in two stages (cholecystostomy followed by cholecystectomy), he advocated primary cholecystectomy. On the other hand, he was a staunch advo-cate of two-stage procedures under appropriate circumstances. Lilien-thal was the first surgeon in this country to perform a successful ab-dominal colectomy for colitis[17] and the first to perform two-stage suprapubic prostatectomy.[18] Other notable achievements included a technique for nephroureterectomy, a method for performing a permanent colostomy that became widely accepted, and a procedure for the repair of ankylosis of the temporo-mandibular joint. He was also an early proponent of open reduction and fixation of fractures. Furthermore, Lilienthal was the surgeon of record on the first patient in America to receive appropriately citrated blood, the solution having been developed at Mount Sinai by Richard Lewisohn.[19]

Many of the early surgery House Staff graduates from 1877–1902 went on to very distinguished careers. William H. Wilmer (1887) would become a world-famous ophthalmologist and would have the Eye Institute at Johns Hopkins Medical Center named after him. Samuel Brickner (1893) and Martin Ware (1894) would become senior gynecologists at Mount Sinai, and Walter M. Brickner (1898) would become the Chief of Radiology. Charles Elsberg (1895), Albert A. Berg (1896), and Edwin Beer (1902) would achieve worldwide recognition in neurosurgery, abdominal surgery, and urology, respectively.

The final decade of the nineteenth century witnessed enormous growth throughout Mount Sinai but especially on the surgical service. Aseptic surgery led to a significant increase in surgical volume, necessitating the building of a second operating room in 1895. This for the first time allowed clean and dirty cases to be treated in separate operating rooms, establishing a custom that would continue for more than seventy-five years. The first report of an operation for strangulated femoral hernia appears in the annual report for 1879; the first bowel resection during hernia repair took place in 1885. From that time on, there was a steady increase in hernia surgery. Abdominal surgery was coming into its own; the first "exploratory incision" (laparotomy) for a sarcoma of the pelvis took place in 1885. The first laparotomy for intestinal obstruction occurred two years later. Thereafter, the number of laparotomies performed annually increased at a significant rate. The first appendectomies were performed in 1890, a year in which a total of 724 operations were performed.

In 1896, following the resignation of Wyeth, Gerster was placed in charge of the entire General Surgery Service, assisted by Lilienthal and William Van Arsdale, who had joined the staff in 1893. A total of 225 beds were now available in the Hospital, an expansion from the original 110 in 1872; sixty-two of these beds were allocated to the surgical service. The more than 1,500 operations performed in 1896 included

820 general surgical procedures. In the ensuing three years, surgical volume increased by more than 30 percent, so that in 1899 there were 2,028 operations in all, including 295 laparotomies. The caseload was overwhelming, and in 1899 Lilienthal was promoted to Attending Surgeon and placed in charge of a second, newly created General Surgery Service.

Coincident with growth was the need for more House Staff. Three House Surgeons completed their training in 1903, and for a number of years thereafter, four men graduated annually. This number held fairly steady until the close of World War I, when there was again an increase in the number of physicians training in surgery. The graduates of those years included many individuals mentioned elsewhere in this book who went on to forge outstanding careers in either surgery, a surgical specialty, or, in some cases (Eli Moschcowitz, 1903; George Baehr, 1910; Nathan Rosenthal, 1915), in the Department of Medicine at Mount Sinai.

The move of the Hospital to its current site in 1904, with more beds and more operating rooms, coupled with the growth of surgery and the surgical specialties, necessitated another reorganization of the Surgical Service. The elevation of Gerster to Consultant in 1914 provided that opportunity, and in that year four separate divisions were created. Lilienthal was placed in charge of the Thoracic Division and from that time on devoted himself almost exclusively to thoracic surgery. The Neurosurgery Service was headed by Charles Elsberg,[20] the Genitourinary Service by Edwin Beer,[21] and Albert A. Berg was placed in charge of the Intestinal Service. The creation of the specialized services proved to be salutary. As Berg would later note, "Mount Sinai became one of the leaders in specialization in general surgery. . . . Developments have followed the specialization which has contributed tremendously to the advance of surgery in these particular fields."[22] Beer, Elsberg, and Lilienthal would all have echoed those sentiments.

Albert Ashton Berg, born in New York of immigrant German Jewish parents, arrived at The Mount Sinai Hospital in 1894. Serving for a period of time as Gerster's assistant after completion of his training, Berg was appointed to the inpatient staff in 1899. A brilliant technician, "his ability in abdominal exploration was fantastic. His long, skinny fingers could disentangle previous operative adhesions from someone else's work, and could lay things bare."[23]

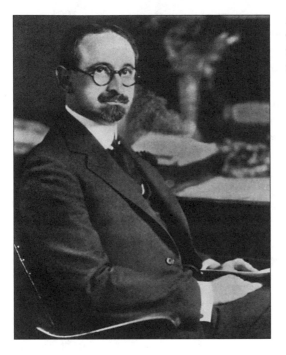

Albert A. Berg, M.D.,
Chief the Gastrointestinal
Service of the Dept. of
Surgery, 1915–1934.

Berg was a workaholic who operated six days a week and frequently on Sundays, as well. It is alleged that he also regularly scheduled an operation for shortly after midnight on New Year's Eve. This
tradition, which tormented the Hospital staff, was, it seems, based on
a superstition that if he began the year with surgery, he would live
through to the next year. Never married, Berg lived with his older
brother Henry, an internist, who created a considerable fortune buying
real estate. The Berg brothers were avid collectors of early editions of
rare books and manuscripts. They are remembered outside the medical profession because of the forty-thousand volumes that they donated to the New York Public Library to form the Berg Collection. At
A. A. Berg's death, a substantial amount of money was bequeathed to
that library for maintenance of the collection; he also made bequests to
both New York University and Mount Sinai. At the latter institution,
funding for the Henry W. Berg Laboratory Building was donated by A.
A. Berg to honor his brother in 1946. The Laboratory Building opened
in 1953.

Although not a prodigious writer, Berg did publish in 1905, a text for students and practitioners. Moreover, he developed operative techniques for the management of malignant tumors of the urinary bladder and of right-sided inflammatory bowel disease; he also originated the retroduodenal approach to the common bile duct. Most notably, he was the surgeon who performed the first gastrectomy for peptic ulcer disease in America. In addition, he was also the surgeon who operated on all of the patients in the landmark report of Crohn, Ginzburg, and Oppenheimer, "Regional Enteritis."[24] In 1934, on his elevation to Consultant status, the surgical staff paid tribute to Berg by publishing *The Surgical Technique of Dr. A. A. Berg.*[25] The chapters detail the techniques devised by Berg that have been carried down through the decades; many are still in use today.

Operating in an era before the advent of antibiotics or the modern knowledge of fluid and electrolyte balance, Berg achieved remarkable results. A staunch advocate of the use of subtotal gastrectomy in the treatment of gastric and duodenal ulcer,[26] Berg reported a mortality rate of 7 percent in more than five hundred primary and secondary operations for ulcer disease.[27] The recurrence rate (gastrojejunal ulcer) was slightly over 1 percent, compared to the recurrence rate of 34 percent after gastrojejunostomy alone; the latter procedure was the one most often employed by others at the time.

Revered by his patients, Berg was not, however, beloved by all the staff. Although all agreed that he had great skill, he was known to tyrannize nurses and assistants, as well as members of the staff. He will always be remembered, however, as the individual who put Mount Sinai's gastrointestinal surgical service on the map in the twentieth century.

Other members of the intestinal service gained worldwide recognition in the years just before World War I, the most prominent being Richard Lewisohn and Alexis Moschcowitz. Born, educated, and surgically trained in Germany, Richard Lewisohn arrived in this country in 1906 and was appointed to the staff of Mount Sinai shortly thereafter. He would remain active at the Hospital almost to the day of his death in 1961. His contributions to medicine fall into four disparate areas. The first was the development of "the citrate method" of blood transfusion in 1915.[28] The second area related to gastric surgery. Learning of the work of Hans von Haberer, in Innsbruck, Austria, advocating gastric resection for peptic ulcer disease, Lewisohn visited von Haberer in 1922.

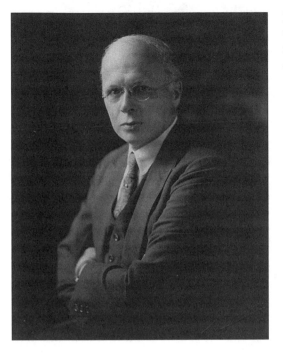

Richard Lewisohn, M.D.,
Chief of the General
Surgical Service, Dept.
of Surgery, 1928–1936.

He, too, became convinced of the justification for using the procedure, a very radical proposal at the time. Associated with Berg on the latter's service, he persuaded Berg to adopt the procedure, and the rest is history. Radical for its time, the work of Berg and Lewisohn in the surgical management of gastric and duodenal ulcer paved the way for the acceptance of resection as the preferred method of surgical therapy. In a major study of gastrojejunal ulcer published in 1925, Lewisohn noted that, after resection, the gastric contents became anacid, whereas gastric acid was unchanged after gastrojejunostomy. He then commented, "Whatever the real etiology of ulcers may be (infection, embolism, or other source), experience has shown that hyperacidity is a contributory factor in the growth of these ulcers."[29] Suggesting infection as a possible etiologic agent in ulcer disease put Lewisohn about 60 years ahead of his time. His third field of interest was cancer research. Following his retirement as an attending surgeon because of the Hospital's imposed age limit, Lewisohn returned to the laboratory and spent ten years in cancer research. These investigations were the first to establish the significance of folic acid in the biology of the cancer cell.[30] Anticancer

Alexis V. Moschcowitz,
M.D., Chief of Surgery,
1915–1927.

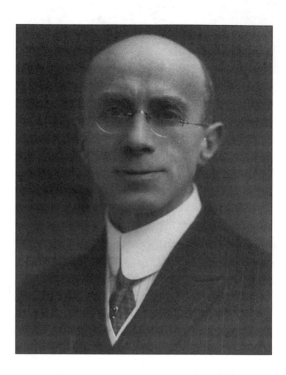

agents were tested, and Lewisohn treated George Herman "Babe" Ruth in 1947 with teropterin, one of the earliest folic acid antagonists, when the latter was suffering from late-stage nasopharyngeal cancer. Finally, as to the fourth area of accomplishment, Lewisohn, at age eighty, created Mount Sinai's first cell research laboratory, in which he worked almost daily for the next five years. Lewisohn died in 1961 at the age of eighty-six years.

Alexis V. Moschcowitz was born in Hungary in 1865 and emigrated to New York at the age of fifteen. Appointed to the staff in surgery at Mount Sinai in 1894, he would be affiliated with the Institution until his death in 1933. One of Moschcowitz's earliest papers was an important study of tetanus and the beneficial effects of serum therapy. Although he published extensively, and "there is hardly an organ in the human body which at one time or another did not receive his attention,"[31] Moschcowitz's major achievements were in the surgery of hernia and rectal prolapse; his name is still associated with both his repair of femoral hernia[32] and his method of repair of rectal prolapse.[33] He also elucidated the pathogenesis and management of epigastric hernia and published a definitive study of sliding hernia.[34] Called into military service in World War I, Moschcowitz served as Chief of Surgical Services at major army hospitals and in 1918 was appointed to the Empyema Commission, which was organized to deal with the devastation of postinfluenzal pneumonia empyema.[35] Moschcowitz died of an acute coronary occlusion in 1933.

As we have seen, the work of many of the well-known Mount Sinai surgeons encompassed the years before and after World War I. And so it was with Leo Buerger, who in 1908 described thromboangiitis obliterans,[36] soon thereafter to become known as Buerger's disease. Although not the first to identify the condition, Buerger provided a highly accurate pathological description that set the disease apart from other vascular conditions. Although Buerger does not mention the association of the disease with smoking in his original report, in 1924 he noted that "Tobacco is probably a predisposing factor. . . . Most of the cases are heavy smokers, although smoking was denied in 1 per cent of the author's cases."[37] Buerger also made significant contributions to urology with the development of the Brown-Buerger cystoscope.[38]

Buerger's work in vascular disease was carried on by Samuel Silbert. Originally appointed to the Neurosurgical Service in 1922, Silbert became interested in thromboangiitis and in 1924 originated the Thromboangiitis Clinic at Mount Sinai. This was the first vascular clinic in New York City and perhaps one of the first of its kind in the world. The Clinic soon expanded its scope and in 1940 changed its name to the Peripheral Vascular Clinic. Silbert was the first surgeon on the staff at Mount Sinai to devote his entire efforts to the field of vascular surgery and established the subspecialty on the Surgical Service. In 1945, Silbert was able to report on more than one thousand patients with thromboangiitis, one hundred of whom had been followed for ten to twenty years.[39] He reconfirmed the importance of tobacco in the etiology of the disease and was able to state that, if the patients stopped smoking, amputation was never required.

On the Surgical Service, as in all other departments, the years between the two world wars were a time of growth as the Hospital's bed capacity expanded. In 1932, Neurosurgery split from Surgery to become a separate department, headed by Ira Cohen.[40] Urology became an independent department in 1942 under the leadership of Abraham Hyman.[41] Many of the surgical House Staff would remain and build their practices at Mount Sinai; other, already established surgeons were given inpatient appointments and moved their practices to Mount Sinai.

Percy Klingenstein began his training at Mount Sinai in 1919 and would serve the institution in numerous capacities for three quarters of a century. When Mount Sinai's Third General Hospital was called to active duty in September 1942, Klingenstein became the Chief of Surgery, serving with the Unit in the African and Italian campaigns. Returning home late in 1945, Klingenstein resumed his practice at Mount Sinai, and the following year he accepted a position as the Chief of Surgery at the Hospital for Joint Diseases, a position he held for twelve years. Active on the Gastrointestinal Service, he was often given the responsibility for the most difficult cases on the service. His presentations on GI problems and in breast cancer were models of accurate statistical reporting. Klingenstein was a highly respected teacher throughout his career and a fine clinician, with outstanding judgment and excellent technical skills. Although formally retired in 1971, he remained a role model for another generation of young surgeons. Attending Surgical Grand Rounds until well into his nineties, he could always be counted on to ask the most incisive question of the session. His legacy remains in the form of the Klingenstein scholarships and the Percy Klingenstein M.D. Scholars program. He died in 1996, several months after his one hundredth birthday.

After completing his surgical training at Mount Sinai and study abroad, Leon Ginzburg became Berg's assistant at a time when the latter was far and away the busiest surgeon in the Hospital. It was in this milieu that Ginzburg and Gordon Oppenheimer, then a fellow in pathology, began their study of unusual lesions of the terminal ileum, work that culminated in the classic description of regional enteritis, shortly thereafter to be given the eponym "Crohn's disease."[42] During World War II, Ginzburg served throughout the North African and Italian campaigns with Mount Sinai's Third General Hospital. Upon his return, he built an extensive practice of his own and, although he never left Mount Sinai, served for two decades as Chief of Surgery at the Beth Israel Medical Center. A true Renaissance man and an outstanding teacher, Ginzburg was equally at home quoting from Shakespeare and from the latest paper on gastrointestinal surgery.

During the 1920s and 1930s, other physicians would come to the fore in the Department of Surgery. Ernest Arnheim would become

Mount Sinai's first pediatric surgeon. Samuel Klein would make significant contributions to the surgery of inflammatory bowel disease and, as a distinguished teacher, play a major role in the resident training program for many years. Sylvan Manheim and, later, Robert Turell would become renowned for their expertise in ano-rectal surgery; both would go on to write definitive texts on proctology and colon and rectal surgery. In 1959, Turell was one of the three founding members of the Society for Surgery of the Alimentary Tract and served as its President in 1966–1967. After his death in 1990, his widow endowed a professorship in his name.

During the 1920s and 1930s, there were also two individuals who trained elsewhere and who would play pivotal roles in the future of the Department and the Hospital. In 1923, Ralph Colp joined Mount Sinai; he was followed a decade later by John Garlock.

Recruited by George Blumenthal, then President of the Hospital, Ralph Colp began an association with Mount Sinai that lasted more than fifty years. The son of a pharmacist who owned Colp's Drug Store in Greenwich Village, young Ralph used to help his father compound prescriptions. Following his medical school graduation, Colp trained at the Presbyterian Hospital and then served two years in the U.S. Army Medical Corps during World War I. Appointed to the staff of the Beekman Downtown Hospital (now NYU-Downtown) in 1919, he helped establish an outstanding Trauma Service there. Concurrent with the appointment at Beekman was an instructorship in anatomy and surgery at Columbia University's College of Physicians and Surgeons. Colp always considered this appointment and his teaching of anatomy to have played a major role in his emergence as an ambidextrous, technically brilliant and remarkably rapid operator.

Colp's interests in surgery were many and varied. His early papers from Beekman were trauma oriented, and his interest in anatomy led to the development of a procedure for bilateral excision of the submaxillary glands for the treatment of Ludwig's angina, a rapidly fatal infectious phlegmon of the floor of the mouth. In 1926, Moschcowitz, Colp, and Klingenstein presented the results of mastectomy for breast cancer at the American Surgical Association, and one year later Ira Cohen and Colp published a series of fifty-nine cases operated on for pancreatic cancer. In 1934, Colp was the first to describe regional enteritis crossing the ileocecal valve to involve the cecum; this was the first description of granulomatous ileocolitis.[43]

Ralph Colp, M.D., Chief of Surgery, 1935–1952, as seen on the cover of *The New Gewalter*, the Alumni Dinner Dance program for the Hospital centennial celebration, 1952.

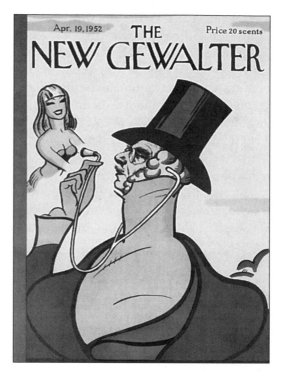

Under Berg's aegis, the Gastrointestinal Service grew to such an extent that upon his retirement in 1934, it was divided; Colp was placed in charge of a Gastric Service, and Garlock took over a Colon Service. Colp was one of the first surgeons to recognize the importance of basic science research to the clinical development of surgeons. In 1940, he was instrumental in establishing the Gastrointestinal Physiology Laboratory, which remained in existence for almost fifty years. In that laboratory, Franklin Hollander, Edward Jemerin, and Vernon Weinstein developed the insulin test to ascertain the completeness of vagotomy,[44] Henry Doubilet did monumental work on bile metabolism and the role of the Sphincter of Oddi, and David Dreiling began his many important studies of pancreatic physiology, which were continued in the Pancreatic Physiology Laboratory, also created by Colp. Colp did much to further investigation, creating a prize for the best published papers in *The Mount Sinai Journal of Medicine* and providing fellowships and lectureships within the Department of Surgery.

Colp was the recipient of every honor that could be bestowed upon a Mount Sinai physician. He was the President of the Medical Board at the time of Mount Sinai's one hundredth anniversary in 1952, and a caricature of him graces the cover of *The New Gewalter*, a publication by the alumni in honor of that anniversary. In that same year he became the holder of Mount Sinai's Gold-Headed Cane.[45] In every way, Ralph Colp can rightfully be called one of Mount Sinai's Giants.

So can John H. Garlock, who joined the Surgical Service in 1933, having moved from the New York Hospital, where he had trained and been on staff. One of the finest surgical technicians the world has known, Garlock was a founding member of the American Board of Surgery, the American Board of Plastic Surgery, and the American Board of Thoracic Surgery. He played an important role in the creation of Mount Sinai's Division of Plastic Surgery. Although he published fundamental studies on the use of free full-thickness skin grafts, hand surgery, the release of burn contractures, and the management of bronchopleural fistula, it was the gastrointestinal tract, and specifically the esophagus, that was his surgical passion. His techniques for management of carcinoma of the esophagus and gastric cardia were creative and unique and have stood the test of time. He was the first to report a successful resection of a middle third esophageal carcinoma with reestablishment of continuity.[46]

A stern taskmaster, Garlock was an excellent but unusual teacher. He said little, whether it was in the operating room or at the bedside; one learned by watching a master at work. Garlock was right-handed, not ambidextrous, but he would always say, "Don't watch my right hand; it's the left that does the work to make it easy for the right." John Madden, a friend and a former Chief of Surgery at St. Clare's Hospital, would frequently visit Garlock's operating room and has commented, "There I witnessed a surgeon whose surgical technique was poetry in motion and literally bloodless. . . . He was a surgeon's surgeon."[47]

But Garlock's hands did more than operate. He was a superb pianist of concert quality who spent many evenings playing chamber music with the greats of the musical world. He also became an accomplished painter. Garlock's publications number more than 165. On June 6, 1965, while working on the final chapters of a single-authored book on gastrointestinal surgery that was devoted to his personal techniques

John H. Garlock, M.D.,
Chief of Surgery,
1937–1952.

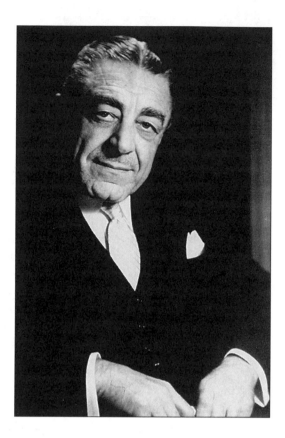

and results,[48] Garlock suffered a vascular catastrophe that rapidly proved fatal.

With the formation of the American Board of Surgery, in 1937, the Department of Surgery's residency was restructured to be compatible with Board requirements. Albert S. Lyons and Bernard Simon were the first individuals to graduate under the new program, in 1942. Both would become vital members of the Surgical Service in the years to come. Lyons became Garlock's assistant and, exposed to the latter's large inflammatory bowel disease practice both in the private pavilion and on the ward service, created the "Q-T Club," the first ever stoma support group. Named after the surgical wards Q and T, the Club was remarkably successful and spawned many similar groups throughout the world that continue to this day. Lyons was also responsible for creating the Mount Sinai Archives and was the institution's first historian and archivist. Bernard Simon would go into plastic surgery and cap a highly successful career as surgeon and teacher with his appointment as Chief of the Division, in which position he served from 1965 to 1982.

The Division of Plastic Surgery was launched in 1952, and Arthur J. Barsky was appointed Chief. During his period of service in the military during World War II, Barsky had established the first independent hand service in the U.S. Army. He was a charter member of the American Society for Surgery of the Hand and served as its President in 1965. In that same year, he founded the International Federation of Hand Societies and served as its Secretary-General for seven years. Immediately after his appointment, Barsky initiated the residency program in plastic surgery. In 1955, he and his practice associates, Sidney Kahn and Bernard Simon, participated in the Hiroshima Maiden Project, the rehabilitation of twenty-five Japanese women who had suffered severe burn deformities as a result of the atomic bomb blast in 1945. In the ensuing years, Mount Sinai surgeons went to Japan and provided training in plastic surgery, leading to the introduction of the specialty in Japan. Barsky retired from Mount Sinai in 1965 and was replaced by Simon as Chief.

The post–World War II years saw the beginnings of the full-time system in the clinical departments of Mount Sinai. Full-time chiefs were in place in Psychiatry (Kaufman, 1945), Medicine (Gutman, 1949), and Pediatrics (Hodes, 1949). Alan Guttmacher would become Chief of Obstetrics and Gynecology in 1952. It was now time to fill the position of Chief of Surgery. At this time, the Surgical Service consisted of three Divisions, the Gastric (Colp) Service, the Colon (Garlock) Service, and the Thoracic Service, now headed by Arthur S. W. Touroff, who had succeeded Harold Neuhof.[49] The Senior General Surgery Attendings were amenable to the change to a full-time Chief. Garlock, Colp, and Ginzburg stated that it was important to have an individual based within the Hospital to direct the teaching program, to oversee the residency on a day-to-day basis, and to build upon the existing research program.

And so, on September 1, 1952, Mark M. Ravitch began his tenure as the first full-time Director of Surgery and Surgeon-in-Chief to the Mount Sinai Hospital. A member of the faculty at Johns Hopkins, where he had trained under Alfred Blalock, Ravitch was a brilliant individual who spoke eight languages fluently and was a prolific writer. He had already made significant contributions to surgery and had pioneered a new technique for the management of pectus excavatum that had become the procedure of choice. His work with David Sabiston in the 1940s on ileo-anal anastomosis, though years before its time, paved the way for the ileo-anal pull-through procedure now used routinely in the management of ulcerative colitis and familial polyposis.

Ravitch made radical changes in the residency program, but in the process he eliminated the divisional structure that had existed and in so doing upset the balance of power with the Voluntary Staff. The only exception was in pediatric surgery, where Jerrold Becker was recruited to the Voluntary Staff to head the Division. With Ravitch's changes, the Residents were given much greater independent responsibility for patient management on the ward service, in the operating room, and in the clinics. Two distinct ward services of about forty-five beds each were created, each led by a Chief Resident, two Assistant Residents, and several Rotating Interns. There were now twenty-two Surgical Residents. The work was long and arduous. Ravitch insisted that his Chief Residents be on call twenty-four hours a day, seven days a week. When he heard that one of the Senior Residents was making out a call schedule for the Junior House Staff that had them working every other night, his comment was, "What, do they want to miss half the cases?"

Ravitch was an exceptional teacher whose concepts were frequently diametrically opposite to those of the prior chiefs of the service, and it was inevitable that friction would develop between the old guard and the Chief. The former felt that they were being disenfranchised, and, in fact, they were. The more junior Attendings were, for the most part, supportive of Ravitch, and those Residents who completed the program under Ravitch felt that they had received excellent training. Robert Paradny, one of the few to graduate while Ravitch was still Chief, became a mainstay of the teaching program for almost forty years.

The situation deteriorated rapidly, and, when Ravitch returned from a vacation in September 1955, he announced that he would be leaving within sixty days. And indeed he did, returning to Baltimore to become the Chief of Surgery at the Baltimore City Hospital. His career would then take him to Chicago and finally to Pittsburgh, where he spent many years as Chief of Surgery at Montefiore Hospital. Ravitch's continuing contributions to surgery were many. Shortly after leaving Mount Sinai, he went on a trip to Russia and returned with a primitive stapling device that he had seen used in Russia. It was to be the forerunner of the surgical stapling "revolution" in the United States. His

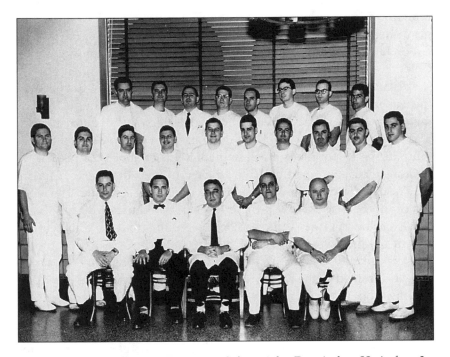

Surgical House Staff, 1954. Front row, left to right: Drs. Arthur H. Aufses, Jr., Joseph M. Levin, Mark M. Ravitch, Chief; Robert Paradny, Philip W. Goldman. 2nd row, left to right: Isidore Mandelbaum, Stuart M. Denmark, Stanley E. Goodman, Arthur Sicular, Milton Glickstein, William Kramer, Robert J. Rubin, Donald R. Weisman, David W. Moss, Sheldon Roger. 3rd row, left to right: Victor Weinberg, Milton L. Levine, Robert J. Wilder, Jack I. Lipman, Horace Herbsman, Sheldon S. Schoen, Arthur G. Ship, Ezra S. Shaya.

two-volume history of the American Surgical Association would become a classic. There are currently two chairs in Surgery named after Mark M. Ravitch, one at Johns Hopkins and one at the University of Pittsburgh. In the 1980s, Ravitch returned to Mount Sinai as a visiting professor in the Department of Surgery. The moderator introduced Ravitch with the comment "Although his tenure here was short and stormy, what he left behind has made the life of subsequent full-time chiefs much easier."[50]

John Garlock became the Acting Chief of Surgery while a search committee looked for a successor to Ravitch. Ivan D. Baronofsky, Associate Professor at the University of Minnesota, was appointed as of

March 1957 and immediately set about instituting an open heart surgery program.[51] Baronofsky's tenure was as short as that of Ravitch; he left on June 15, 1959, at which time Samuel H. Klein became the Acting Chief.

Allan E. Kark arrived from South Africa in early 1961 to take over the leadership of the Department. The former Chairman of the Department of Surgery at the University of Wittwatersrand in Durban, Kark was greeted warmly by Klein and the staff, all of whom yearned for stability in the Department. Kark immediately set about the task of rebuilding the Department, and, with the recruitment of Chiefs of Cardiac and Vascular Surgery, he returned it to a divisional structure. The modern cardiothoracic surgery program was initiated under the able leadership of Robert Litwak, who had been recruited from the University of Miami along with his colleague Howard Gadboys.[52]

Kark recruited Julius Jacobson II to head the Division of Vascular Surgery. Trained at the Presbyterian Hospital, Jacobson had done pioneering work in microvascular surgery while on the faculty of the University of Vermont,[53] work that he would continue at Mount Sinai and for which he would become known as the father of microsurgery. Jacobson went on to develop Mount Sinai's hyperbaric chamber, for which a separate building was constructed on the corner of Fifth Avenue and 101st Street, just to the north of the Housman Pavilion. One of the largest such facilities on the East Coast, the chamber was a cylinder measuring forty-five feet long and twelve feet in diameter, capable of pressurization to forty-five pounds (the equivalent of a sixty-six-foot dive below sea level.) It was accompanied by a recompression chamber, able to pressurize to a dive level of 165 feet, for treatment of diving accidents. The chamber was in operation for twenty-two years (1966–1988); some thirty-six thousand treatments were given for gas gangrene, necrotizing infection, radiation necrosis, and other conditions, and 1,700 operations (primarily vascular surgery procedures) were performed in it. The Chief of Vascular Surgery for almost thirty-five years, Jacobson endowed a professorship in the Department in 1992.

Other vascular surgeons had made their mark in the Department before the Division was formalized. Lester Blum had made a singular contribution to open heart surgery with the development of a parabiotic pump that excluded the heart from the circulation.[54] In the 1960s, Robert Nabatoff, who had performed many of the earliest cardiac surgical procedures in the Hospital, began to specialize in the surgery of varicose veins. Recognizing that hospitalization was not required,[55] Nabatoff persuaded Blue Cross and other insurance carriers to pay hospital charges for ambulatory surgery, paving the way for the explosion of ambulatory surgery that would follow.

Almost immediately after his arrival, Kark recognized the need to widen the scope of the resident experience, which by the very nature of Mount Sinai was overweighted with gastrointestinal surgery and deficient in areas such as trauma. He sought out and worked with Ray Trussell, the Commissioner of Health of New York City, to arrange an affiliation with Greenpoint Hospital in Brooklyn and to staff it with Attendings and Residents. Kark was able to overcome the expected reluctance of the other Chiefs, and, in 1962, David A. Dreiling, known worldwide for his studies in pancreatic physiology, became Chief of Surgery at Greenpoint. The success of the venture led Trussell and the City to pursue affiliation agreements for the staffing of all of its hospitals by the major centers in New York. Among the City hospitals, City Hospital Center at Elmhurst was the prize, and, in 1964, Dreiling and the staff moved to Elmhurst and quickly structured an excellent teaching program for residents.

In 1963, Mount Sinai received its charter from the State to start a medical school, and Kark was on the original small committee set up to establish the structure and requirements of the school. Although Kark was never totally in favor of a four-year medical school for Mount Sinai, he took on the challenge of preparing the Department for the eventual opening of the medical school in 1968. The task of expanding the full-time faculty was difficult because of inadequate salary support, lack of an adequate practice plan for income supplementation, and the entrenched referral patterns of the voluntary staff. Despite many obstacles, Kark persisted. William Shoemaker was recruited to plan, build, and direct a Surgical Intensive Care Unit in conjunction with the Department of Anesthesiology. A kidney transplant program was started under the direction of Lewis Burrows, who had been sent to England by Kark to study with Peter Medawar, the Nobel laureate. The first kidney transplant at Mount Sinai was performed in 1967; that patient was still alive thirty-four years later.

With the encouragement of Kermit Osserman, who oversaw one of the largest myasthenia gravis clinics in the country, and assisted by Angelos Papatestas, Kark initiated a comprehensive program in the use of transcervical thymectomy in the management of this complex disease. Numerous publications written in conjunction with the medical and anesthesiology staff proved the validity of the procedure over the long term. The program would continue under the aegis of Papatestas after Kark left and would be carried on by Paul Tartter after Papatestas's untimely death in 1989.

Gastrointestinal surgery remained a mainstay of the Department and was strengthened even further by the recruitment of Adrian Greenstein and Jack Rudick. The former would, over more than twenty-five years, make fundamental contributions to the understanding of the natural history of inflammatory bowel disease. Rudick would continue his innovative studies in gastric physiology in collaboration with Dreiling. Chang-Yul Oh, a graduate of the House Staff, would become the Department's leading proctologist. His anatomical studies of the ano-rectum and perineum would lead to greatly increased utilization of the posterior approach for surgery of the rectum.

Kark was invested as the first Franz W. Sichel Professor of Surgery in December 1967, eight months before the Medical School admitted its first students. After eleven years at the helm, Kark left on a sabbatical to London in 1972 and, while there resigned his position at Mount Sinai. Shoemaker became the Acting Chair of the Department, until he too left in 1973. Dreiling took over until a permanent Chair was appointed the following year.

On September 1, 1974, Arthur H. Aufses, Jr., assumed the Chair of the Department of Surgery, returning to Mount Sinai after three years as Chief of Surgery at the Long Island Jewish Medical Center. No stranger to Mount Sinai, Aufses had trained at the Columbia-Presbyterian Hospital and completed his residency at Mount Sinai in 1956. He then went into practice, at first geographic full-time and then voluntary. In 1964, he and Isadore Kreel formed a partnership that built a successful general surgical practice. While still a Resident, Kreel had described the "postperfusion syndrome" that followed open heart surgery.[56] In 1970, they were joined by Irwin Gelernt; one year later, Aufses left the practice. Now charged by the Hospital and School administration to increase the productivity of the Department in both arenas, Aufses set out to expand the full-time faculty while at the same time trying to eliminate the town-gown issues that unfortunately existed in Surgery as well as elsewhere on the campus.

The early years of Aufses's tenure were (in his view) an ideal time to be the chairman of a department at Mount Sinai. Thomas Chalmers, the President and Dean, constantly sought excellence and stimulated his chairmen to do likewise. In a time of fiscal prosperity for hospitals (it unfortunately didn't last long), the Directors of the Hospital, S. David Pomrinse, M.D., and his successor, Samuel Davis, were able to contribute support in the way of money and equipment. The Annenberg Building was about to open and supplied the necessary space for the expansion of the Department.

Aufses was also blessed with remarkable people in the Department. To their credit, the full-time and voluntary faculties became a cohesive unit, working for the betterment of the Department in all of its activities. David Dreiling, the Chief at Elmhurst under Kark, was appointed Vice Chairman of the Department for research and education and was instrumental in developing a notable student clerkship. At the same time, he continued his own bench research and stimulated countless Residents and students to become engaged in the laboratory. Un Sup Kim was appointed to replace Dreiling at Elmhurst and provided the Department with inspiring leadership at that institution. A highly skilled surgeon and scholar, Kim received numerous teaching awards from the students and house officers; his papers on biliary tract disease and gall stone pancreatitis were important additions to the literature. He has brought stability to Elmhurst Hospital for more than twenty-five years, a feat few could have accomplished.

During Aufses's first year, the integration of the residency program with that of the Bronx Veteran's Administration Hospital Department of Surgery was completed. Here, too, the appointment of James McElhenny as Chief in 1975 to replace E. Converse Peirce would provide singular leadership and teaching for more than a quarter of a century. The combined residency (Mount Sinai, Elmhurst, and the Bronx VA) was approved for a total of seventy-two house officers and was stabilized to graduate six Chief Residents each year. Each Chief would spend two months on each of three general surgery teaching services at Mount Sinai, four months at Elmhurst, and two months at the VA. The mix of the university hospital, the municipal hospital, and the VA hospital provided the Chief Resident with an excellent blend of major surgery, trauma, and independent responsibility. In 1976, on his return from military service, Gary Slater joined the full-time faculty with responsibility for day-to-day management of the residency program. Slater ran the program with aplomb and resourcefulness; for example, each Resident returning from research always had a place waiting for him or her, regardless of how many years the Resident spent in the laboratory.

For the first time in the Department's history, women were recruited and graduated from the program. The first, Karen Arthur, would have a successful career with the Kaiser-Permanente Group. Alisan Goldfarb would join the voluntary faculty and play a valuable role in the development of the breast service and the Breast Resource Center. Elizabeth Harrington and Victoria Teodorescu joined the full-time faculty after fellowships in vascular surgery. They would both contribute to the teaching program in vascular surgery in many meaningful ways.

The tradition of collaboration between the Department of Medicine's Gastroenterology Division and the gastrointestinal surgeons established in the early part of the twentieth century at Mount Sinai continued to flourish; the volume of GI surgery was extraordinary. For many years, more colon resections (for benign and malignant disease) were performed at The Mount Sinai Hospital than at any other comparable academic institution. Many significant innovations and publications ensued. Irwin Gelernt and Isadore Kreel developed refinements of the Kock pouch for continent ileostomies. Joel Bauer, Barry Salky, Michael Harris, and Stephen Gorfine would join them in practice, and the group subsequently collected one of the largest series of ileo-anal pouch procedures for ulcerative colitis in the country. Kreel and Gelernt were stimulating and brilliant teachers both in the operating room and at the bedside. Bauer would also make a vital contribution to the educational program as Director of the surgical clerkship for many years. Arthur Sicular, who had worked with Garlock, acquired extensive experience in esophageal surgery. Aufses and Slater were principal investigators in early trials of postoperative chemotherapy and radiotherapy in colorectal cancer as part of the Gastrointestinal Tumor Study Group. The hypothesis of Burrows and Tartter[57] that perioperative blood transfusion reduced immunity and led to increased recurrence in colorectal cancer was confirmed in several studies and extended to other malignancies and to the development of postoperative complications. Tomas Heimann published significant findings on the consequences of immunologic deficiencies in cancer and inflammatory bowel disease.

Heimann also published a well-received book on familial polyposis and related syndromes.

The twenty-two years of Aufses's tenure were marked by consistent growth in all of the existing divisions and by the institution of major new programs. On the vascular service, Harry Schanzer, who had been responsible for starting a transplant immunology laboratory, innovated a unique procedure for managing the "steal syndrome" associated with arterio-venous access procedures.[58] The breast service, under the leadership of Gerson Lesnick, Angelos Papatestas, and then Paul Tartter was at the forefront of the change in breast cancer management from radical to modified radical mastectomy and then to breast conservation. Their papers relating to risk factors of both cancer development and prognosis are often quoted. Eugene Friedman and Arthur Schwartz provided noteworthy long-term oversight of the head and neck and soft tissue service. Friedman introduced the laser into the armamentarium of the operating room. In 1991, a departmental professorship was named in his honor.

No history of the Department encompassing the second half of the twentieth century would be complete without mention of Arthur Wallen. A technician in the animal facility, Wallen, an inspiring teacher, taught surgical technique to students and Surgical Residents for more than twenty-five years, not retiring until he was in his late eighties. In 1983 he was awarded an honorary Doctor of Pedagogy degree by the Mount Sinai School of Medicine.

The Surgical Intensive Care Unit (SICU), established jointly by the Departments of Surgery and Anesthesiology, would become a crucial component of the patient care, teaching, and research efforts of both departments. Directed by Shoemaker and Christopher Bryan-Brown, the anesthesiologist, the unit opened in 1971. Bryan-Brown would take over after Shoemaker's departure. In 1979, Koing Bo Kwun joined the unit after completing his surgical residency and became Director the following year when Bryan-Brown left Mount Sinai. Three years later, Thomas Iberti, just out of his internal medicine residency and critical care fellowship, joined the unit and in 1983 became Director when Kwun left to return to his native Korea to become Chairman of the Department of Surgery at the Medical School in Taegu. Young and irrepressible, Iberti was a driving force in the expansion of critical care services at Mount Sinai. Also in 1983, Ernest Benjamin, trained in internal medicine, anesthesiology, and critical care, joined Iberti, and for ten years the two worked hand in hand until Iberti's tragic death in 1993. Iberti played a preeminent role in the design of the remarkably functional SICU in the new hospital building that opened in 1992. The SICU became a favorite site for elective rotation, not only for Mount Sinai students but also for students from many other schools. The critical care fellowship was highly regarded, and the surgery resident rotation through the ICU provided a unique learning experience. The unit's contributions to critical care medicine and surgery have been extraordinary.[59] Since 1993, Benjamin, as Director, has expanded the staff, increased research and funding, and provided exemplary leadership in a vital area of the Department.

In 1984, Stephen E. Dolgin joined the full-time faculty as Chief of the Division of Pediatric Surgery. A charismatic teacher, Dolgin not only expanded the service in an impressive way but also came to play a leading role in medical student teaching, first as Director of the first-year course in embryology and then as Director of the surgical clerkship.

After four years on the faculty, Steven T. Brower created a Division of Surgical Oncology in 1990. Dedicated to bench to bedside research, Brower forged links with Mount Sinai's Institute for Gene Therapy to undertake exciting studies in pancreatic cancer and other malignancies. Michail Shafir, a long-time member of the Department, who for his entire career has been involved in the Cancer and Leukemia Group B clinical trials group, has been a major contributor in the field of surgical oncology.

For more than forty years, Demetrius Pertsemlidis has exemplified the ideal faculty member and clinician scientist. Following his residency at Mount Sinai, Pertsemlidis spent several years in very productive research in biliary and lipid metabolism at the Rockefeller Institute. Returning to Mount Sinai, he established the Lipid Research Laboratory in the Department, which over a period of ten years produced important studies relating to the clinical use of lipid-lowering drugs, the effects of rapid weight reduction on the lithogenicity of bile, and the relation of lipid metabolism to the risk and prognosis of breast cancer. A revered and respected teacher, Pertsemlidis later became involved in the management of pheochromocytoma and accumulated one of the largest personally operated series of adrenalectomies extant.

In 1982, Saul Hoffman replaced Simon as Chief of the Division of Plastic Surgery. A gifted surgeon and teacher, Hoffman guided the division through a difficult period with great skill. Six years later, Lester Silver became the first full-time Chief of the Division. Well known internationally for his surgical missions to disadvantaged countries, Silver expanded the full-time faculty, increased both the clinical and the research output of the division, and added strength and stability to the training program.

As noted earlier, Lewis Burrows instituted a renal transplant program in 1967 that grew steadily, held back by the ever-present shortage of cadaver organs. After the advent of laparoscopic surgery, the program was bolstered by a most successful laparoscopic live-donor nephrectomy program. An immunology laboratory was established and became a favored site for Residents interested in the field to spend one or more years in research. In the early 1980s, after Thomas Starzl's early experiences with liver transplantation in Denver and in Pittsburgh and then the development of cyclosporine, it became evident to Aufses that a liver transplant program would prove to be a major asset to the Department and the Medical Center. Although it took a bit of time to persuade administration of that value, the approval was eventually given. It is to the everlasting credit of Barry Freedman, Director of the Hospital at the time, that, once he was on board, he saw to it that the necessary resources were allocated wherever needed to ensure the success of the program.

Charles M. Miller, a Mount Sinai School of Medicine graduate who had trained in general and vascular surgery at Mount Sinai and had recently joined the full-time faculty, was chosen to direct and develop the program. Arrangements were made with Starzl, and Miller spent one year as a member of the former's faculty at the University of Pittsburgh. While there, Miller devised a new technique of organ harvesting that became standard practice.[60] During that year, teams of anesthesiologists, operating room nurses and critical care personnel all spent time in Pittsburgh learning the nuances of peri-operative care. On Miller's return, he instituted extensive laboratory training for the team before the first successful transplant was performed in September 1988. Under Miller's stellar leadership, the program achieved immediate local, regional, and national success and within a few years was one of the largest programs in the country. By the end of November 2000, 1,941 transplants had been performed in 1,651 patients. A byproduct was an enormous increase in the volume of liver surgery performed under the outstanding guidance of Myron Schwartz, himself Mount Sinai trained.

Patricia Sheiner joined the group in 1992 and played an important role in all aspects of the program. The group has also been at the forefront of the development of live donor liver transplants.

A successful pancreas transplantation program was instituted at Mount Sinai under the leadership of Richard Knight. A transplant fellowship was established; the graduates of the program have gone on to extraordinarily successful careers throughout the world, and several have remained on the faculty. Sukru Emre was appointed Chief of the pediatric liver transplant program, and Thomas Fishbein initiated a highly successful small-bowel transplant program. In 1999, Jonathan Bromberg, formerly at the University of Michigan, joined the Department as Surgical Director of Kidney and Pancreas Transplantation and Surgical Director of Transplantation Research. Endowed by a former liver transplant recipient, the Recanati/Miller Transplantation Institute was inaugurated in 1998, providing critical support for the ever-expanding program.

The laparoscopic "revolution" of the late 1980s provided the Department with an unusual opportunity. Thoracoscopy had been frequently performed during the tuberculosis era by Arthur H. Aufses, Sr. In the late 1950s, Aufses, Jr., utilizing an ancient, nonmagnifying, eyepiece lighted scope, had performed guided liver biopsies with Fenton Schaffner, of the Department of Medicine. Pneumoperitoneum, in those days, was introduced utilizing a 50 cc. syringe, a three-way stop-cock, and room air. By 1988, when laparoscopic cholecystectomy took the surgical world by storm, Barry Salky, a gifted associate of Kreel and Gelernt, had already been performing diagnostic laparoscopy for years and had utilized the technique for some therapeutic procedures. Salky performed the first laparoscopic cholecystectomy at Mount Sinai in 1989. In 1992, Salky was recruited to the full-time faculty, placed in charge of a newly formed Division of Laparoscopic Surgery, one of the first such divisions in an academic medical center, and given the responsibility for training and credentialing advanced laparoscopic procedures. The venture proved highly successful, and the Department developed one of the earliest programs to perform large-volume advanced laparoscopy. Michael Edye, Salky's first recruit to the new Division, was in charge of the live-donor nephrectomy program and also added significant overall expertise to all aspects of the Division.

Another watershed change in surgical management that occurred during Aufses's tenure was the dramatic shift to ambulatory and day-of-admission surgery. The former received its impetus when, as noted earlier, Nabatoff was able to convince Blue Cross and other insurers to pay hospital charges for ambulatory surgery, saving the cost of in-hospital care. Day-of-surgery admissions became ever more frequent following the shift to diagnosis-related group reimbursement. By the end of 2001, ambulatory and day-of-admission surgery accounted for about 85 percent of all surgical cases in the Hospital.

Aufses retired from the Chair in 1996 and handed over leadership to Larry H. Hollier, a world-renowned vascular surgeon, who had previously served as Chairman of the Section of Vascular Surgery at the Mayo Clinic, Chairman of the Department of Surgery at the Ochsner Clinic in New Orleans, and Chief of Surgery and Executive Director of Clinical Affairs at Health Care International Ltd. in Glasgow, Scotland. Almost immediately, Hollier recruited Michael Marin from Montefiore Hospital to initiate an endovascular stent program. Marin, a Mount Sinai School of Medicine graduate, quickly built a comprehensive and highly successful clinical and research program and in 2001 was named the Chief of Vascular Surgery.

A separate Division of Colo-Rectal Surgery with an approved residency was established; in 2001, Randolph Steinhagen, a long-time member of the full-time faculty and a stimulating teacher of students and Residents, was named Chief. A large clinical and research program in wound care was instituted. The recruitment of Michel Gagner, his associate Alphonse Pomp, and W. Barry Inabnet greatly expanded the Department's capabilities in minimally invasive surgery and endocrine surgery.

In 1997, as a result of a major gift from Ruth J. Hauser, the Department was named the Ruth J. and Maxwell Hauser and Harriet and Arthur H. Aufses, Jr., M.D., Department of Surgery. Today, 150 years after patient No. 1 had his surgery at the Jews' Hospital, the Department looks forward to many years of continued success in its patient care, teaching, and research activities.

PART II

THE LATER DEPARTMENTS

14

Department of Anesthesiology

THE SUCCESSFUL DEMONSTRATION of ether anesthesia by William Morton in 1846 was followed one year later by the introduction of chloroform by Sir James Simpson. These events set the stage for all patients who might require anesthesia to obtain it when the Jews' Hospital opened its doors in 1855. Although it is not recorded in the casebook, we may assume that patient No. 1, admitted June 8 with a rectal fistula and successfully operated on by Israel Moses, was "put to sleep" with one or the other anesthetic agent. The first recorded use of anesthesia in the Hospital occurred on September 30, 1855. The patient was a young female with cervical gland tuberculosis. Alexander Mott removed "20 enlarged glands of various sizes, requiring more than two hours to complete the operation, the patient being under the influence of chloroform."[1]

It would be almost half a century before "professional anesthetists" would be appointed to the staff. In the intervening years, anesthesia was given by either the untrained House Staff or by other members of the surgical staff. Most anesthetics were administered in the patients' rooms or on the wards, and major problems frequently occurred. This led Samuel Brickner, the gynecologist, to publicly criticize anesthesia services and to stress the need for the training of young anesthetists: "Make the young men who act as controllers of life and death read some standard work on anesthesia [and he named two], and pass a rigorous examination before a committee of attending surgeons before the lives of patients are entrusted to their willing but helpless care."[2]

Following a patient death in 1898, the Medical Board decided that "anesthetization in the future shall be carried out by two members of the house staff in place of one unless otherwise ordered by the operator."[3] The Trustees remained concerned and pressed the Medical Board for further action. After prolonged consideration, the position of Anesthetist was created in March 1902, and within a month two physicians, M. L. Maduro and C. P. Denton, were appointed, each to spend the equivalent of six months a year on duty. Their role was to instruct incoming House Staff in "the principles and administration of the various general anesthetics" and to be on call "to administer anesthetics to such ward and private patients as the surgeon may desire."[4] By 1903, two anesthetizing rooms and two recovery rooms were built opposite the operating rooms, and the administration of anesthetics in private rooms and wards was eliminated.

Maduro and Denton preferred nitrous oxide and ether to chloroform as the technique of choice because of the safety of the former combination. The two men quickly gained credibility within the institution for their service, as well as for their research. Conducting an investigation into the causes of postoperative pneumonia, they found that body cooling during or after surgery and unclean rubber breathing bags in the anesthesia apparatus were important factors in the development of postoperative pneumonia. They recommended maintaining body heat with blankets and sterilizing the rubber bags.[5] Thomas Bennett was added to the staff in 1905. Already well known for designing the Bennett apparatus for the administration of nitrous oxide and ether, and an excellent clinical anesthesiologist and teacher, he would remain on the staff until his death in 1932.

In 1884, cocaine was introduced by Carl Koller in Vienna for clinical use as a local anesthetic.[6] It has been stated: "The reading of his [Koller's] first paper on the subject at an ophthalmological congress in Heidelberg marks the inception of the modern period in anesthetic practice."[7] Not surprisingly, cocaine became a very popular local anesthetic at Mount Sinai, since Koller joined the Mount Sinai staff in 1890, serving for many years as Chief of Ophthalmology. In 1903, Maduro noted that "local anesthesia in the general surgical service has been made use of in such operations as herniotomies, colostomies, and gastrostomies. A number of such operations begun by this method have been finished under general anesthesia."[8]

Spinal anesthesia did not fare as well at Mount Sinai. It was first performed successfully in a human by August Bier of Kiel, Germany, in 1899. Maduro commented four years later: "We are happy to say that subarachnoid cocainization has been performed but once within the past two years. The dangers attendant on the use of this method have influenced our surgeons to consider it as still in the experimental stage of development."[9]

William Branower was appointed as an anesthetist in 1908, serving simultaneously as a surgeon in the Out-patient Department. Named a

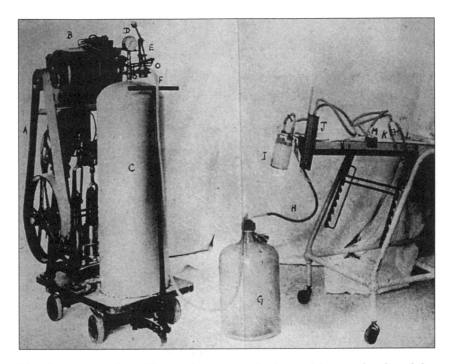

The first practical positive pressure anesthesia machine as developed by Charles Elsberg, M.D., 1910.

"Supervising" Anesthetist in 1923, Branower would serve with Bernard Eliasberg as the nominal heads of the Anesthesia Service for twenty years until his retirement. In 1936, Branower developed a respirator that was widely accepted and used for many years.[10]

Described as "the starting point of endotracheal anesthesia,"[11] a singular event occurred at Mount Sinai on February 20, 1910, that would change anesthesia and surgery forever. On that date, Charles Elsberg, a member of the Surgical Service since completing his training in 1895, administered the first intratracheal insufflation of anesthesia in humans. Relying upon the experimental work of Meltzer and Auer, of the Rockefeller Institute, and using a portable anesthesia apparatus designed with the help of Eliasberg, Elsberg, after extensive animal studies,[12] tested the technique by successfully administering oxygen to a comatose patient with advanced myasthenia gravis. Although that patient died, the technique proved feasible, and shortly thereafter Elsberg administered intratracheal anesthesia for the drainage of a lung abscess by thoracotomy performed by Howard Lilienthal. This success was followed by use of the technique on another patient, who had surgical drainage of an empyema. Elsberg presented the work before the New York Surgical Society on May 11, 1910. The last sentence of a paper subsequently published in the *Annals of Surgery* presages the development of thoracic surgery: "If the future will show that it is as safe for the human being as it is for the animal—and our experiences seem to point in that direction—then surgery will have a very simple method for the prevention of the dangers from acute pneumothorax, a danger which has been the chief hindrance to the development of intrathoracic thoracic surgery."[13] Lilienthal, in reporting the surgical aspects of the case, commented: "The most notable feature of the anaesthesia . . . was the total disappearance of the rattling respiration which existed during the administration of the ether by the usual method."[14] In a series of papers over the next two years, Elsberg would report on almost five hundred cases of intratracheal anesthesia administered for general and thoracic surgical procedures; Eliasberg administered the anesthetic for most of the cases. Elsberg, a man of many talents and trained in general surgery and neurosurgery, would go on to even greater fame in the field of neurosurgery.[15]

In 1910, Bernard Eliasberg was appointed Resident Anesthetist to the Private Pavilion. Working with Branower, the two gradually expanded the corps of trained anesthetists so that by 1940 the staff consisted of more than ten physician and nurse anesthetists. In 1943, upon the death of Branower, Eliasberg was appointed Anesthetist to the Hospital, a position he held until 1950; the Service was represented for the first time on the Medical Board. A founder of the New York State Society of Anesthesiologists and an original member of the American Board of Anesthesiology, Eliasberg was also responsible for the training of the first Resident in anesthesiology at Mount Sinai, Gerda J. Weil, who graduated from the program in 1943. Two years later, Irma Back served in the program and was joined in 1946 by a second resident. A gentleman of great knowledge, wisdom, and humor, Eliasberg was a superb teacher of a generation of anesthesiologists, and beloved by all. He played a pivotal role in the development of anesthesiology at Mount Sinai.

Milton Adelman was named Director of Anesthesia and Anesthesiologist to the Hospital in 1950 upon the retirement of Eliasberg. Appointed to the staff in 1942, Adelman was called to military service in World War II almost immediately thereafter and served with distinction as a regional consultant in Anesthesia to the European Theater of Operations. An astute observer, Adelman authored early papers on the potential fatal interaction of epinephrine given during cyclopropane-ether anesthesia, on allergic reactions during anesthesia, and on the use of promethazine. Adelman developed an automatic controlled respirator that, by relieving the anesthesiologist of the burden of manually inflating the lungs, proved of inestimable value in the management of endotracheal anesthesia.[16] The technique also greatly simplified anesthesia in the experimental laboratories by allowing for continuous endotracheal anesthesia without the presence of an anesthesiologist.[17]

Adelman formalized the residency training program, which had five positions in 1950 and which, as it grew, gradually replaced the nurse anesthetists who had been on staff. A second year was added to the residency in 1951. In that year, the Anesthesiology and Physics Departments developed an electro-shock machine for the treatment of ventricular fibrillation. In 1957, the Inhalation Therapy Department became part of the Anesthesiology Department. Many of the graduates of the anesthesiology residency would remain on staff as the Department expanded to keep up with the increasing volume of the Surgical Services. Joseph Jagust became one of Mount Sinai's premier anesthesiologists. In his honor after his early retirement due to illness, the Joseph A. Jagust Award in Anesthesiology was endowed and is presented annually to a graduating medical student who excelled in the anesthesiology clerkship.

Morris Bien, a most valued colleague of Adelman, was appointed to the staff in 1943 and would serve Mount Sinai for more than three decades. A proponent of and a pioneer in the development of techniques for regional anesthesia, Bien was also at the forefront of chronic pain management. He recognized the need for preoperative medication to allay patient apprehension[18] and the need for the anesthesiologist to visit the patient preoperatively, once again to allay fear.[19] Bien symbolized the partnership that existed in Mount Sinai operating rooms between the surgeons and the anesthesiologists. In 1946, he stated:

> The anesthesiologist has two responsibilities—to the patient and to the surgeon. While he is selecting the best anesthetic agent and the procedure best suited to the patient, he must always bear in mind that the

anesthetic risk can be equal to, or less, than the surgical risk; but it can never be greater. The anesthetist makes the surgeon as comfortable as possible, gives him a clear field in which to work, and enables him to devote his entire attention to the operation.[20]

Bien also had the distinction of being the first faculty member of the Mount Sinai School of Medicine to have a family member in the School. His son Ralph, now a psychiatrist, graduated with the Class of 1973.

Following the trend to the appointment of full-time Chiefs of Service, Leslie Rendell-Baker was named Chairman of the Department in 1962, a position he would hold for seventeen years. Trained in England, Rendell-Baker came to Mount Sinai from the faculty at Case-Western Reserve University. Instrumental in setting standards for anesthesia equipment and for the safety of the operating room, Rendell-Baker chaired the International Standards Committee of the American Society of Anesthesiologists for many years. He also played a major role in the development of special equipment for the pediatric population.

The years of Rendell-Baker's tenure, spanning as they did the opening of the Medical School, saw enormous growth in the role of the anesthesiologist within the institution. In a major collaborative effort with the Department of Surgery in the late 1960s, Rendell-Baker and Allan Kark, Chairman of the Department of Surgery, proposed the establishment of a Surgical Intensive Care Unit (SICU) to be operated jointly and staffed with full-time faculty who would be engaged in patient care, teaching, and research. A five-bed unit already existed, but, in this small unit, each surgeon was responsible for the care of his own patients. Considerable resistance to the new unit was encountered from both the surgeons, who felt they would lose control of their patients, and the administration, which did not want to absorb the cost of the unit and the salaries of the faculty. The plans were eventually embraced, and the unit opened in 1970 with William Shoemaker of Surgery as the Director and Christopher Bryan-Brown of Anesthesiology as Co-Director. Over the years, the SICU would become a jewel in the crown of Mount Sinai.[21]

The creation of the Division of Cardiothoracic Surgery within the Department of Surgery necessitated the formation of a Division of Cardiac Anesthesia. Barbara Lipton was recruited to head the Division and, with her colleagues, made major contributions to the management of these patients, especially as related to the neurological sequelae of open heart surgery.[22] George Silvay, an early member of the Division, would go on to become an international leader in the field, especially in the area of anesthesia education.

Lipton would also became the senior anesthesiologist to work in Mount Sinai's hyperbaric chamber when it was operational. In conjunction with her colleague Avram Weinreich and with Julius Jacobson, of the Department of Surgery, she conducted a series of elegant experiments on the physiology and role of hyperbaric oxygen.[23,24] Lipton's career was tragically cut short by her untimely death from breast cancer in 1974 at the age of forty-six years. A letter she wrote to the graduating residents just three weeks before her death epitomizes the compassion and humanistic view of the specialty of anesthesiology that has characterized this Department throughout its existence. In it, she states:

> The patient must always be uppermost in your thoughts, his welfare the most important thing for you to care about; you must be patient with him and gentle; his anesthetic and surgical procedure may be routine to you, but to him he is experiencing one of the most vital and traumatic days of his life. As an anesthesiologist practicing your profession with skill, you, as a matter of course, will deprive him of his consciousness, respiration, autonomic reflexes. You take him into the great unknown and you are as responsible as any one person can ever be for anyone else, including a parent for a child.[25]

The divisional structure established by Rendell-Baker during his tenure created an academic environment that stimulated research productivity. Robert Roberts's and Michael Shirley's work on the prevention of aspiration pneumonitis during Cesarean section was classic.[26] A major collaborative effort involving Medicine and Surgery in the treatment of myasthenia gravis by thymectomy produced important publications on the anesthetic management of this challenging group of patients. Digvijay Girnar and Weinreich, in a large series of cases, demonstrated for the first time that tracheostomy was not needed for the vast majority of these patients.[27]

Case volume increased consistently. In 1977, eighteen thousand patients, including three thousand obstetrical cases, were cared for by the Department. The Gaisman Surgical Pavilion, dedicated in 1974, provided nineteen new operating rooms and recovery facilities for general and specialty surgery in the newly opened Annenberg Building. For the first time in Mount Sinai's history, there would be a recovery room available twenty-four hours a day.

With the growth of the Medical School, the teaching program of the Department evolved to include a fourth-year elective for medical students. The residency expanded, and a third year of training in either cardiothoracic or neurosurgical anesthesia was introduced. In 1962, after the death of Bernard H. Eliasberg, a library was created and named for him in the Department, and the Eliasberg Memorial Lecture was established. The Lecture grew to be a full-day symposium in 1971.

David C. C. Stark, Assistant Director of the Department since 1970, succeeded Rendell-Baker in 1979. At the time of the transition, there were forty-four residents in the Department. Although Stark emphasized the importance of research in the Department, his forte was as a superb clinical anesthesiologist. Stark and Roberts's book, *Practical Points in Anesthesiology*,[28] went through three editions. With the aging of the population, anesthetic management of the older patient came to occupy the interest of the Department for many years. More recently, of cognitive function during the perioperative period has been studied, both clinically and in the laboratory.

The appointment of Joel Kaplan as Chairman in 1983 brought to Mount Sinai a nationally and internationally known clinician and researcher in cardiac and thoracic anesthesia. Recruited from Emory University School of Medicine, where he had been Chief of Cardiothoracic Anesthesia, Kaplan converted the members of the Department to a totally full-time faculty in a very short time. A prolific writer, Kaplan edited *Cardiac Anesthesia*,[29] the primary textbook in the field, now in its fourth edition, and authored fundamental papers on nitroglycerin infusion during coronary artery surgery; the value of the precordial electrocardiographic lead in patients with coronary artery disease; the optimal management of patients with ischemic heart disease for noncardiac surgery; and the early diagnosis of myocardial ischemia using the pulmonary artery catheter.

In 1986, Kaplan was named to the newly created Horace W. Goldsmith Chair in Anesthesiology. In that same year, he became the founding Editor-in-Chief of the *Journal of Cardiothoracic Anesthesia*, the only journal in the field. He published another seminal paper in 1988, this one on the role of ultrashort-acting beta blockers in the perioperative period.[30] One of Kaplan's earliest priorities was to obtain a mandatory anesthesia clerkship for all third-year medical students. This rapidly became a most popular clerkship and increased the number of Mount Sinai School of Medicine students who chose careers in the specialty.

The recruitment of Randall Griepp and M. Arisan Ergin in the Division of Cardiothoracic Surgery in 1985 significantly increased volume in the specialty, and the Cardiothoracic Anesthesiology Division became ever more active, both clinically and in the research arena. Steven Konstadt and David Reich, the Co-Directors of Cardiac Anesthesia, and their colleagues championed the intraoperative use of transesophageal echocardiography (TEE) and were the first to validate left ventricular function with this modality.[31] They helped define the guidelines for the use of TEE and established its usefulness in identifying atherosclerosis of the ascending aorta during cardiac surgery, as well as in detecting a patent foramen ovale. TEE became a sensitive indicator for the detection of cardiac preload changes induced by transfusion and phlebotomy in the pediatric population. An algorithm was designed to assess intraoperative mean arterial pressure lability, and predictors of failure of pulse oximetry data were identified.

The Department created a Division of Thoracic Anesthesia, and, under the leadership of Edmond Cohen, its staff produced a number of important papers relating to one-lung ventilation. Cohen's book *The Practice of Thoracic Anesthesia*[32] has become one of the leading texts in the field.

The 1980s saw a dramatic increase in ambulatory and day-of-admission surgery and the need to develop, test and provide anesthetics for short-term procedures that allowed the patient to return home the same day in a stable condition. At the same time, computers and automation began to play an increasing role in the Department's activities. Databases of anesthetics and outcomes were constructed, and work was begun on creating proficient computer systems in anesthesiology.

The institution of the liver transplant program in 1988 provided yet another opportunity for the newly created Division of Transplant Anesthesia to make significant contributions to the literature in this area. Collaborating with the transplant surgeons, George Gabrielson and his colleagues showed that flushing the donor liver with autologous blood improved intraoperative hemodynamic stability and early graft function. Gabrielson was also the senior author of a primary paper on the use of continuous infusion of phentolamine and esmolol in the management of patients with pheochromocytoma.[33] This technique has been adopted by almost all centers that manage these patients.

As noted earlier, Morris Bien was the first of the anesthesiologists at Mount Sinai to be involved in pain management; at that time, pain management consisted primarily of regional blocks for both acute and chronic conditions. Many years later, the value of sympathetic blockade as a diagnostic and therapeutic modality was recognized, and the use of nerve blocks in the relief of cancer pain was started. A formal pain service was organized in the mid-1980s with both inpatient and outpatient components. Postoperative pain therapy with intravenous patient-controlled analgesia (PCA) was begun in 1988. Shortly thereafter, continuous epidural fentanyl infusion was added as a therapeutic option.[34] Both techniques gained rapid acceptance by both patients and surgeons.

Under the leadership of Joel Kreitzer since 1991, the Pain Management Service has experienced exponential growth. In 1999, almost five thousand postoperative patients were treated with either intravenous or epidural PCA. A recently instituted program uses continuous axillary and interscalene catheters for postoperative pain in upper extremity surgery. The volume of the Chronic Pain Service has also grown in dramatic fashion. Between 1996 and 1999, patient census doubled, and almost four thousand procedures were performed on the entire population in 1999. The Service has published multiple articles dealing with postoperative and chronic pain management by the use of new drugs, new delivery systems, and improved techniques of management. In 1994, an approved Pain Fellowship was created and now trains four Fellows per year.

In 1994, with an effort led by Kaplan, Mount Sinai acquired the first computerized simulated patient in its geographic area and has since acquired two more. The mannequin simulators provide a realistic operating room environment for students, Residents, and Attendings to practice intubation and the administration of anesthetic agents and injected drugs and to manage intraoperative complications. The program represents the Mount Sinai Medical Center's commitment to advancing education and patient safety. In 1992, the new Guggenheim Pavilion, with a twenty-two-room surgical suite, a large recovery area (now called the Post-Anesthesia Care Unit), and sixty-six specialized Intensive Care Unit beds, was completed.

The Clinical Service flourished under the leadership of Raymond Miller and Ian Sampson. Superb teachers and mentors of Residents, students, and junior faculty, they assumed responsibility for the ever-increasing patient volume and the ever-increasing complexity of the cases operated upon. In 1999, thirty-five thousand anesthetics were administered by a faculty of seventy-five at Mount Sinai. There were, in addition, thirty- six Attending Anesthesiologists at Elmhurst Hospital Center, the Bronx VA, Mount Sinai of Queens, and Queens Hospital Center. In the 1999–2000 academic year, there were forty-two Residents and twelve Fellows in training.

Paul Goldiner was recruited to the faculty in 1992. The former Chairman of the Department of Anesthesiology at the Memorial Sloan-Kettering Cancer Center and at the Albert Einstein College of Medicine, Goldiner had previously served as President of the New York State Society of Anesthesiology and was widely known and respected for his abilities as a leader and teacher. When Kaplan left Mount Sinai in 1997, Goldiner became the Interim Chair and succeeded to the Chairmanship in 1999. When Goldiner was installed as the second Horace W. Goldsmith Professor of Anesthesiology at the School of Medicine's convocation in 2000, Dean Arthur Rubenstein stated:

> You have made seminal contributions to anesthesia and critical care medicine emphasizing the improvement of perioperative care of cancer patients. Initiatives which you have spearheaded in your Department at Mount Sinai, such as the expansion of clinical trials; have produced enormous benefits. Under your direction the residency training program in anesthesia has become one of the leading programs in the country. For your leadership in all three components of the tripartite mission of academic medicine—research, education, and patient care—I am delighted to invest you as the second Horace W. Goldsmith Professor of Anesthesiology.

With these words, Goldiner assumed the leadership of an outstanding Department of Anesthesiology and will lead it to new heights in the coming decade.

(Adapted from an article by Arthur H. Aufses, Jr., M.D., published in *The Mount Sinai Journal of Medicine*, 69 (2002): 3–11.)

15

Department of Cardiothoracic Surgery

FROM 1914 UNTIL 1990, the Thoracic Surgical Service and, later, the Division of Cardiothoracic Surgery were an integral part of the Department of Surgery. In 1990, an independent Department of Cardiothoracic Surgery was established in the Medical School and in the Hospital. Rather than have part of this story told in the chapter on surgery and part of it here, it is all recounted in this chapter.

The seeds of thoracic surgery at Mount Sinai were planted by Arpad C. G. Gerster, a Hungarian emigre, shortly after his appointment to the staff in 1880.[1] Seven years later, those seeds began to germinate when Howard Lilienthal, a native-born American and a Harvard graduate, was appointed to the House Staff.[2] Different as these two were in family origins, education, medical training, and extracurricular talents, they combined to become a potent force in the creation of thoracic surgery at Mount Sinai. The primitive state of thoracic surgery in those early days is best illustrated by the case history of L. S., a Mount Sinai Trustee whom Gerster was called to see in consultation in 1882. The patient presented with chills and fever, a draining purulent sinus alongside the sternum, an irregular pulse, and physical findings of cardiac displacement by a mediastinal mass. Successful curative surgery was carried out, consisting of debridement and resection of osteomyelitis of the sternum, along with drainage of a mediastinal abscess, and the patient did well. The event took place long before the discovery of x-ray (1895), the use of the electrocardiogram (1903), or the availability of intratracheal anesthesia (1910) or citrated blood transfusion (1915), and long before Intensive Care Units became the vogue. In gratitude, the patient exercised his influence in facilitating Gerster's election to the prestigious New York Surgical Society.

This story is related by Gerster in his autobiography, *Recollections of a New York Surgeon*.[3] The case was never published in the medical literature. Although Gerster's bibliography lists more than eighty publications, only one, relating to the esophagus, deals with thoracic surgery.

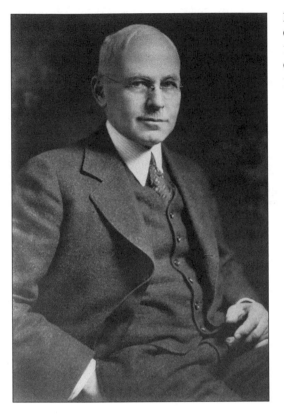

Howard Lilienthal, M.D.,
Chief of Surgery,
1898–1914, Chief of the
Cardiothoracic Service,
1914-1922.

Born in Albany, New York, in 1861, Howard Lilienthal was the oldest child of immigrant parents from Germany. He attended schools in upstate New York, matriculated at Harvard College, graduating cum laude in 1883. After earning his medical degree from Harvard in 1887, he took the Mount Sinai internship examination, ranked first, and became the first house officer to choose surgery in the ten years that the House Staff had been separated into Medical and Surgical divisions. He archly recounts the story: "When I expressed a preference for the surgical service I found that I had committed what seemed to be the equivalent of a social error for, apparently, no one had ever thus slighted the medical departments. It was not, however, disrespect for Medicine but sincere love for Surgery and I have never regretted my choice."[4]

After completing his training, Lilienthal went into practice and became Gerster's assistant. Appointed to the staff in 1890, he was elevated to the rank of full Attending in 1899. The Surgical Department was then divided into two Services led by Gerster and Lilienthal, respectively. It was at this time that Lilienthal began to develop the expertise in cases of pleural and pulmonary suppuration that would ultimately lead to his world-acclaimed accomplishments in pulmonary resection for these conditions. However, rapid growth of the field was stymied until 1910, when Lilienthal became the surgeon of record[5] in the first operation (drainage of an empyema) performed under intratracheal anesthesia devised and administered by Charles Elsberg.[6] From that moment on, thoracic surgery became safer and, therefore, was performed more frequently; it was only natural that, with the reorganization of the Surgical Service in 1914, a Thoracic Service was created with Lilienthal as Chief. In that same year, he performed the first successful pulmonary lobectomy in the United States for suppurative disease of the lung.

Each of the four Surgical Services became the nucleus of multidisciplinary, collaborative specialty groups. The thoracic disease group included pulmonologists, otolaryngologists, radiologists, and pathologists. This group in somewhat altered form, content, and scope, continues to function today as a highly successful entity and represents one more example of the multidisciplinary collaborative efforts that have been the hallmark of Mount Sinai throughout its existence.

Shortly after this reorganization took place, World War I began, and the Hospital was involved with the war effort. U.S. Base Hospital No. 3 was constituted with Major, later Lieutenant Colonel, Howard Lilienthal as its Chief Medical Officer. Lilienthal was eager to be involved in the surgery of the severely wounded and for a time was on detached service with advanced surgical teams, assigned to Evacuation Hospital No. 8 and U.S. Army Hospital No. 101. He received the Distinguished Service Medal. Tragically, his son, an infantry officer, was killed in action just a few weeks before the Armistice.

After his return from overseas, Lilienthal resumed his hospital activities and published his large series on lobectomy for suppurative lung disease.[7] In 1921, at the meeting of the American Surgical Association, Lilienthal presented an epochal report on carcinoma of the esophagus.[8] Mark Ravitch, in his classic publication *A Century of Surgery*, has commented that this was unique, a "striking report of tortuous extrapleural resection of the esophagus for carcinoma with the construction of a skin-flap tube connecting the two ends of the esophagus still lying in the mediastinum"[9] without a complementary gastrostomy.

Outside the Hospital, Lilienthal was active in the thoracic surgical community. He, along with Willy Meyer of the Lenox Hill Hospital and others, founded the New York Society for Thoracic Surgery in 1917, the oldest thoracic surgical society in the world. With this organization as its base, the national American Association for Thoracic Surgery (AATS) was launched later that year. Through the years, Mount Sinai thoracic surgeons continued to be active in the New York Society of Thoracic Surgery. Those who have served as President have included Paul Kirschner, Robert Litwak, Randall B. Griepp, M. Arisan Ergin, and Steven Lansman. Lilienthal served as the fifth President of the AATS, in 1922. His presidential address was entitled "Malignant Tumor of the Lung: Necessity for Early Operation."[10] In it, for the first time, he made a clear distinction between the two main topographical types of lung cancer, the central large bronchus type and the peripheral parenchymal type, and stressed the need for early diagnosis and surgery. This paved the way for the staging system so widely used today. In a journal article in 1925, Lilienthal clearly delineated the rationale for thoracic surgery as a specialty,[11] antedating the Specialty Boards by more than twenty years.

Lilienthal published his classic two-volume text *Thoracic Surgery*[12] in 1926, the first such publication of its kind in the United States. In addition to providing comprehensive discussions of pulmonary and esophageal pathology and surgery, Lilienthal devoted four chapters to the management of cardiac and great vessel problems. He described his experiences with pericardiostomy and pericardiectomy and approaches to aortic aneurysms and pulmonary embolism. The book also revealed the author's insight in anticipating the role of surgery in the management of cardiac valvular pathology. Moreover, Lilienthal authored more than sixty additional publications after his retirement until his death in 1946.

Between 1923 and 1930, the Chiefs of the Thoracic Service were Alexis V. Moschcowitz and Richard Lewisohn. Noted for his contributions to the surgery of hernia and the management of rectal prolapse,[13] Moschcowitz also did important work in thoracic surgery. In 1918, while in the U.S. Army Medical Corps, Major Moschcowitz served on the Empyema Commission at Camp Lee, Virginia. The Commission was seeking the explanation for the very high postoperative mortality rate for empyema in the Army. A worldwide epidemic of influenza (Spanish Flu) was raging. Contagion was rife in the crowded barracks

Harold Neuhof, M.D.,
Chief of the Cardiothoracic
Service, 1930-1946.

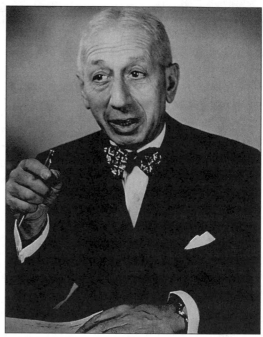

of the Army training camps. Empyema was a common complication of postinfluenza pneumonia. Standard treatment at the time was open drainage, which was attended by a horrendous mortality rate, often exceeding 50 percent. The Commission determined that the cause of death in most instances was not the empyema per se but "anoxemia" secondary to the collapsed lung, which was also the seat of pneumonia. By changing from "open" to "closed" drainage using only a chest tube and maintaining lung expansion, doctors decreased the mortality rate to low single-digit numbers.[14] In 1918, Moschcowitz also published a pivotal paper on the treatment of diseases of the costal cartilages.[15]

The bulk of the thoracic surgery during these years, however, was performed by Harold Neuhof. A New Yorker, Neuhof began his internship at Mount Sinai in 1905. Appointed to the staff immediately upon completion of his training, Neuhof always exhibited a wide range of medical and surgical interests, especially confronting the challenges of life-threatening diseases. An early interest in transplantation led to his performing a xenotransplant of a lamb's kidney to a young woman suffering from acute renal failure. The patient survived nine days. This experience and a large number of clinical and laboratory studies led to the publication of *The Transplantation of Tissues*[16] in 1923.

Appointed Chief in 1930, Neuhof had boundless energy, was an ever-productive source of new ideas, and, much like Lilienthal, was small and wiry in physique. Although the origin of Neuhof's nickname, "Skippy," remains obscure, it accurately denoted his personality. Although he published major works on venous thrombosis and pulmonary embolism, mediastinitis, and lung cancer, Neuhof's most significant work, however, was in the management of acute putrid lung abscess in the pre-antibiotic era. His first paper on the subject, in collaboration with Harry Wessler in 1932,[17] was followed by more than twenty-five papers on the subject over the next fifteen years. A paper by Neuhof and Arthur S. W. Touroff, in 1936,[18] describing the one-stage procedure for drainage of putrid lung abscess and the results in thirty-seven cases, has been acknowledged as one of the "classics in thoracic surgery."[19]

In collaboration with Neuhof and members of other departments, all of the thoracic surgeons contributed new knowledge to the rapidly expanding field. Using the topographic classification of lung cancer, Arthur H. Aufses, Sr., established lobectomy as a curative therapy for many lung cancers.[20] Irving Sarot demonstrated the value of pleuropneumonectomy in tuberculosis, and Gabriel P. Seley continued Neuhof's work in lung cancer and lung abscess.

In 1940, two years after the first successful ligation of a patent ductus arteriosus by Robert Gross in Boston, Touroff reported the first survivals in two of four patients who underwent ductal obliteration in the presence of active *Streptococcus viridans* infection.[21] After serving in the military for an extended period of time during World War II, Touroff returned a much decorated hero and became Chief of the Service upon Neuhof's retirement in 1946. Three years later, Touroff performed the first shunt procedure for cyanotic heart disease at Mount Sinai.[22]

The years after World War II saw intracardiac surgery become a reality. At Mount Sinai, Robert Nabatoff initiated a highly successful series of mitral commissurotomies. Irving Sarot and, later, Mark Ravitch were also involved in mitral valve surgery, as well as ligation of patent ductus and correction of coarctation of the aorta.

The appointment of Mark M. Ravitch in 1952 as the first full-time Chief of Surgery and the changes that he introduced altered the character of the department.[23] The Divisional Services, including the Thoracic

Surgical Service, disappeared; all of the components were amalgamated into one Service headed by Ravitch, with the Attending Surgeons being assigned to cases on an ad hoc basis. Ravitch remained at Mount Sinai for only thirty-eight months and in 1957 was replaced by Ivan D. Baronofsky.[24]

Baronofsky promptly initiated an aggressive canine experimental laboratory effort, utilizing the University of Minnesota system, the goal being to begin clinical open heart surgery as soon as both a reliable pump-oxygenating system and a support staff could be established. He assigned three Surgical Residents to the project, which culminated with the inception of the clinical program in January 1958, when a successful repair of an atrial septal defect in a ten-year-old boy was performed.

Approximately one hundred open heart procedures were performed over the next two years. Isadore Kreel, one of the original Residents on the team, noted that each case was a "logistical nightmare," since the protocol required twenty units of fresh heparinized blood to be drawn on the morning of surgery. The lack of a cardiac surgical recovery room or Intensive Care Unit made postoperative management difficult, to say the least. Kreel and his colleagues were the first to observe and to report on the "postperfusion syndrome."[25] The open heart surgical program was temporarily discontinued after Baronofsky's resignation in 1960.

The appointment of Allan E. Kark as Director of Surgery in 1961 not only provided a period of growth and stability in the Department of Surgery but also led to the rejuvenation of cardiac and thoracic surgery with the establishment of a formal Division of Cardiothoracic Surgery. Recruited by Kark from the University of Miami, Robert Litwak and his talented colleague Howard L. Gadboys began work in 1962 as Chief of the Division and Director of Research, respectively. To help ensure the success of the new venture, major resources were committed by Hospital administration to provide for a dedicated cardiac surgery operating room and personnel and for a Cardiothoracic Surgery Intensive Care Unit. Within two months of the new team's arrival, open heart surgery resumed, the first patient being a six-year old child who underwent a pulmonary valvotomy.

Litwak organized the Division into thoracic and cardiac sections and received approval for a cardiothoracic surgery resident training program. The noncardiac thoracic surgeons (all of whom were members of the voluntary staff) accepted responsibility for the thoracic surgery portion of the training, which was also strengthened by rotations to the Bronx Veterans Administration Medical Center under the leadership of A. James McElhinney and Hideki Sakurai. In 1979, an officially designated Section of General Thoracic Surgery was created under the direction of Paul A. Kirschner. A member of the thoracic surgical group for more than half a century, Kirschner has been the epitome of the ideal surgical scientist. His surgery was meticulous; his teaching was always based on the latest available knowledge; and each of his many publications demonstrated the ultimate in scholarship.

Shortly after the early descriptions of mediastinoscopy, Kirschner adopted the procedure in cases of mediastinal tumors and lung cancer. Early reports by Kirschner[26] led to widespread adoption of mediastinoscopy in the routine management of lung cancer, and it quickly became one of the foundations upon which the current staging of lung cancer is based. This experience also led to the "rediscovery" of the long-forgotten technique of transcervical thymectomy that had been performed in infants and children in the early part of the twentieth century. The technique was applied in myasthenia gravis, a disease in which Mount Sinai has always been a leader. Under the direction of Kermit Osserman, Mount Sinai's Myasthenia Clinic had become one of the largest in the world. Although controversial, thymectomy had previously been carried out by either a thoracic or sternal splitting approach. An early report[27] led to the adoption of the transcervical procedure throughout the world; more than one thousand operations have been performed at Mount Sinai, the majority by Angelos Papatestas.

Litwak moved quickly to expand the clinical open heart program and to establish a research initiative. Support staff included nurse clinicians and the first physician assistants to be hired at Mount Sinai. A major bioengineering collaboration was initiated with The Artificial Organs Research Laboratory of Columbia University and with the Institute of Medical Sciences at The Presbyterian Medical Center in San Francisco. Led by Richard de Asla, a bioengineer, and Roy A. Jurado, an early graduate of the training program, a bedside sensing and data acquisition unit was constructed and utilized to acquire online, real-time computerized surveillance studies of cardiac, hemodynamic, and pulmonary variables. In 1977, Jurado and his colleagues documented for the first time that computerized surveillance could significantly reduce sudden, unexpected life-threatening events in postoperative cardiac surgical patients.[28] The data were so impressive that, when a new

Cardiac Surgery Intensive Care Unit was constructed within a few years of the publication, all eight beds were computerized.

During the 1960s, the clinical program expanded slowly but steadily, held back to a certain extent by the reluctance of some of the cardiology group to refer patients, especially for coronary artery bypass grafting (CABG) until documented proof of its efficacy was published. Eventually the program flourished under the direction of Salvador B. Lukban. Manuel R. Estioko's employment of a "no blood" approach in the management of Jehovah's Witnesses led to Mount Sinai's being designated a regional referral cardiac surgical center for members of this religious group.

In the early years of the program, intra-aortic balloon pumping was the procedure of choice for management of the failing heart. A second circulatory support system, the left heart assist device, developed at Mount Sinai and one of the earliest systems of its kind, was used with considerable success both here and throughout the world.[29]

The Cardiothoracic Surgical Research Laboratory provided several examples of outstanding "bench-to-bedside" research. Studying the postoperative hypovolemia of patients undergoing cardiopulmonary bypass, researchers undertook animal investigations that clearly incriminated homologous blood as the etiologic factor in producing these reactions. Subsequent confirmatory studies in humans were the basis for important changes in the conduct of bypass procedures.

An institutional commitment in the early 1980s to expand Mount Sinai's solid organ transplant program to include heart and liver transplantation provided Litwak and the Department of Surgery the opportunity to recruit and/or develop the required expertise. Randall B. Griepp, then Chief of Cardiothoracic Surgery at Downstate Medical Center, well known for his early work in heart transplantation with Norman Shumway at Stanford, as well as for his expertise in pediatric cardiac surgery and surgery of the aorta, was recruited to serve as Chief in August 1985. Having been Chief of the Division for twenty-three years, Litwak viewed the opportunity to recruit Griepp as a propitious time for a change of leadership. Litwak, a distinguished Chief of Cardiothoracic Surgery and a true gentleman and scholar, was responsible for the training of a generation of cardiac surgeons who have become leaders in their own right. His preeminence as a cardiac surgeon is matched by his accomplishments as an acclaimed jazz musician. Litwak has continued on in the Department, accepting responsibility for undergraduate and resident teaching.

Griepp brought with him M. Arisan Ergin and Steven Lansman, both former trainees and colleagues. Ergin, a brilliant surgeon, investigator, and teacher, became a mainstay of the clinical open heart surgery program, which grew rapidly under his leadership. Lansman, also a gifted surgeon, assumed responsibility for the heart transplant program. The first heart transplant was performed in August 1986; the patient was alive and well fifteen years later.

Under Griepp's able leadership, pediatric cardiac and aortic surgery volume grew rapidly. A pioneer in the use of hypothermic circulatory arrest, Griepp undertook laboratory initiatives that have translated into improved patient care and surgical outcomes. Studies on the factors underlying the paraplegia associated with surgery of the descending thoracic aorta have prompted significant modifications in the operative approach to these cases.

A lung and heart-lung transplant program was commenced in 1990 and has grown slowly, in large part held back by the shortage of organs. In that same year, with enthusiastic support from the Department of Surgery, the Executive Faculty, and the Board of Trustees, cardiothoracic surgery became an independent Department in both the School and the Hospital.

The appointment of Paul F. Waters as Chief of the Division of General Thoracic Surgery and Director of the lung transplant program in 1999 brought to Mount Sinai a surgeon with one of the world's largest experiences in lung transplantation. In July 2001, Griepp stepped down from the Chair to devote more time to research. Six months later, David H. Adams, recruited from the Brigham and Women's Hospital in Boston, began his tenure as the new Chairman of the Department.

When Howard Lilienthal performed his first open chest procedure employing intratracheal anesthesia in 1910, he could not have foreseen the incredible advances and seminal contributions in both general thoracic and cardiac surgery that have been made by the Mount Sinai staff in the intervening years.

(Adapted from essays by Robert Litwak, M.D., and Paul Kirschner, M.D.)

16

Department of Dentistry

ALTHOUGH THE SCOPE of modern dental training and practice embraces all the diseases and abnormalities of the mouth and jaws, it is the core identification with the decay, infection, and loss of teeth that established dentistry's importance in public health. This was officially recognized at the Mount Sinai Hospital in 1910 with the appointment of Milton Simon as Dentist and Samuel M. Getzoff as Adjunct Dentist, thus establishing the Dental Department.

In the beginning, the attending dental staff, which included Maurice Green and Louis Bieber, conducted an inpatient clinic and made ward rounds twice weekly to care for the dental needs of hospitalized patients. During these early years, the dental staff exemplified one of the goals of the institution, namely that all staff members be active participants in medical research. Mount Sinai dentists were among the first in the United States to use procaine, synthesized in Germany by Alfred Einhorn in 1905, as a local anesthetic. Guido Fischer was a leader in testing the principles and methods in the administration of procaine. When Fischer later came to the United States, Leo Stern, who joined the Mount Sinai staff as an Assistant Dentist in 1915, traveled the country with him to demonstrate the use of procaine to dentists.[1] Stern had served as Director of the Commission on Standardization of Local Anesthesia of the Dental Society of the State of New York from 1913 until 1915. The early use of procaine by dentists at The Mount Sinai Hospital signaled the beginning of a medical approach to pain control and the widespread use of local anesthetics within the specialty. Mount Sinai would continue to be at the forefront of advances in hospital dentistry throughout the history of the department.

The Dental Service played a significant role in Mount Sinai's overseas effort during World War I. The table of organization of Base Hospital No. 3 called for two dentists; Leo Stern and Jacob Asch would serve in France with the unit until May 1919. The fifty-bed facial fracture ward ("jaw service") became one of the largest and most active dental centers in the Allied Expeditionary Force, receiving a special commendation for the development of oral surgery techniques for trauma management. In May 1919, Harry Goldberg was appointed Dentist to the Hospital. Stern joined him as Assistant Dentist a few weeks later, and together they organized a comprehensive dental service staffed by five voluntary clinicians to care for the dental needs of the hospitalized patients. Space, operating equipment, and nursing assistance were provided in the basement of the Administration Building on the north side of 100th Street. At the time, the theory of focal infection and its role in the pathogenesis of many systemic diseases had wide credence, and large numbers of patients were referred from the medical and surgical services for dental roentgenographic examination and for the removal of all teeth that might be presumed to harbor sepsis.

In 1924, enlarged dental quarters were constructed and equipped on the third floor of the Administration Building. In addition, an Out-Patient Clinic housing six dental units was located on the second floor of the Out-Patient Building. As the role of the Dental Department expanded, areas of specialization emerged, attracting prominent dentists and teachers: Joseph Schroff in oral surgery, Harry Shapiro in anatomy and numerous others. Clinical training programs in oral surgery, orthodontics, periodontics, and prosthetic dentistry brought considerable attention with an augmentation of the staff to more than forty dentists by 1935. Goldberg established a dental House Staff in 1932, appointing Marvin Freid and Herbert Goodwin as the first Interns.

During the decade prior to World War II, departmental research was multifaceted. Auto-polymerizing methyl methacrylate was clinically tested as a replacement for silicates for cosmetic fillings and as a vehicle to permit rapid prosthetic repairs, as were alginate impression materials. Interdepartmental collaboration increased, and studies of lesions of the mouth, jaws, and associated structures were published. Major contributions were made to identifying the role of dental calculus aspirated during sleep or anesthesia in the pathogenesis of lung abscess.[2,3] The manifestations of oral side effects of the anticonvulsant phenytoin, or dilantin sodium, were described in an original study by Stern and Leon Eisenbud (who first joined the staff as an Intern in 1940)[4] and by Stern, Eisenbud, and Jack Klatell.[5] Metastatic carcinoma to the maxilla, a rarely reported lesion, was described.[6]

The staff of the Dental
Clinic at the Third General
Hospital in North Africa,
1943 or 1944.

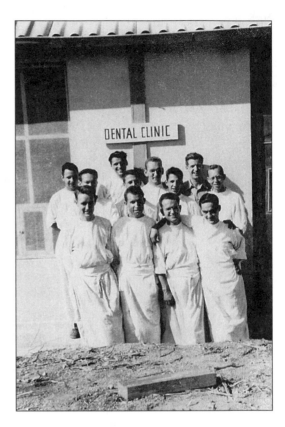

With the advent of World War II and the establishment of Mount Sinai's Third General Hospital, six members of the Department served during the African and Italian campaigns.

Following Harry Goldberg's retirement in 1943, Leo Stern was appointed Director, and the Dental Department was reorganized as the Dental and Oral Surgery Service. In 1946, Mount Sinai became a pioneer by granting hospital admitting privileges to its dentists. Stern went before the Medical Board to request an inpatient facility for the Dental Department in order "to ensure appropriate hospital care for patients who require dental and oral surgery, and to provide for clinico-pathologic studies of significant and problem cases."[7] The Board agreed, and a six-bed unit was created, two on the pediatric ward and four on the surgical wards. The Service would have responsibility for the scope of oral surgery, including "swellings of dental origin, fractures of the jaw, deformities of the jaw, dental anomalies, neuralgias of dental origin, and temporo-mandibular abnormalities."[8]

At this time, a comprehensive reconstruction of the oral surgery treatment and operating rooms was undertaken and a recovery room for ambulatory general anesthesia cases created. As a Hospital Department, the Service was represented on the Medical Board for the first time.

In the pre-antibiotic era, dento-alveolar abscess was the leading cause of admission to the Dental Service. Presentation could be relatively benign, but, too frequently, the patient would arrive with a fulminating cellulitis of the face and neck. In either event, early diagnosis was critical to allow for dental extraction and intraoral drainage before rapid spread of infection necessitated more radical surgery. The advent of penicillin and then the tetracyclines totally revamped the therapy of these life-threatening infections. Stern published one of the earliest papers on the role of penicillin in dentistry,[9] the first of several by the staff. Antibiotics and subsequent technical advances in endodontic therapy permitted the saving of teeth, and the edentulous patient requiring full denture replacement slowly began to vanish from the American scene.

In 1946, Lester R. Cahn was appointed Associate Dentist for Oral Pathology, a move prompted by the rapid emergence of this specialty as a diagnostic and teaching entity. Stanley L. Lane, M.D., D.D.S., fully trained in general and head and neck surgery, was appointed Associate in Oral Surgery and shared the teaching role for the inpatient service with Eisenbud, Freid, Klatell, and Leo Stern, Jr. Jacob Salzmann, appointed Associate Dentist to head an enlarged outpatient program in orthodontics, conducted a number of studies in facial growth and development.[10] In conjunction with the New York State Department of Health, Salzmann also published studies of fluorine in the water supply.[11] Others who began service in the Out-Patient Department at this time were Kenneth Adisman in prosthodontics and David Mossberg in orthodontics; both later became Chiefs of their respective Divisions.

Closer liaison with the Columbia University School of Dental and Oral Surgery led to undergraduate and graduate teaching courses being conducted at Mount Sinai. As Chief of Service, Leo Stern was appointed Clinical Professor of Dentistry at Columbia. Eight members of the dental staff were invited to join the teaching staff of the Guggenheim Dental Foundation in 1947, where they presented courses in oral medicine, oral surgery, and clinical oral pathology until the closing of the foundation in 1967.

The Board of Oral Surgery of the State of New York was established in 1947 with Stern as its first Executive Secretary. With the goals of setting standards for practice as well as training, the Board certified 245 diplomates prior to its discontinuation in 1959. Many of these diplomates organized the Society of Diplomates of the Board in order to maintain the academic environment that had been created. Dedicated to education, Stern also played a role in the development of the Metropolitan Conference of Hospital Dental Chiefs in the late 1930s, an organization committed to the advancement of dental education and to strengthening the role of dental departments within hospitals.

The staff was especially productive during Stern's sixteen-year tenure, from 1943 to 1959. Eisenbud and Ralph Brodsky devised clinical cameras for intraoral and facial photography, enabling them to record the clinical progress of cases for teaching and analysis. Interest in the oral manifestations of systemic disease grew, and collaborative studies with Hematology, Dermatology, and other medical departments were undertaken. Leo Stern, Jr., published an extensive series of pemphigus cases presenting with either the primary lesion or the majority of the lesions in the mouth.[12]

Cahn's oral pathology seminars and lectures to the dental staff attracted many medical visitors and were an academic highlight. A world-renowned oral pathologist, Cahn amassed an extraordinary number of honorary degrees in the United States and abroad. He published extensively and was a founder of the American Academy of Oral Pathology, the American Board of Oral Pathology, and the New York Institute of Clinical Oral Pathology. In 1980, Cahn became the first dentist to receive Mount Sinai's prestigious Jacobi Medallion.

Although the management of infection and trauma remained the bedrock of the service, the oral surgeons provided an ever-widening range of surgical procedures to both ambulatory and hospitalized patients. Deformities of the mouth, salivary gland obstruction, oral cysts, and benign tumors were diagnosed and treated with expertise. Conservative management of large jaw lesions proved eminently successful.[13]

Led by Salzmann and Stern, a major collaborative effort culminated in Mount Sinai's designation, in 1952, as the first pilot Cleft Palate Rehabilitation Center in New York State. Dentistry, Pediatrics, Psychiatry, Anesthesiology, Otolaryngology, Plastic Surgery, Nursing and Social

Services joined forces to form a unique multidisciplinary service. Salzmann and Arthur J. Barsky, Chief of Plastic Surgery, were appointed the
first Co-Directors of the Center.

The achievements of the group in cleft lip and palate care were outstanding in offering balanced choices of therapy and rehabilitation.[14,15]
In the first year alone, more than two hundred cases of cleft palate and
cleft lip were seen. The Mount Sinai clinic emphasized team scheduling
to coordinate services, allowing for comprehensive care with a minimum number of visits. Surgical procedures were divided among the
plastic surgeons and the oral surgeons, the former managing the cleft
lip cases and a third of the palate cases; this was a singular sharing
agreement that continued, with only minor changes, until just prior to
the retirement of Leo Stern as Chief of Service. New operative techniques were introduced so that children who required extensive repair
could be treated in a single operative session, thereby minimizing multiple exposures to general anesthesia. Jerry Markowitz, a prosthodon-
tist, introduced the use of a palatal obturator in the earliest days of life
as a temporary therapy to assist feeding until surgical closure of the
palatal cleft could be performed at about two years of age.[16]

Other areas of active research in the department during the 1950s
included the placing of subperiosteal implants for tooth replacement
and early clinical trials of lidocaine versus procaine as a local anesthetic.

In 1953, a residency in oral surgery as a second postgraduate year
following internship was instituted and approved by the American
Dental Association.

In 1957, upon reaching the age of retirement for his rank, Lester
Cahn was appointed Attending Pathologist for Oral Pathology in the
Department of Pathology. His continued liaison with the Dental Department led to American Board of Oral Pathology certification for a
number of the dental staff.

Alvin Nathan succeeded Leo Stern in 1959 upon Stern's retirement
and continued the expansion of the service. The oral surgery residency
program was extended to a three-year term, which included a year of didactic study, a new requirement of the specialty board. The staffs of the
dental specialties were expanded. A dental anesthesiology residency
was initiated under the direction of William Greenfield and, later, David
Valauri. The number of oral surgery Interns increased from three to six
and the number of general practice Interns from two to four in 1963. A
brief affiliation of Mount Sinai with Greenpoint Hospital was followed

in 1964 by Mount Sinai's affiliation with Elmhurst Hospital, which has continued to the present. Roger Gerry, Director of the Department of Dentistry at Elmhurst, was appointed head of the joint residency program in oral and maxillofacial surgery. Shortly thereafter, the Bronx Veterans Administration Hospital and later Queens General Hospital became affiliates and were incorporated into a strengthened training program and into the postgraduate courses offered to the profession.

In 1964, Jack Klatell was appointed Director, and the Department changed its name to the Department of Dentistry. Having joined the Department in 1941 as a Dental Intern, Klatell completed a residency at Seaview Hospital and served in the Army Dental Corps during World War II from 1943 until 1946, finally rejoining the Attending Staff at Mount Sinai.

As Director of Service, Klatell defended and strengthened the role of the Department of Dentistry and was frequently called upon to adjudicate disputes with other departments relating to the specialty of oral surgery and patient care. Dedicated to the advancement of hospital dentistry, Klatell expanded dental care to patients with severe comorbidities such as hemophilia, cardiac disease, and pregnancy.[17–19] With the assistance of Marvin Freid, Jack Hirsch, and Melvin Blake, Klatell stressed the general practice training program, which was enlarged to fourteen residents. The Department's great success in attracting outstanding residents through the resident matching program is directly attributable to the superlative didactic program of lectures and chairman's rounds, extensive clinical practice under the supervision of outstanding Attendings, and rotations to all the dental specialty clinics.

In 1965, during the formation of the Mount Sinai School of Medicine, the Department of Dentistry was made a full Department in the School with Klatell as Chairman and Professor. This was the first time in the United States that a school of medicine without an affiliated dental school had an independent department of dentistry as part of its faculty of medicine. In an initial effort to formulate preliminary plans for a school of dentistry, Klatell recruited a large number of voluntary faculty for various subdivisions. Although the dental school never materialized, the high quality of the faculty was invaluable for clinical care and teaching in the enlarged general dentistry training program. Also in 1965, the dental clinic was restructured to run on an appointment basis, with patients seeing the same dentist at every visit, providing the continuity of care that patients normally receive in a private practice.[20]

A Temporo-Mandibular Joint Clinic headed by Andrew Kaplan was inaugurated, became highly successful, and received numerous referrals, leading to the publication of a textbook,[21] a book for laymen, and numerous articles. In 1979, J. Gordon Rubin conducted what is said to be the first dental phobia program to be administered and staffed by dentists, rather than psychologists. This clinic developed a behavioral and cognitive approach to "desensitize" patients to their fears, allowing them to undergo comprehensive dental care without resorting to general anesthesia. An oral and maxillofacial pathology residency program (later to become a fellowship within Otolaryngology) was established under the direction of Harry Lumerman and Marie Ramer. In 1991, the Department published *The Mount Sinai Medical Center Family Guide to Dental Health.*[22] In response to the AIDS crisis and in collaboration with the Division of Infectious Diseases in the Department of Medicine, the Department conducted studies on needle-stick prevention and the universal adoption of gloves and masks. In 1990, Klatell became the second dentist to be awarded the Jacobi Medallion.

Daniel Buchbinder became Mount Sinai's first full-time Chief of the Division of Oral and Maxillo-Facial Surgery (OMS) and director of the residency program in 1988. Two years later, the residency became a six-year integrated program, with the Residents attending the Mount Sinai School of Medicine and receiving the M.D. degree. They then completed one year of general surgery training, followed by the oral and maxillo-facial residency. Not to be outdone by his trainees, Buchbinder enrolled in the Mount Sinai School of Medicine and received his M.D. degree in 1999. The contributions of George Anastassov at Elmhurst Hospital added significantly to the strength of the division. Technical innovations in orthognathic reconstruction, microvascular techniques, free flaps for reconstruction of massive craniofacial defects, and maxillofacial grafting were intensively pursued in collaboration with other departments.[23–25]

Historically, the dental profession has prospered as a separate and autonomous profession since the first dental degrees were awarded by the Baltimore College of Dental Surgery in 1840. In recent decades, dental education has pursued a more rigorous foundation in the basic biologic sciences; many dental schools now offer a preclinical curriculum nearly identical to that of medical schools. The oral surgery/medical degree initiative of Klatell and Buchbinder brings dentistry at Mount Sinai to the forefront in uniting the two professions. As noted earlier,

Leo Stern obtained recognition for dentistry's coequal status with medicine at Mount Sinai. It is in oral and maxillofacial surgery that the affinity with medicine and surgery is closest, standing as it does between dentistry (of which it is a specialty and where it evolved) and the regional specialties of otolaryngology and head and neck reconstructive surgery.

Klatell stepped down as Chairman in 1999, and Buchbinder was appointed Acting Chairman, the first time the position has been held by an individual with both D.M.D. and M.D. degrees. Associated with a highly qualified team of hospital dentists and oral and maxillo-facial surgeons, Buchbinder has the exciting task of leading the Department into the twenty-first century.

17

Department of Dermatology

AT THE TIME The Mount Sinai Hospital was founded in 1852, there was no formal dermatology department. Dermatology as a specialty was not officially recognized by the American Board of Medical Specialties until 1938, when the American Board of Dermatology and Syphilology was established, although the field had long been recognized in Europe. The fields of dermatology and syphilology were united because of the numerous dermatologic manifestations of syphilis.

By 1872, when The Mount Sinai Hospital moved to its second location, at Lexington Avenue between 67th and 68th streets, there were many dermatologic cases. At the time, many dermatalgic conditions were treated with preparations that were derivatives of arsenic, mercury, sulfur, and tar.[1] Psoriasis was treated with carbolic acid in glycerine, tar, oil of cade, or mercury ointment. Eczema was treated with 10 percent oil of cade. Basal cell carcinoma was treated by arsenic paste or cautery. For syphilis, "the great imitator," as the saying went, "One night with Venus, and the rest of your life with mercury."

In 1891, a Clinic for Skin and Venereal Disease was created in the Out-Patient Department of the Hospital. In 1893, Sigmund Lustgarten was appointed Consulting Dermatologist for the patients on the Hospital wards. In 1900, a small number of beds were set aside for dermatology patients, and Lustgarten's position was changed to Attending Dermatologist, the equivalent of Chief of Service. Lustgarten was a student of the great European dermatologists Ferdinand von Hebra and Moritz Kaposi. He came to the United States from his native Vienna in 1889 and became active in medical circles, quickly gaining a reputation as a skilled clinician and diagnostician. He did not—and could not, in these early years of specialization—limit his diagnostic work to dermatology alone, however, and he was frequently called to attend the general wards.

At the time, diagnosis depended almost entirely on clinical knowledge. On one famous occasion, Lustgarten made the diagnosis of leprosy in a patient on the general wards. His diagnoses were usually preceded by a mysterious approach. In this case, he asked to have a "pimple" pricked on the lip of the patient. He made a smear that could be used to test for the tubercle bacilli, as well as for leprosy. Many thought he was testing for tuberculosis, although everyone was sure this was not the correct diagnosis. Instead, the smear proved that the patient had leprosy. On another occasion, he visited a syphilitic patient who had broken out with a fiery, red rash, which was diagnosed as scarlet fever. The patient was put in isolation. Lustgarten examined the patient and diagnosed the rash as a case of overdose of mercury, which had been given to treat the syphilis. Associates claimed that Lustgarten was the first to give Salvarsan as a treatment for syphilis in the U.S.[2]

Lustgarten was a man of extreme discretion and tact. In going through a hotel lobby one day with another dermatologist, Richard Hoffman, Hoffman saw and greeted a man they both knew. Lustgarten did not acknowledge the acquaintance. When Hoffman pointed out that the person was someone they both knew, Lustgarten explained that he rarely greeted people in public because his reputation as a syphilis expert might embarrass some of his acquaintances.[3] Lustgarten was also a man of culture and erudition, a lover of music, and a connoisseur of art. He was a good draftsman and a collector of fine engravings and etchings. Soft spoken and dignified, he was considered a man of great intellectual stature and commanded universal respect.

On Lustgarten's death in 1911 at age fifty-three, Hermann Goldenberg became the Chief of Service. Goldenberg had trained in Munich and did postgraduate work for several years in Europe. During his tenure as Chief of Dermatology, Mount Sinai was among the first to introduce modern methods in the treatment of syphilis. Goldenberg received some of the original allotment of Salvarsan before the drug was released for general use. It was said that he treated patients with early syphilis with miraculous results.[4] As the years passed, the Department had eight allocated beds, with the privilege of also utilizing beds on the pediatric wards. These beds were always occupied. Many interesting cases from the ward and clinics were presented at the various grand rounds. As was noted later:

> In the early part of the twentieth century the skin clinics of Mount Sinai Hospital were outstanding for their large and interesting material. Dermatologists and other interested physicians from all parts of the country visited the clinics for weeks at a time to see the unusual

cases and listen to the illuminating discussions carried on by Dr. Lust-garten, Dr. Goldenberg and other members of the staff.[5]

When Goldenberg retired in January 1929, Walter J. Highman and Isadore Rosen became Attendings in Dermatology. Highman did two years of postgraduate work in Berlin, Paris, Freiberg, and Vienna and in Bern under Josef Jadassohn. It was during his years at Mount Sinai that Highman established the first dermatopathology section at Mount Sinai.[6] Highman published more than seventy articles and was the author of the textbook *Dermatology*, published in 1921.[7]

On the death of Highman in 1934, Isadore Rosen became the sole Chief of Dermatology. A New Yorker, Rosen made groundbreaking advances in the standardization of modern treatments of acquired syphilis.[8] He was among the first in America to organize a clinic for the systematic treatment of congenital syphilis. Rosen was also among the first to apply fever therapy in the treatment of chronic, recurrent dermatoses and to conduct chemical and biologic studies of the blood and sweat of these patients.[9]

During Rosen's tenure, the dermatopathology facilities were used for dark field examinations for the recognition of early syphilis and for the microscopic examination of hairs and scales for the diagnosis of fungal diseases. The Syphilis Clinic had two full-time Medical Assistants who administered treatment. By the 1930s, many skin diseases were treated by radiotherapy, which was administered by radiologists in the Hospital, not by dermatologists, a fact that concerned Rosen deeply.[10]

During the 1930s, a breakthrough made by staff members caused a major sensation: a five-day treatment for syphilis developed by Louis Chargin, Harold T. Hyman, and William Leifer.[11] Chargin first suggested that the slow-drip method might be used for the injection of large amounts of arsenicals in syphilitic patients. Patients received four grams of neoarsphenamine in five days, reducing the cost of treating syphilis to less than ninety dollars. For a time, it looked as if Hyman, Chargin, and Leifer had realized Erlich's hope for the "magic bullet." However, the course of treatment of syphilis was soon changed forever with the discovery of penicillin, and the Mount Sinai contribution was eclipsed.

Louis Chargin was born in Minsk in 1881, grew up in New York, and graduated from the University of Maryland School of Medicine in

1902. Following postgraduate study abroad, he began a long association with Mount Sinai. A skilled practitioner, he maintained a prestigious practice on Central Park West. Chargin had his quirks: he wore white gloves, bedroom slippers, and a visor in his office. He would never touch the fees he received. Patients were to slip the fees through a slit in a shoebox fashioned by Chargin. Mindful of the future, he bequeathed to the Hospital the Chargin Fund for Dermatologic Research in the Department.

Over the years, dermatologic advances were made at Mount Sinai by nondermatologists. Koplik spots of measles were first characterized in 1896 by Henry Koplik.[12] Jacob Churg and Lotte Strauss, the pathologists, described allergic granulomatosis.[13] The Kveim Test, which involves the intradermal testing and a skin biopsy for the diagnosis of sarcoidosis, was refined by Louis Siltzbach.[14,15]

On Rosen's retirement in 1946, Samuel Peck assumed the position as Director of Dermatology, a post he held until 1971. During Peck's years as Chairman, a residency program was established for the training of dermatologists. The first Residents "graduated" in 1948. Peck was also Chairman during the formation of the Mount Sinai School of Medicine and was responsible for developing an undergraduate curriculum in dermatology for the medical students. Peck himself was a role model for the Residents and students, maintaining a busy practice and teaching while doing research and publishing extensively.

Born in 1900, Peck trained with John Fordyce in New York, as well as in Berlin and Zurich under Professor Bruno Bloch. His studies in the field of contact and industrial dermatoses, insect-bite reactions, melanin, and mycology proved invaluable. His article on the introduction of the use of moccasin venom for the treatment of bleeding symptoms caused a sensation in 1932.[16] In 1938, Peck was also among the first to show data on the use of undecylenic acid, the first available antifungal agent.[17]

Peck published more than one hundred articles and co-authored several books, including *Occupational Diseases of the Skin*, with Louis Schwartz and Louis Tulipan.[18] He also maintained an active clinical practice with an extensive following. His office was crowded with patients from before five in the morning until the early afternoon. He continued his private practice until nearly his ninetieth year. He attended Grand Rounds in the Department for a few years after this, contributing actively to the clinical discussions.

On Peck's retirement in 1971, Arthur Glick was named Acting Chairman, a position he held for four years. Glick published several papers on industrial dermatoses and expanded the dermatologic surgery clinic. An avid fisherman, jazz enthusiast, and cigar aficionado, Glick brought in many new Attendings and was the first to send Residents in dermatology to the Bronx Veterans Administration Hospital. Glick exerted a strong presence in the clinic with his sonorous voice and dapper bow tie. He also maintained an elegant practice on East 67th Street on the top floor of a brownstone.

Another outstanding Attending during these years was Orlando Canizares. He was born in Cuba and studied medicine in Paris and dermatology in Madrid but settled in New York after World War II. His most important writings were on tropical dermatology, venereal diseases, the treatment of parapsoriasis with vitamin D2, and atrophoderma of Pasini and Pierini. He was regarded as dermatology's goodwill ambassador to tropical countries. Canizares published several volumes of *Clinical Tropical Dermatology*,[19] which became a classic. He was also an accomplished artist and found time to draw caricatures of many dermatologists.

On Glick's retirement in 1975, Harry Shatin became the first full-time Chairman of the Department. He placed a special emphasis on the teaching of Residents—Shatin was credited with the organization and re-credentialing of the residency program—and worked on integrating the residency programs at Mount Sinai, Elmhurst Hospital, and the Bronx Veterans Administration Medical Center. (During this time, Leonard Kornblee, a long-time Mount Sinai Attending, became the full-time Chief of Dermatology at the Bronx VA.) A noted venereologist, Shatin was an astute and witty clinician. On one occasion, Shatin presented a case of bullous pemphigoid to his residents. He told his orderly of the diagnosis before the conference. During the conference, when none of the residents was able to diagnose the patient's condition with certainty, Shatin asked the orderly, who promptly proclaimed, "Bullous pemphigoid!" At this, Shatin exclaimed, "You see, even the orderly knows the diagnosis."

On Harry Shatin's retirement in 1979, Raul Fleischmajer was appointed Chairman of the Department. Fleischmajer was research oriented and made crucial breakthroughs in collagen vascular diseases, scleroderma, and dyslipidoses. He was the first to measure collagen in a quantitative fashion in the skin. He was also instrumental in

Four Chiefs of Dermatology, left to right: Raul Fleischmajer, M.D. (1979–1995), Harry Shatin, M.D. (1975–1979), Samuel M. Peck, M.D. (1946–1971), and Arthur Glick, M.D. (1971–1975). Photo courtesy of Douglas Altchek, M.D.

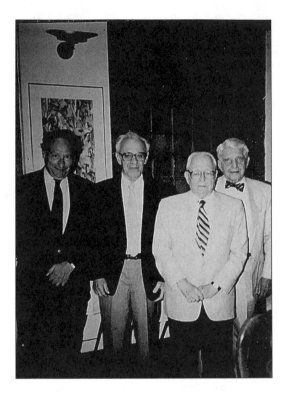

designating scleroderma as a disease of inflammatory origin and in documenting the association of scleredema and diabetes mellitus. In his years at Mount Sinai, he was extensively involved in the study of the nature of collagen fibrillogenesis. Fleischmajer's findings greatly enhanced our knowledge of how different connective tissue components interact to form the dermal matrix. He brought to Mount Sinai's Department of Dermatology a level of respect in the dermatologic scientific community that has remained as his legacy. One of his notable publications was an article on lipoid proteinosis (hyalinosis cutis et mucosae),[20] an extremely rare disease recognizable by the "string of pearls" nodules of the eyelids and hoarseness of voice. On one occasion, Douglas Altchek, a perceptive clinician, identified the condition in a subway rider and convinced him to come to Mount Sinai for skin biopsies and treatment. The patient was very cooperative and even returned for a repeat biopsy. Because of the unusual nature of the lesion, the specimens were sent to the Max Planck Institute in Munich for further study.

Fleischmajer was also a skillful clinician and maintained an active, hospital-based practice. He was widely traveled and had a worldwide reputation. His lectures were most compelling from the scientific standpoint and also quite entertaining. He would share with Residents and Attendings alike his research ventures in places like Reims, which is, by no coincidence, the champagne capital of the world. Fleischmajer was also a connoisseur of opera and fine food.

During the Fleischmajer years, several prominent dermatologists joined the full-time staff. Brian Berman, known for his studies of the Langerhans cell and interferon, joined the Department, established a laboratory, and, as a superb clinician, took charge of the consult service. Also joining the Department under Fleischmajer was Philip Prioleau, who was trained in general surgery, plastic surgery, general pathology, and dermatopathology. He took charge of the Service's fledgling dermatopathology service. While his task was to read the dermatopathology slides, his natural abilities in clinical dermatology and dermatologic surgery made him a master teacher in all aspects of dermatology.

Others were added over these years. Mark Lebwohl, who had already completed a residency in internal medicine, was recruited by Fleischmajer as a Resident and then as a faculty member. Irwin Kantor, a long-time associate of Peck, joined the full-time faculty and added his vast experience to the Department. Robert Phelps became the first full-time dermatopathologist and greatly expanded the division of dermatopathology. By the early 1990s, more than twenty-five thousand skin pathology specimens were being read annually. Marsha Gordon, a fine teacher and clinician, joined the Department, as well as Donald Rudikoff, a board-certified internist and dermatologist. An outstanding clinician, he was placed in charge of the Dermatology-HIV Clinic. Ronald Shelton also joined the Department as its first Mohs chemosurgeon.

Mark Lebwohl became Chairman of the Department in 1996. By that time, he had written the first *Atlas of the Skin and Systemic Disease*[21] and had edited two additional books, *Difficult Diagnoses in Dermatology*[22] and *Psoriasis*.[23] He serves on many editorial boards and has been a leader in professional organizations. He has authored or co-authored hundreds of articles with an emphasis on psoriasis and on pseudoxanthoma elasticum (PXE). Lebwohl has identified new techniques of diagnosing PXE[24] and was the first to report its cardiac complications.[25,26] He also played a major role in elucidating its pathophysiology[27] and was part of the team that identified the genetic defect in PXE—mutations in an ABC-C transmembrane transporter protein.

The Department has been at the forefront of psoriasis management. Many treatment protocols and regimens have been formulated by Lebwohl and his co-workers, and treatment interactions and systemic drug therapy for the condition are continuous works in progress. Many of these agents are now being studied for the treatment of arthritis and other inflammatory diseases. Lebwohl is the founding Editor of *Psoriasis Forum* and Medical Editor of *The Bulletin* of the National Psoriasis Foundation.

Two other key contributions made in the Department include the first description of reactive perforating collagenosis occurring with diabetes and renal disease[28] and the observation that many patients diagnosed with eosinophilic fasciitis had taken L-tryptophan, the agent that causes eosinophilia myalgia syndrome.[29]

The Department flourished under Lebwohl's able chairmanship. James Spencer was recruited to take over the Division of Dermatologic Surgery, which has expanded into one of the leading surgical programs in the nation. Spencer established a cosmetic and dermatologic surgery fellowship program and a lecture series that is attended by dermatologists from around the City. With Albert Lefkovits and Rudikoff, Spencer co-directs the highly popular Mount Sinai Winter Symposium: Advances in Medical and Surgical Dermatology. This annual December program attracts a worldwide audience. It is one of the largest dermatology meetings in the world and one of the largest meetings held at Mount Sinai.

Spencer also expanded the use of lasers at Mount Sinai. He made seminal observations on the use of the 308NM laser for the treatment of vitiligo. This treatment repigments patients with this disfiguring disease more quickly than any other therapeutic modality available and is rapidly becoming one of the most common therapies for the disorder. Heidi Waldorf was recruited to oversee the rapidly growing laser surgery program.

Huachen Wei was also recruited to head the Dermatology Research Laboratories. Wei is a pioneer in the use of genistein for the prevention of chemical and ultraviolet light-induced squamous cell carcinomas.[30] This agent, which has been patented by Mount Sinai, is a tyrosine protein kinase inhibitor that intercalates between DNA strands and prevents replication of damaged DNA. The agent not only prevents carcinogenesis but also prevents other consequences of ultraviolet light-induced damage, including photo aging and sunburn. Wei has won numerous awards for his work, including an award from the American College for Cancer Research, The Dermatology Foundation, and the American Academy of Dermatology's prestigious Young Investigator Award.

The Department is currently involved in the investigation of aging of the skin, the molecular mechanisms in ultraviolet light skin aging, and in pseudoxanthoma elasticum as a model for accelerated aging. Additionally, the Department has been involved in the classification of the structure and function of connective tissue. Numerous clinical trials are under way in the management of psoriasis, acne, atopic dermatitis, herpes simplex, and fungal disorders. The dermatopharmacology program is one of the largest in the country, and the skin cancer research and psoriasis therapy programs are universally recognized. An international fellowship training program, directed by Suhail Hadi, trains individuals from around the world, who then return to their native country to provide much-needed dermatology services.

The voluntary Attending staff has contributed greatly to the teaching program and to the specialty. Robert Berger, Hillard Pearlstein, and Douglas Altchek are all notable dermatologic surgeons and excellent teachers. Stephen Kurtin, whose father, Abner Kurtin, pioneered dermabrasion at Mount Sinai,[31] and David Orentreich, whose father originated hair transplantation, have both continued in the tradition. Ronald Sherman has been an innovator in combining the fields of cosmetology and dermatology. Michael Kalman has been creative in dermatologic surgery and dermatopharmacology. Albert Lefkovits, a fine clinician and teacher, is very active in hospital affairs. Michael Fellner, an expert in immunodermatology, has helped bridge the gap in our understanding of the immunology of the skin. Susan Bershad was the lead author on the study examining hypertriglyceridemia and isotretinoin, which is used for the treatment of nodulo-cystic acne.[32]

In this age of technology, the practice of dermatology continues to expand in many exciting directions. While meeting the challenges of the future as innovative researchers, teachers, and clinicians, the Department's faculty continues to maintain the meticulous traditions of the past.

Adapted from an article by Douglas D. Altchek, M.D., published in *The Mount Sinai Journal of Medicine*, 63, (1996): 263–272.

18

Department of Emergency Medicine

ON JUNE 3, 1855, two days before the opening of the doors of the Jews' Hospital on West 28th Street, the Board of Directors (today's Trustees) decreed that "the Visiting Committee be instructed not to receive any patients other than Jews except in cases of accident, until further notice."[1] At the outbreak of the Civil War, the federal government asked for help, and the Hospital set up extra cots as beds to accommodate wounded Union Army soldiers. In 1862, when the Hospital was still located on 28th Street, Civil War draft riots erupted immediately outside the Hospital's doors, and Hospital personnel administered aid to victims of the riots. These two events were important factors in convincing the Directors that the Hospital was nonsectarian in nature and that the name should be changed to The Mount Sinai Hospital, an event that took place in 1866. Five years later, the Orangemen riots also broke out near the Hospital, and a number of casualties were treated at Mount Sinai.

In 1872, the Hospital moved to Lexington Avenue and 67th Street, and over the years there was a small but steady increase in the number of emergencies and accident cases, the latter caused mainly by traffic and machinery. In 1889, a fire broke out at the Presbyterian Hospital, then located at 70th Street and Park Avenue, and Mount Sinai immediately accepted forty of their patients. The first reference to an actual emergency room (ER) appears in the Annual Report for 1888, when the House Staff treated 301 emergency cases. This tiny ER was often referred to as "the accident closet" and was located in the entrance hall of the main Lexington Avenue building. When the Hospital moved uptown to its current location, in 1904, the ER was given larger quarters on the lower level of the medical ward building. An ambulance entrance on 100th Street near Madison Avenue provided an entryway separate from the main Hospital entrance.

Mount Sinai began its own ambulance service in 1902. The service picked up patients, transported them to different hospitals, and

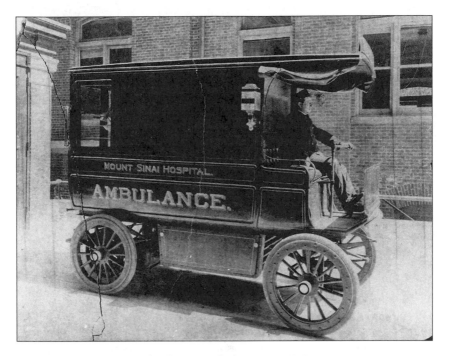

One of Mount Sinai's early electric ambulances, c. 1910.

brought them home. Initially, a member of the House Staff rode along in the ambulance. As the use of private ambulance services expanded, Mount Sinai's own ambulance service was slowly phased out and was terminated by the end of World War II.

What came to be known as Emergency Services continued to develop and expand throughout the years. An admitting physician was assigned to cover the reception area. On weekdays and weekend mornings, any patient could present himself or herself for admission to the hospital, regardless of the nature of the illness. Urgent and emergent cases were seen in the ER at all hours and either admitted or treated and released, usually with a return visit scheduled for one of the clinics or a referral to their private physician. Residents in the various specialties were called to the ER to treat patients as needed. In 1947, 33,192 emergency cases were treated. In 1967, a separate pediatric emergency area was created and staffed by the Department of Pediatrics. In 1985, with the ER now under the direction of Barbara Richardson of the

Department of Medicine, the Hospital was designated as an Emergency Medical Services (EMS) ambulance destination site and a level II trauma center. That same year, a separate walk-in referral area was created for the more efficient treatment of patients with minor ailments. In 1989, Emergency Services moved into the new Guggenheim building, essentially doubling its space. However, by the time the building opened, the number of visits had almost doubled from the number recorded when the facility was planned; the space was inadequate from the outset, and Richardson had major problems with physician coverage. A similar situation existed at Mount Sinai's principal academic affiliate, the City Hospital Center at Elmhurst.

At this point, some knowledge of the development of the specialty of emergency medicine (EM) is necessary to understand the evolution of the EM program at Mount Sinai. Between 1955 and 1970, visits to emergency departments quadrupled throughout the United States, and the public began to recognize that, for the most part, these facilities were understaffed. During the 1960s, a few physicians in disparate locations began to give up their office practices and to staff ERs in an attempt to improve care. The American College of Emergency Physicians was formed in 1968, and, two years later, the University Association for Emergency Medical Services was established. The first formal (but unapproved) residency in EM began in 1972; it would be seven more years until the American Board of Medical Specialties approved the American Board of Emergency Medicine. By 1989, there were eighteen academic departments of emergency medicine in medical schools in the United States.

In 1993, the Medical Board and the Administration of Mount Sinai were convinced that the best, and probably only, way to attract and retain the highest quality staff would be to create a separate department. Consequently, an academic Department of Emergency Medicine was established. At the time, Mount Sinai was only the second voluntary institution in the metropolitan area to have such an academic department. The following year, Sheldon Jacobson was appointed Chairman of the Department. Jacobson had previously designed the emergency medicine residency at Albert Einstein College of Medicine, as well as the first paramedic training program in New York City. Jacobson forged the Department with a dedication to excellence in patient care, professional education at all levels, community service, and research. Divisions were created in Research, Prehospital Care and Disaster Medicine, Pediatric

Emergency Medicine, Toxicology, Geriatric Emergency Medicine, Informatics, and Medical Economics.

In 1995, a three-year Emergency Medicine residency program with ten Residents per year was initiated, with Residents receiving training at both Mount Sinai and Elmhurst, as well as at the New York City Poison Center at Bellevue Hospital. In addition, the Department is responsible for the required emergency medicine subinternship for fourth-year medical students and also teaches prehospital and emergency care, including basic life support, to incoming first-year medical students.

Research plays a vital role in the overall teaching and patient care activities of the Department. The recent formation by the Department of a computer-assisted training program accessible via the Internet has been analyzed and evaluated.[2] With each Division responsible for developing its own research projects, a number of articles have recently been published on informatics, complementary and alternative medicine, prehospital care of stroke and head trauma victims, postsexual exposure prophylaxis, spousal abuse, post-traumatic stress in children, and geriatric emergency medicine.[3] There is also an active drug trials program, with several trials ongoing. Another innovative departmental activity provides training and coordination to help companies and organizations establish automatic external defibrillator (AED) programs to treat victims of cardiac arrest.[4]

Under the direction of Andy Jagoda, members of the Department have traveled to a number of foreign countries, including Chile, Madagascar, the Netherlands, and Guyana, to aid in education and the formulation of emergency medicine programs. The Department is also involved in a number of community service activities in New York. The Department has a close working relationship with the Yorkville Common Pantry, which provides counseling, shelter, and meals to the needy. Part-time paid work experiences are offered for junior and senior high school students on a variety of research topics.

The Department has responsibility for the full-time academic clinical management of four emergency departments: The Mount Sinai Hospital; the City Hospital Center at Elmhurst, a level I trauma center; and the Jersey City Medical Center and The Mount Sinai Hospital of Queens, both level II trauma centers. For the twelve-month period ending June 30, 2001, the four sites had almost 300,000 patient visits; The Mount Sinai Hospital treated 84,250 patients, 20 percent of whom were admitted. A fifth institution, Queens Hospital Center, became part of the academic enterprise early in 2002.

Mark Blumenthal, the first and only Attending and Resident physician, saw every patient when the Jews' Hospital opened its doors 150 years ago. He would surely be amazed if he were alive today, at the activity now taking place in Mount Sinai's Department of Emergency Medicine.

19

Department of Geriatrics and Adult Development

ESTABLISHED IN 1982 as the first academic geriatrics department in the country, the Department of Geriatrics and Adult Development is a relative newcomer to the Mount Sinai scene. Mount Sinai's pioneering tradition of geriatric medicine, however, can be traced back to the beginning of the twentieth century. As early as 1909, Ignatz Leo Nascher, former Chief of Clinic in the Mount Sinai Outpatient Department and a "Father" of geriatrics in America, coined the term "geriatrics" in his first paper on geriatric medicine.[1]

Ahead of his time, Nascher suggested this new term—from *geras*, "old age," and *iatrikos*, "relating to the physician"—as "an addition to our vocabulary, to cover the same field in old age that is covered by the term pediatrics in childhood, to emphasize the necessity of considering senility and its diseases apart from maturity and to assign it a separate place in medicine."[2] Five years and more than thirty articles on geriatrics later, Nascher, in 1914, wrote the first American textbook on geriatric medicine, *Geriatrics: The Diseases of Old Age and Their Treatment, Including Physiological Old Age, Home And Institutional Care, and Medico-Legal Relations.*[3] The introduction to this landmark text was written by another Mount Sinai giant, Abraham Jacobi, one of the founders of pediatrics in the United States. Still, many tried to dismiss Nascher's work, and, although it was initially refused by a number of publishing houses, *Geriatrics* enjoyed a second printing in 1916 and several more editions in the years to follow. Nascher's foresight was that much more impressive when one considers that at the time he was practicing, only 4 percent of the United States population was over the age of sixty-five, and the average life expectancy was forty-five years.[4]

A champion of geriatrics throughout his professional life, Nascher wrote more than fifty articles on various subjects relating to geriatrics. He also lectured, provided clinical leadership, and founded the New

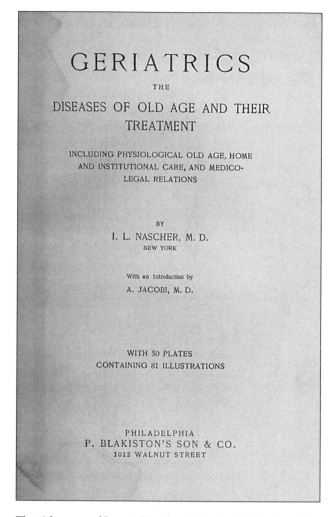

GERIATRICS

THE

DISEASES OF OLD AGE AND THEIR TREATMENT

INCLUDING PHYSIOLOGICAL OLD AGE, HOME
AND INSTITUTIONAL CARE, AND MEDICO-
LEGAL RELATIONS

BY

I. L. NASCHER, M. D.
NEW YORK

With an Introduction by
A. JACOBI, M. D.

WITH 50 PLATES
CONTAINING 81 ILLUSTRATIONS

PHILADELPHIA
P. BLAKISTON'S SON & CO.
1012 WALNUT STREET

The title page of Ignatz Nascher's book, which coined the
term "geriatrics." Nascher was on the Mount Sinai staff.

York Geriatrics Society. Nascher accomplished all of this despite the in-
difference and, often, the outright censure of both the medical establishment and the general public; he remained hopeful that "geriatrics
would soon be taught and practiced as one of the major specialties of
medicine."[5] This hope was somewhat premature, however, for in the

years following Nascher's retirement in 1929, geriatrics seemed to all but disappear.

Just prior to the onset of World War II, there was increasing interest in geriatric research and education, particularly at nursing homes and chronic disease hospitals. In 1939, a group of scientists and physicians formed the Club for Research on Ageing. The American Geriatrics Society was established in 1942. In 1945, members of the Club for Research incorporated the Gerontological Society of America to "promote the scientific study of aging."[6] A growing number of journals addressing geriatric concerns also began cropping up at this time, but, while there was occasional talk of the need for a geriatric specialty, no serious propositions ever materialized.

Closer to home were the efforts of Frederic D. Zeman, a 1921 graduate of the Mount Sinai House Staff. While still a member of the active staff at Mount Sinai, Zeman concentrated his efforts on developing a patient-centered model of care for the aged at the Home for Aged and Infirm Hebrews, later known as the Jewish Home and Hospital for Aged (JHHA) and now the Jewish Home and Hospital (JHH). He served there as Medical Director for forty-five years. Then, in 1962, at the JHHA, Zeman formed the first experience-based instructional facility for training in geriatrics in this country, supported by a government grant. Shortly after his death in 1970, the training center was renamed the Frederic D. Zeman Center for Instruction.

Following World War II, acceptance of geriatric medicine in America increased. Alvin Goldfarb of the Mount Sinai Department of Psychiatry, while working at the Home for Aged and Infirm Hebrews, designed the first screening test to measure the psychological states of the elderly in 1953.[7] Goldfarb also played a substantial role in creating the field of geriatric psychiatry in the United States.

Although 1965 brought the creation of Medicare and Medicaid and the passage of the Older Americans Act, none of the federal appropriations were earmarked for the training of geriatricians. A significant advance toward such training occurred in 1972. At that time, Leslie Libow initiated the first nationally recognized geriatric fellowship (later residency) in the United States, approved by the American Board of Internal Medicine (ABIM) and located at the City Hospital Center at Elmhurst, Queens, a major teaching affiliate of the Mount Sinai School of Medicine. Libow negotiated the fellowship's approval with the ABIM so that a year of geriatric training could follow a full medical residency or would be accepted in lieu of a third and final year of an internal medicine residency. Most Fellows trained for a period of twenty-four months. The ABIM insisted upon, and received, full support for the innovation from Solomon Berson, the Medical School Chairman of the Department of Medicine, and from Stanley G. Seckler, the Director of Medicine at Elmhurst.[8,9] After the success of the fellowship at Mount Sinai and at Elmhurst, other institutions followed suit, and, between 1975 and 1980, at least ten other fellowship programs in geriatrics were created throughout the United States.

Around the same time, the first academic nursing home in America was also established at Elmhurst, linking residency and fellowship training, medical and nursing student training, and research. Years later, this model of the academic nursing home was termed the "teaching nursing home," in recognition of the significant role these nursing homes played in the university- affiliated teaching hospital.[10]

Because of Mount Sinai's affiliation with Elmhurst, medical Interns and Residents, as well as medical students rotating through on elective, all received training in geriatric medicine. Still, it was not until 1979, when Fred Sherman was recruited to the Department of Medicine from the Jewish Institute for Geriatric Care in New Hyde Park, New York (where he had worked with Libow), that Mount Sinai had its own Division of Geriatrics. Sherman, however, did not just set up the Division; he *was* the Division. One of Sherman's most visible accomplishments was to obtain sixteen hours of geriatrics lecture time during the pre-clinical years. Although the Division of Geriatrics had no curriculum hours of its own, Sherman approached other departments to request curriculum time to teach geriatric topics relating to each respective field, and in general these requests were well received. One particularly successful course, Human Growth, Maturation, and Senescence, was taught through the Department of Pediatrics and notably gave equal attention to growth, development, aging, and senescence.

Another milestone for the Division was the formation, in 1980, of an interdisciplinary Geriatric Consult Team, made up of Sherman, Jane Morris, R.N., and Susan Blumenfield, D.S.W. The team saw patients on both the medicine and the psychiatry floors and, using a team-based approach, created programs that addressed the psychosocial needs particular to aging. Nurse Practitioner students worked closely with older patients on the ward, and, in 1981, a formal Geriatric Nurse Practitioner Training Program was initiated at the Long Term Care Gerontology

Center by the Hunter-Bellevue School of Nursing. The program, taught by faculty from Mount Sinai and JHH, continues to this day.

Mount Sinai was quickly emerging as a leader in geriatric medicine, and this reached a peak in 1982 when Mount Sinai became the first medical school in the country to establish a freestanding Department of Geriatrics.

These early developments in geriatrics at Mount Sinai, while remarkable, were not the reason the Department was created. In 1975, Robert N. Butler was selected as the first Director of the National Institute on Aging (NIA), and he quickly established a program to develop academic geriatrics. Fred Sherman won one of the first NIA awards.

Encouraged by Stephen Schwartz, of the Brookdale Foundation, Thomas C. Chalmers, President and Dean of The Mount Sinai Medical Center, invited Butler to establish an institute of gerontology at Mount Sinai. Desiring to introduce geriatrics in American medical education, Butler proposed a full-scale academic department instead. Hans Popper, former President of Mount Sinai, encouraged Butler to come. Butler then recruited Libow, who had worked with Butler at the National Institutes of Health (NIH) in 1960–1961 and brought Judith Howe and Malvin Schecter from NIA to help establish the Department.

While the Department's ensuing success resulted from the outstanding faculty, staff, and administrators who were quickly brought on board, the Department owes its existence to the vision and insight of Chalmers. Recognizing that true power in an academic health center depended on the creation of a Department rather than a Division, Chalmers backed Butler and pushed for a freestanding Department of Geriatrics, despite staunch opposition from certain quarters. Chalmers realized the far-reaching potential for a Department that would not only bring clinical prominence but would also serve as a national resource center.

Chalmers had actively sought out Butler to come to Mount Sinai. Butler, a Pulitzer Prize–winning author and internationally recognized figure in the field of aging, was originally brought to Mount Sinai as a consultant. Butler soon found himself aggressively courted for the Chairmanship. While Butler had no intention of leaving his position at the NIA or moving to New York City, Hans Popper advised him to write out a request for the "most outrageous and comprehensive department" he could possibly imagine. If Mount Sinai accepted his terms, then the offer of Chairman would be too good to pass up; if not, Butler would have convenient grounds for refusal.[11] Butler submitted his proposal, with contributions by Libow and Schecter, in December 1981; it became the first mission statement of the Mount Sinai School of Medicine's Department of Geriatrics and Adult Development.

Knowing there was strong resistance to the idea of a Department of Geriatrics at Mount Sinai and anticipating potential problems garnering resources from the Medical School and the Hospital, Butler, Libow, and Schecter drew up a rigorous proposal. They demanded that the Department be granted mandatory medical student curriculum time, including an obligatory four-week clerkship in geriatric medicine for all fourth-year students, two weeks of which were to be spent either at the Jewish Home and Hospital (JHH) or at Mount Sinai's Geriatric Evaluation and Treatment Unit (GETU). They also required an institutional affiliation with a teaching nursing home such as JHH, a provision requiring faculty to evenly divide their time between Mount Sinai and the JHH (later the two campuses would develop their own full-time faculties), and the allocation of sixteen acute hospital beds at Mount Sinai to the Department of Geriatrics. Their proposal called for four full professorships, as well as research initiatives in molecular biology, neurobiology, and immunology. The proposal stressed inpatient, outpatient, and long-term care, strong research and teaching components, and a need to move beyond exclusively hospital-based training and education.

Among the most contentious of these issues were the mandated curriculum time and the designated geriatric acute care beds. Mount Sinai's Curriculum Committee insisted there was no available time for the Department to get its own curriculum hours. A strong contingent within the Committee further felt that, because most patients in the acute care units were over sixty-five, there was no need for specific geriatric beds. As for the medical students, many resented having to do a geriatrics rotation in the first place, and when the Department decided that fourth-year students had to spend two weeks of their mandatory geriatrics rotation in a nursing home, students actually sent a letter of protest to the Deans.

The greatest resistance, however, came from the Department of Medicine. Many in Medicine felt not only that a separate Department of Geriatrics was unnecessary but also that the Department's very existence posed a serious threat by implicitly suggesting that internists were ineffective or deficient in the care of their elderly patients. These objections ran so deep that for years the Department of Medicine refused to make referrals to the Department of Geriatrics. Most patients who found their way into the geriatrics practice were self-referred, often because of Butler's reputation as an advocate and educator on the medical and social rights and needs of the elderly.

Board certified in psychiatry and later in gerontology, Butler, while working at the National Institute of Mental Health (1955–1966), had conducted physiological research that helped to distinguish aging from disease and showed that senility and decreased libido were not an inevitable part of the aging process. At the NIA, Butler also established Alzheimer's disease as a national research priority and introduced the terms "life review," "ageism," and "productive aging" into our lexicon. A founding member of the Alzheimer's Disease Association, the American Association of Geriatric Psychiatry, the American Federation for Aging Research, the American Geriatrics Society, and the Alliance for Aging Research, Butler was also Medical Editor-in-Chief of *Geriatrics* from 1986 to 2000. These accomplishments and others were reflected in the strong leadership he brought to the Department, and, in his work as consultant and oft-quoted source for the television, radio, and print media, Butler brought with him the kind of visibility that prompted patients to seek out care at Mount Sinai's new Department.

Other key players in the Department included Christine Cassel, the first Fellowship Director, Fred Sherman, who joined as an Associate Professor upon the Department's inception, and Diane Meier, an Assistant Professor. As Libow remembers, when the new faculty arrived, "there was no plate on the door, no computer, not even a typewriter. Just a space, the legacy of Elmhurst, and Fred Sherman."[12]

With the creation of the Department came Mount Sinai's own geriatric fellowship program, which remains to this day one of the largest such programs in the country, enrolling seven Fellows in each of the two years of the program. The fellowship program's components include education, research, and clinical care for a range of geriatric patients, from the healthy elderly to the acutely ill or frail to institutionalized patients. In a program that was unique from the very start—particularly given that there were no standardized guidelines for a geriatric fellowship at the time—Mount Sinai's Geriatrics Fellows were all either board certified or board eligible in internal medicine or family medicine. In a marked shift from the earlier reluctance of clinicians to become associated with geriatric medicine, the applicant pool for this program far exceeded the number of available positions.

By July 1983, the Coffey Geriatrics Outpatient Clinic had opened its doors, and Department members were able to begin seeing ambulatory patients. Around the same time, the inpatient Geriatric Evaluation and Treatment Unit (GETU)—later renamed the Acute Care for the Elderly (ACE) Unit—was established. Both programs, and indeed all branches of the Geriatrics Department, utilize a team-based multidisciplinary approach and focus on helping patients to regain and/or maintain the highest level of functional independence possible. At the Jewish Home and Hospital, the Rehabilitation of the Frail Elderly Program strives to achieve similar goals and includes a home visit by an occupational or physical therapist prior to discharge to ensure that a patient will be able to function in his or her home environment.

Additional programs created between 1983 and 1985 include the Osteoporosis and Metabolic Bone Disease Program, the first osteoporosis clinic in New York, started in collaboration with the Department of Obstetrics, Gynecology, and Reproductive Science; the Gait, Falls, and Immobility Program; the Urinary Incontinence Program, staffed by the Departments of Geriatrics, Urology, and Obstetrics, Gynecology, and Reproductive Science; and the Geriatric Psychiatry Program, a joint effort to ensure continuity of care between clinical departments and research centers within the Departments of Geriatrics and Psychiatry. Butler sought to combat the prevailing concept of ageism among medical students by exposing them to healthy, vigorous older persons. To accomplish this, he created Ronald Adelman's Well Elderly Program with members of the senior division at the 92nd Street Y. This program offers fourth-year medical students the opportunity to gain a more well-rounded understanding of the elderly in their community by working once a week with active, independent older people, while teaching them about various aspects of healthy living and disease prevention.

The year 1985 marked the fiftieth anniversary of Social Security, the twentieth anniversary of Medicare, and the tenth anniversary of the NIA. This was also a year in which Mount Sinai graduated its first geriatrics Fellows, created a position for the first geriatrics cardiology Fellow, and initiated the Center for Productive Aging, which became operational a year later. On the research front, Mount Sinai, in a collaborative effort with the Department of Psychiatry and the Bronx Veterans Administration Medical Center, established one of the first five Alzheimer Disease Research Centers in the country and became one of the first medical centers in the country to receive federal funding for the study of Alzheimer's disease.[13]

By July 1986, Mount Sinai's affiliation with the Bronx VA had extended to the inclusion of the VA facility as a teaching nursing home site. As Libow's responsibilities both as Vice Chairman at Mount Sinai and as Chief of Medical Services at the Jewish Home and Hospital for Aged continued to grow, Myron Miller joined the Department as Vice Chair of Acute Care, thus enabling Libow to focus his energies as Vice Chair of Long-Term Care.

Geriatrics now had a secure enough footing to expand its services within the community in other ways, as well. In one example, the Departments of Geriatrics and Adult Development, Social Work Services, and Nursing established, in 1986, the Elder Abuse Assessment and Assistance program, which sought to train medical, nursing, and social work staff to identify and assist victims of elder abuse. Barbara Paris, by this time co-director with Diane Meier of the outpatient clinic, oversaw the project, the first hospital-based, interdisciplinary elder abuse program in New York. Another far-reaching program developed around that time was the East Harlem Living-at-Home Program, chaired by Judith Howe, Ph.D., which endeavored to find alternatives to institutionalized care of the elderly. Perhaps the Department's largest undertaking, and the brainchild of Butler and Howe, was Linkage House, federal HUD section 202 housing on 118th Street for lower-income elderly, created to help address the substandard living conditions of many geriatric patients living in East Harlem. The Department secured a grant for Linkage House in 1991, broke ground in 1996, and, under the direction of Howe, spearheaded the formation of a still vibrant partnership with community-based organizations to create an innovative seventy-unit building, modeled on the principles of shared living with enhanced on-site social and health care services.

In a turn of events that affected the entire Mount Sinai medical community, and the Department of Geriatrics and Adult Development even more profoundly, John W. Rowe, Professor of Geriatrics and Medicine, became President of The Mount Sinai Medical Center in 1987. While Chalmers had been the founder and was always a friend and advocate of the Department, Rowe's position as President, with a joint appointment in Medicine and Geriatrics, even more firmly cemented the Department's place at Mount Sinai. Rowe's involvement in the national geriatric community included the Presidency of the American

Federation for Aging Research (AFAR), as well as the Chairmanship of the Committee on Leadership for Geriatric Medicine of the Institute of Medicine, National Academy of Sciences. Rowe also directed the MacArthur Foundation's National Research Network of Successful Aging and was President of the Gerontological Society of America in 1988–1989.

In 1987, stimulated by the Mount Sinai program, the first nationally recognized formal guidelines for geriatric fellowship training programs were published. The certifying examination for a Special Certificate of Competency in Geriatric Medicine was developed jointly by the American Board of Internal Medicine and the American Board of Family Practice in 1988. All Fellows subsequently took this examination to obtain geriatric certification. Those pioneers, of whom there were many at Mount Sinai, who had been practicing geriatric medicine for years but who had not completed a formal fellowship because they were the creators of the existing fellowship programs, were certified through a "grandfather" provision.

In 1990, Butler inaugurated the United States branch of the International Leadership Center on Longevity and Society, now the International Longevity Center (ILC), the "first private, non-partisan, non-profit, international center of research, education, and policy development, devoted exclusively to longevity and population aging."[14] Importantly, while ILC is a freestanding nonprofit 501-C3 organization, it remains a unit of the Mount Sinai Department of Geriatrics and Adult Development, and the Chair of the Department and the Dean of the School are automatically members of the ILC board.

As the climate nationally was warming to the idea of an academic specialty in geriatric medicine, so too was the environment at Mount Sinai. Students had gone from their earlier protest letters over forced time in a teaching nursing home to the founding of a Geriatrics Student Interest Group at the Medical School. At the Hospital, the educational and clinical components of the GETU were integrated with the Department of Medicine through the Division of Clinical Geriatric Medicine, allowing Medicine House Staff to take on a primary-care role in the GETU, while Fellows assumed more teaching and supervisory roles. By 1991, all Mount Sinai Medicine Residents were required to rotate through the geriatric inpatient unit; within a year similar rotations were required of Internal Medicine Residents throughout the United States. Recognizing, however, that there was a need to offer geriatric training to clinical specialists beyond those in internal or family medicine, the Department established the Commonwealth Fund Scholars Program, which enables specialists in other fields to become experts in the geriatric aspects of their own areas.

In 1995, Butler decided to leave his position as Chairman of the Geriatrics Department to become President and Chief Executive Officer of the International Longevity Center. The torch was passed to Christine Cassel. After serving as Chief of the Division of Primary Care Medicine and building up a geriatrics program at the University of Chicago, Cassel returned to take over as Chair at Mount Sinai because she admired the Department's approach to geriatric medicine and its creation of "a national platform through visibility and visionary work."[15] Cassel ushered the Department into a new era, with a reinvigorated emphasis on research and policy change, as well as new directions in patient care. One indicator of this change was Cassel's insistence that her acceptance of the Chair be contingent upon the creation of a Vice Chair for Research, to which she appointed John Morrison, Ph.D., Co-Director of the Arthur M. Fishberg Center for Neurobiology. Later, Morrison also became director of the newly formed Laboratory for Neurobiology of Aging, a venture jointly sponsored by the Department of Geriatrics and the Fishberg Center.

In addition to holding the Chair of the Department of Geriatrics and Adult Development, Cassel became Director of the Geriatric Research, Education, and Clinical Center (GRECC) at the Bronx Veterans Affairs Medical Center and Director of the Center to Advance Palliative Care, a national program office of the Robert Wood Johnson Foundation. Cassel's many appointments included membership in the prestigious Institute of Medicine of the National Academy of Sciences. She also served as President of the American College of Physicians in 1996–1997 and as the Chairman of the American Board of Internal Medicine in 2001–2003, distinctions even more notable because she is the first woman to hold either of these leadership positions.

One of the first major events after Cassel took over as Chair was the merging of the Coffey Outpatient Geriatrics Clinic with the Geriatrics Medicine Associates, the faculty practice group of the Department. This move allowed for further integration of resources and enabled both private and clinic patients to benefit from an interdisciplinary team approach. Barbara Paris took over as Medical Director of the Clinic, and Diane Meier became Chief of the Division of Geriatrics within the Department of Medicine, as well as the Director of the Palliative Care Center. Fred Sherman also returned to Mount Sinai in 1996 as Vice Chair for Clinical Affairs and soon became the Medical Director of the Program for All-Inclusive Care for the Elderly (PACE). PACE has enabled nursing home–eligible patients with Medicare and Medicaid to receive long-term care at home, rather than being forced into a nursing institution.

Keeping abreast of the Department's continued expansion, in 1996, the ACE Unit increased in size from seventeen to thirty-four beds and moved from the Klingenstein Clinical Center to the new Guggenheim Pavilion. The following year, Barbara Paris took over as Chief of the Geriatric Consult Service, ensuring continuity of care for patients who need to be admitted to the Hospital but who are placed in units other than ACE. Rosanne Leipzig, M.D., Ph.D., also joined the faculty that year as Director of Medical Education and Training, which included direction of the Fellowship Program. An internationally recognized leader in the movement for evidence-based medicine, Leipzig established the Center for Evidence-Based Medicine and Aging, in collaboration with Albert Siu, Chief of the Division of General Internal Medicine, who has joint appointments in Geriatrics and in Medicine. Along with Leipzig, the current Co-Director of the Center is Jane Sisk, a well-known health economist who is a Professor of Health Policy.

In 1995, Diane Meier and Sean Morrison, a Mount Sinai geriatrics Fellow in 1993 and a new addition to the faculty in 1995, began to lay the groundwork for a program in palliative care with the active support of both Butler and later Cassel. By 1997, the Palliative Care Clinical Consultation Service was established, and, in January 1988, Mount Sinai's Palliative Care Unit opened. The Department of Geriatrics has since remained at the forefront of academic palliative care, actively promoting hospital-based palliative care, clinical research, and education. The staff is drawn from a broad range of specialties, including Infectious Disease, Oncology, and Critical Care. Among the Program's most pressing objectives is the integration and normalization of palliative care. Consequently, Sean Morrison has been leading one of the most active academic research initiatives in palliative care in the country. He has addressed such issues as palliative care and nth-stage dementia, cross-cultural issues as they relate to palliative care and to end-of-life care, and inequalities in healthcare, including the failure of pharmacies based in underserved communities to stock opioid analgesics.[16] Meier has been a leader in creating a national model for palliative care and for improving the care of patients and was the first author on a groundbreaking and daring paper on physician-assisted suicide.[17] Meier, Morrison, and others in the program are deeply invested in examining health care in a larger context and in looking at clinical research issues that have the potential to drive social policy.[18]

Other research initiatives in the Department cover a wide range of topics and encompass both basic science and clinical work. In the Kastor Neurobiology of Aging Laboratories (KNAL), researchers are currently examining the basis for age-related changes in memory, led by the studies of John Morrison, Matthew Shapiro, and Peter Rapp. Hormone-brain interactions in aging is another key area of research at KNAL, including Andrea Gore's study of the neurobiological and behavioral effects of estrogen in the aging brain. Charles Mobbs has developed evidence that neurological and metabolic impairments during aging correlate with an age-related decline in the hormone leptin and is currently researching the effects of replacing leptin during aging. In the Division of Experimental Diabetes and Aging, Director Helen Vlassara has identified glycoxidation as one of the major mechanisms that can lead to diabetes-related complications and has conducted studies on small molecules that prevent such complications by inhibiting and/or reversing the glycoxidative damage.

In October 2001, Cassel announced that she would leave Mount Sinai to become Dean of the Oregon Health and Science University School of Medicine, where she had earlier been a Fellow in Geriatrics and a member of the faculty. Bruce Vladeck, Ph.D., Professor of Health Policy and Geriatrics and Director of Mount Sinai's Institute for Medicare Practice, was named the Acting Chairman.

The Brookdale Department of Geriatrics and Adult Development has come a long way since its inception in 1983. Governed by a holistic sense of health and wellbeing, the Department believes that medicine has an obligation to care for both the individual and the community in all aspects of health. As the first and still one of only three freestanding departments of academic geriatric medicine in the country, the Mount Sinai Department has more than proven that geriatrics is not simply a branch of another specialty. Rather than caring only for the very frail or the very ill, the field of geriatric medicine encompasses an "understanding [of] aging as part of the life cycle, and [is] working to improve the quality of life for individuals throughout the life cycle."[19]

20

Department of Neurology

NEUROLOGY HAD ITS ORIGIN as a specialty at Mount Sinai in June 1890, when a clinic for neurologic cases was created in the newly opened dispensary building at 67th Street and Lexington Avenue.

Three years later, Bernard Sachs was appointed as "Consultant" Neurologist to the Hospital and placed in charge of the Clinic. Attracted to neurology while still an undergraduate, Sachs pursued postgraduate study with a number of eminent neuropsychiatrists both in America and abroad, including Sigmund Freud. In 1887, Sachs described the syndrome of "arrested cerebral development,"[1] which he later termed "amaurotic familial idiocy."[2] As Warren Tay had previously described the ophthalmologic features of the same condition, the eponym Tay-Sachs disease became synonymous with what would become recognized as one of the most important of the "Jewish genetic diseases." Sachs also published important works on muscular dystrophies and cerebral palsy.[3,4] In 1885, he opened his own practice and became Co-Editor, then Editor of the *Journal of Nervous and Mental Diseases*. He wrote the first pediatric neurology textbook in America, entitled *Nervous Disease of Children*, in 1895.[5] As Sachs's reputation grew, so did his practice. He acquired a large "society" clientele and was said to have made house calls in the 1890s in a high silk hat. An astute social observer and far ahead of his time, Sachs, as early as 1892, also expressed his concern over the evils of medical expert testimony in trials.[6]

As the Mount Sinai clinic became more widely known, and in recognition of the growth of neurology and the importance of Sachs' work, six male and six female beds were assigned in 1900 for an inpatient service, constituting the first neurologic wards in New York City. Very steady in temperament, very proper and formal in attitude, Sachs, as Chief, stressed that house officers and all physicians must look neat, be scrupulously clean, use good English, and articulate distinctly. A dedicated teacher, Sachs espoused the principle of bedside diagnosis made by a good history and complete physical examination. During

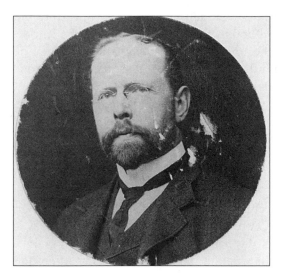

Bernard Sachs, M.D., Chief
of Neurology, 1900–1925.

Sachs's many absences on professional business, Isadore Abramson
was the principal teacher on the service.

Shortly after the Hospital's move to 100th Street, epidemics of poliomyelitis and encephalitis led to a major report by a New York
City–sponsored investigation committee chaired by Sachs.[7] After a period of study in Berlin, in August von Wassermann's laboratory, Sachs
introduced the new Wassermann test for syphilis at Mount Sinai, and
the Department critically assessed its use.[8] The establishment of the
Neuropathology Laboratory in 1920, directed by Joseph H. Globus, led
to a growing emphasis on clinico-pathologic correlations. With the
ever-increasing volume of patients, the bed allocation of the service was
increased to thirty-six in 1922.

Sachs was a world leader in the field of neurology. Elected President of the American Neurological Association in 1894, he was again
elected to the position thirty-eight years later, one of only three men to
have twice held the position in the history of the organization. Sachs
was also responsible for initiating, organizing, and serving as President
of the First International Congress in Neurology, in 1931. "His personal
acquaintance with neurologists all over the world, his universal popu-
larity, delicate diplomacy, and his personal generosity made the Congress a great success."[9]

Sachs achieved great renown in the field of neurology, but his fame
was surpassed by that of an old acquaintance and colleague, Sigmund

Freud. The two had been fellow students in Vienna while studying under Theodor Meynert. Although Sachs acknowledged the importance of Freud's ideas of the unconscious and the subconscious, he strongly disagreed with Freud's theories of infant sexuality and erotic dreams.[10] In fact, in the 1920s, when a number of doctors on the Mount Sinai staff were analyzed by Freud, Sachs voiced intense frustration. The pro- and anti-Freud sentiments raging among the neurologists of the day made for lively debates during meetings of The New York Academy of Medicine.

In 1925, Israel Strauss succeeded Sachs as Chief of Neurology. An Intern at Mount Sinai in 1898, Strauss later pursued postgraduate study in neurology and psychiatry in Vienna, where he developed an interest in psychoanalysis. On his return to the United States, he was appointed Assistant Adjunct Physician and Associate in Neuropathology at Mount Sinai, where he rose through the ranks of the Attending staff.

Strauss was convinced that New York needed an institution for mentally ill patients who were too sick to be treated as ambulatory patients, yet not sick enough to be admitted to a state hospital. Therefore, Strauss organized the Committee of Mental Health among Jews in 1917. Eventually, this led to the establishment of the Hillside Hospital in 1927, where patients were treated with psychodynamic and psychoanalytic methods. In 1919, Strauss and Leo Loewe[11] were the first to succeed in the experimental transmission of encephalitis lethargica.[12]

As Chief, Strauss assigned four of the thirty-six service beds to psychiatry and in 1923 established a new residency program. In the ensuing years, the staff was expanded, and its activities remained chiefly clinical. Moses Keschner, appointed in 1920, contributed to the understanding of the dyskinesias. Globus continued his work on the pathology of brain tumors. Always interested in the malignant gliomas, Globus and Strauss introduced the term "spongioblastoma."[13] Cushing and Bailey, at Harvard, named the same tumor "glioblastoma," and this difference in nomenclature created spirited discussions at various neurological society meetings and ultimately led to the modern classification of brain tumors. Without question, Globus's most important contribution to Mount Sinai was as the founding Editor of the *Journal of The Mount Sinai Hospital* in 1934, a position he held for eighteen years. Globus also founded the *Journal of Neuropathology and Experimental Neurology* in 1942.

Neurological therapy during the 1920s and 1930s consisted chiefly of the treatment of syphilis of the central nervous system and the management of the psychoneuroses. More psychiatrists were added to the staff, the best known being Clarence Oberndorf, Sandor Lorand, and Dudley Schoenfeld, each a pioneer in the psychoanalytic field. Most of their activities were in the outpatient clinics.

Strauss flourished at a time when the discipline of neurology was becoming increasingly concerned with clinical and pathological relationships and specific treatments. During this period, Strauss was interested in the psychiatric aspects of head injuries and brain tumors and published major works on these topics in association with Nathan Savitsky[14] and Keschner.[15] Strauss served as President of the American Neurological Association in 1934.

Israel S. Wechsler succeeded Strauss in 1938. A Romanian immigrant, Wechsler was educated in America and joined Mount Sinai in 1916 as Clinical Assistant in Neurology. About this time he also became Instructor of Neurology at the Columbia University College of Physicians and Surgeons, where he would eventually become Professor. From 1921 to 1925, Wechsler served as Adjunct Attending in Neurology at Mount Sinai. He then left to work at Montefiore Hospital before returning to Mount Sinai as Chief in 1938.

By that time, his classic book *Textbook of Clinical Neurology*[16] had become the standard text on the subject and had been translated into many languages; it would go through nine editions. Wechsler was also well known for his work on movement disorders.[17] In 1936, Richard Brickner's publication, *The Intellectual Functions of the Frontal Lobe*, created much interest, and his monograph is still quoted.[18] In 1939, psychiatry was placed under the leadership of Lawrence Kubie, whose thinking was physiologically as well as psychoanalytically oriented. Kubie and his group of well-known psychoanalysts became nationally prominent and greatly influenced modern psychiatry. Kubie believed that psychiatry should stand on its own feet and, when thwarted in his ability to separate from neurology, resigned. This led, rather promptly, to the formation of a committee, chaired by the Trustee Joseph Klingenstein, which recommended that a new Department of Psychiatry be created.[19]

During his thirteen-year tenure, Wechsler set the stage for the future growth of the Department by procuring substantial funds from the federal government and from private benefactors to support research,

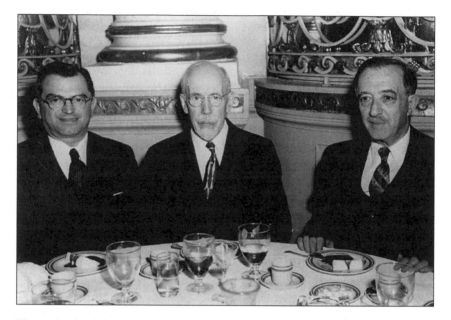

Three chiefs of Neurology, left to right: Morris B. Bender, M.D.(1951–1973), Israel Strauss, M.D.(1925–1938), and Israel Wechsler, M.D.(1938–1951).

fellowships, and Residents in Neurology. Later in his career, in 1958, Wechsler served as President of the American Neurological Association.

In the decade before World War II, two men, Morris B. Bender and Edwin Weinstein, joined the Department. Engaged in neurophysiology research, they kept a small colony of monkeys in a small basement animal room and studied the physiology of brainstem functions and eye movements, especially on the median longitudinal fasciculus.[20] On the lighter side, one day a monkey escaped from the laboratory and perched on the windowsill of a very frightened female patient, who let out the expected scream. As Weinstein later recollected, "That poor little monkey; by the time the rumors had stopped flying, it was the size of King Kong."[21]

Called into the military, Bender and Weinstein were given the opportunity to do research, work that they would continue after their return to civilian life. Weinstein, a major in the U.S. Army Medical Corps, studied the behavioral and emotional disorders associated with brain lesions, culminating in his book *Denial of Illness*.[22] Weinstein also penned a fascinating book on Woodrow Wilson, whose life and presidency were marked by a series of minor strokes and subsequent personality changes.[23]

Bender, a commander in the U.S. Navy, conducted a series of studies on disorders of perception and on visual field defects caused by shrapnel injuries of the brain.[24] After the war, he continued with his investigations on perception of double, simultaneous stimulations in healthy individuals, as well as in brain-damaged subjects.[25] Bender and his colleagues made numerous contributions in the area of determining eye movement. These included a study of the representation of eye muscles in the oculomotor nucleus; discovery of the basis of the various types of eye muscle paralysis; mapping of the regions of the cortex, cerebral hemispheres and brainstem, which are important in oculomotor function; and identification of regions of the brainstem, where even tiny lesions can cause weakness of gaze.[26]

With the introduction of electroencephalography and neuroradiology in the immediate postwar years, a clear trend developed toward the use of laboratory methods in clinical neurology. Research moved toward basic science; psychiatry, while still practiced by some staff members, gradually became extinct within the Neurology Department.

In 1951, Bender succeeded Wechsler as Chief of Service. The next few years saw major changes in the Department, with an emphasis on research and training. The residency program was expanded with the aid of federally sponsored training grants. The Department grew rapidly in all areas. There was greater emphasis on the medical care of neurologic patients. An arch proponent of the nonoperative management of subdural hematomas[27] and malignant cerebral neoplasms, Bender treated these lesions with steroids and/or chemotherapy, rather than surgery.

Research also accelerated. Between 1952 and 1962, laboratories in experimental and clinical neurophysiology, visual function, oculomotor physiology, neurochemistry, cellular physiology, and neuroendocrinology were opened as Divisions within the Department. Later, laboratories in neurovirology and clinical neurophysiology were added. Special clinics for myasthenia gravis and neuromuscular disorders, headaches, seizures, aneurysms, dyskinesias, and vestibular dysfunctions were established. Neuro-ophthalmology was introduced as a subspecialty based on oculomotor system and visual function research.

Pediatric neurology, first introduced by Bernard Sachs, became fully developed within the Department in 1961 under the direction of Nicholas Christoff. Since 1967, the division has been under the direction of Alan Aron, whose major research interests are seizure disorders in children, hydrocephalus, and neurofibromatosis (for which Mount Sinai has the largest clinic in the United States).

In 1956, Bender was the first to classify what he called "transient circulatory disturbance of the brain," which came to be known as transient global ischemia.[28] By 1968, there were between eighty and 110 patients with neurologic disorders in the Hospital at any given time.

With the creation of the Mount Sinai School of Medicine, all members of the Hospital attending staff were appointed to the faculty in 1966. In 1968, the Henry P. and Georgette Goldschmidt Chair in Neurology was endowed by Mrs. Lucy Moses and was first occupied by Bender. The staff, which then consisted of thirteen full-time and a large number of part-time members, participated in the teaching of neurosciences and clinical neurology to medical students and gave special courses in the newly established Page and William Black Post-Graduate School of Medicine. The Mount Sinai group continued to maintain its tradition of prominence in American neurology. As evidence of this excellence, eighteen members of the staff were members of the American Neurological Association in 1972–1973, the year Bender served as its President.

Bender retired in 1973, having been responsible for the training of more than 250 neurologists and having earned the title "Father of Neuro-Ophthalmology in the United States."[29] He continued to conduct his renowned phenomenology rounds on Saturday mornings, often lasting into the afternoon. In fact, he conducted the last one on the day before his death in 1983. During the span of four decades, he created a tradition of patient management that combined observation, diagnosis, treatment, and compassion and that many of his colleagues characterized as "Benderian Neurology." A well-known anecdote has a young colleague asking Bender why he never cultivated any outside interests, such as golf. Bender is reported to have responded, gesturing toward a patient floor, "This is my golf."

In 1974, Melvin D. Yahr was appointed Chairman and Goldschmidt Professor of Neurology. Yahr came to Mount Sinai with a previously established international reputation for excellence in research on Parkinson's disease.[30] While at Columbia University's Neurological Institute,

Yahr and his team played a pioneering role in the development of L-dopa therapy in the treatment of Parkinson's and conducted one of the earliest controlled trials of the drug.[31] In 1969, he served as President of the American Neurological Association, the fifth individual associated with Mount Sinai to lead that organization. Yahr brought the Clinical Center for Parkinson's Disease with him, making Mount Sinai one of the world's leaders in the research and clinical care of this disease.

During Yahr's tenure, notable advances were made by the faculty not only in the diagnosis, pathophysiology, genetics, natural history, biochemistry, behavioral aspects, and treatment of Parkinson's disease but also across a wide spectrum of other neurological diseases. Roger Duvoisin investigated the role of genetics in Parkinson's; Teresita Elizan studied the neurovirology of Parkinson's, Alzheimer's, and amyotrophic lateral sclerosis; Andreas Plaitakis also investigated amyotrophic lateral sclerosis; and Joan Borod researched brain/behavior relationships for emotion in stroke, aphasic, Parkinson's, and psychiatric patients. Borod also established and directs the Neuropsychology Testing Service at Mount Sinai, which provides neuropsychological assessment on cognitive and affective functioning in a variety of patients.

A number of Bender's appointees have remained at Mount Sinai and have had distinguished careers in neurology and the neurosciences. For more than four decades, Tauba Pasik and Pedro Pasik have studied the oculomotor system of primates, utilizing physiologically induced lesions. Their discoveries have led to a more precise localization of brain lesions that cause disturbances of gaze in humans. This research has paved the way for the exploration of "blindsight" in human patients with visual field defects and for the possibilities of improving their vision through training.[32] Computer models were developed to simulate neuronal circuits with the goal of better understanding the role of the lateral geniculate nucleus in processing visual information. In these and other studies, the advanced computer-assisted stereologic methods utilized by the Pasiks have served as a model for other laboratories. In addition, using the hemiparkinsonian monkey, the Pasiks have studied the use of human sympathetic ganglia as a source of brain implants to improve the clinical picture of Parkinson patients. They have demonstrated a long survival time for these implants, as well as the growth of presumably dopaminergic processes into the host tissue, where they establish synaptic connections.[33]

A vital member of the Department, whose work has spanned the tenure of three Chairs, is Bernard Cohen. Known for his work on the vestibular and oculomotor systems, Cohen and his colleagues defined the specific eye movements and patterns of muscle activation produced by individual semicircular canals[34] and demonstrated the neural basis for saccidic eye movements. Later, with Theodore Raphan, of Brooklyn College, Cohen discovered "velocity storage," a process in the vestibular system that is responsible for important characteristics of the vestibulo-ocular reflex.[35] Active in projects relative to the NASA space program and involving interplanetary exploration, Cohen began conducting space studies in 1988 on how eye movements respond to gravity and how balance is organized and maintained in the brain. Later, in 1998, Cohen was involved in the Space Shuttle Neurolab Mission, in which astronauts were centrifuged in space. The researchers found that centrifugation is an effective countermeasure for otolith-ocular deconditioning that occurs during adaptation to microgravity.[36] In February 2001, Cohen was chosen to be Associate Team Leader for the Neurovestibular Adaption Team of the National Space Biomedical Research Institute. The team will research solutions to space motion sickness and body-orientation problems experienced during and after space missions and will later apply these techniques to the treatment of balance disorders here on earth. Cohen founded the Graduate Program in Neurobiology in the Medical School in 1980 and directed it for ten years.

In 1986, the Fishberg Center for Neurobiology was established as a basic science division to investigate the molecular mechanisms for various neurobiological phenomena and to provide continuing interaction with the Department of Neurology and the basic sciences.

At the time of Yahr's retirement in 1991, Mount Sinai was one of the largest neurological training centers in the country. Howard Lipton was chosen to succeed Yahr but left after a brief tenure, and Cohen became the acting Chairman until the appointment of C. Warren Olanow in 1994.

Canadian by birth, Olanow came to Mount Sinai from the University of South Florida. As each Chairman in turn has taken the Department to a new plateau, so it has been with Olanow. With a major interest in Parkinson's disease and the movement disorders, Olanow and his colleagues have continued studies on the iron-infusion model of Parkinsonism, fetal nigral transplantation, and treatment with L-Deprenyl. A program for neuropsychological investigation of deep brain stimulation in movement disorder patients has shown favorable early results.[37]

The Department's established investigators and newly recruited faculty have continued to make major clinical and laboratory contributions. There has been a significant increase in extramural grant support and philanthropic support.

Stuart Sealfon's laboratory pursues the interdisciplinary study of G-protein coupled neurohormone and neurotransmitter receptors. Specific areas of interest include the receptor determinants of hallucinogen effects, structure/function studies of the gonadotropin-releasing hormone receptor, and the function of dopamine receptors in vivo.

Mitchell Brin's dystonia program has expanded and has been involved in early research on the use of botulinum toxin as therapy.[38] Recently, Brin and Pullani Shashidharan have investigated the role of the protein torsinA in neuronal dysfunction in Parkinson's disease and dystonia.

David Simpson was the lead investigator of one of the first randomized, placebo-controlled clinical trials to demonstrate the efficacy of botulinum toxin in the treatment of upper extremity spasticity following stroke. Simpson is currently Director of the Neuro-AIDS Research Program that works to develop treatments for nervous system complications of HIV infection.[39] Simpson has also served as Chairman of the Neurology Subcommittee of the AIDS Clinical Trials Group.

Senior clinicians have long played a major role in the Department. David Coddon directed the Headache Clinic for decades. In 1996, Seymour Gendelman, a member of the Department since the beginning of his residency in 1965 and an outstanding clinician, was recruited to the full-time faculty and given responsibility for the training program. Under his leadership, the educational program has been strengthened to become one of the most sought-after residency programs in the nation.

With the opening of the Neuroscience and Restorative Care Center in the new Guggenheim Pavilion in 1996, Neurology has forged a closer relationship with neurosurgery, neurobiology, psychiatry, and rehabilitation medicine, placing the neuroscience program at Mount Sinai in a position of excellence as it moves into the twenty-first century.

(Adapted from an article by Morris B. Bender, published in *The Spectrum*, no. 3 (spring 1973), pp 4–5, a publication of the Associated Alumni of Mount Sinai.)

21

Department of Neurosurgery

ALTHOUGH THERE IS little doubt that Charles A. Elsberg deserves the accolade "Father of Neurosurgery" at Mount Sinai, neurosurgical procedures were performed in the last decades of the nineteenth century, before his time. In 1885, William Fluhrer, best known as a urologist, successfully extracted a "pistol-ball" from the brain, tracing it with a probe.[1] Arpad Gerster and Bernard Sachs first reported on the surgery of epilepsy in 1892[2] with a follow-up paper four years later.[3] In 1895, Leopold Stieglitz, Gerster, and Howard Lilienthal reported three operated cases of brain tumors.[4] Known primarily as a general surgeon, Gerster was responsible for the early training of two men who would go on to fame in neurosurgery—Elsberg and Ernest Sachs, the nephew of Bernard Sachs, Mount Sinai's first Chief of Neurology. Ernest Sachs would later achieve eminence as the Chair of Neurosurgery at Washington University in St. Louis. In 1896, William Van Arsdale reported on "temporary resection of the skull," utilizing a circular saw and trephine that he had devised.[5]

Born and educated in New York, Charles A. Elsberg had his early training at Mount Sinai and then studied abroad. In 1896, he was appointed First Assistant Pathologist to Frederick S. Mandlebaum, the newly appointed Director of the laboratory. Elsberg's first publication on the use of the Widal reaction in typhoid fever diagnosis was subsequently responsible for tracing an epidemic of typhoid fever among the nursing staff to a probable carrier. He also was responsible for the first animal experimental study to come out of the new laboratories.[6] Although Elsberg's first neurosurgical publication, reporting two cases of cerebello-pontine angle tumors, appeared in 1904,[7] it would be six years before his next neurosurgical paper appeared. But he was far from idle. He maintained his interests not only in general surgery but also in the laboratory. In that interval, he published extensively on general surgical subjects and, in 1909, described an ingenious cannula for direct artery-to-vein transfusion.[8] On the basis of extensive experimental work,

Elsberg administered the first successful endotracheal anesthetic in 1910;[9] over the next several years, he played a major role in the development of this technique. In 1909, Elsberg helped to found the Neurological Institute, at first an independent entity. The first site of the Institute was at 145 East 67th Street, a leased building that had originally been the Mount Sinai Out-patient Department building and Nurse's Home. When the Institute became part of Columbia University's College of Physicians and Surgeons and moved to Washington Heights in 1929, Elsberg took an active part in planning the building and its operating rooms. During construction, he was known to climb the unfinished building at 168th Street to watch its progress.

Elsberg developed an overriding interest in the surgery of the spinal cord and in 1910 recommended that all cord tumors be operated on in two stages.[10] In the first stage, after opening the dura, a small incision was made in the pia over the tumor, allowing the tumor to extrude itself from the cord so that it could be more easily removed at the second stage. In 1912, Elsberg reported a series of forty-three cases of laminectomy for various spinal cord lesions.[11] In that same year, Pearce Bailey, of New York, in discussing another presentation by Elsberg,[12] commented, "Intramedullary surgery has been done previously.... But Elsberg, as far as I know, is the first to take the matter up systematically."[13] Bailey also made a strong case for the emerging specialty of neurosurgery, noting that "Neurologists should be insisting that experienced neurologic surgeons should do all the operations."[14]

Originally assigned to the Surgical Service of Howard Lilienthal, Elsberg was placed in charge of the Neurosurgical Service in 1914 when a major reorganization of Surgery took place. As Chief of the Service, Elsberg was responsible for instituting the changes (special instruments and drapes, nurses with special training in neurosurgical procedures, and, eventually, a separate operating room)[15] that set the stage for the superb Service of today. In collaboration with Harvey Cushing, of Harvard, and Charles H. Frazier, of Philadelphia, Elsberg helped establish the Society of Neurological Surgeons in 1920. In 1929, Elsberg left Mount Sinai to work full-time at the Neurological Institute, where he remained until his retirement in 1937. The following year, he was elected President of the American Neurological Association. He died in 1948, having championed the growth of his specialty locally, nationally, and internationally. Not only did he play a major role in the establishment of two leading neurosurgical services in New York, but also he

Ira Cohen, M.D., Chief of
the Neurosurgery Service,
1932–1950.

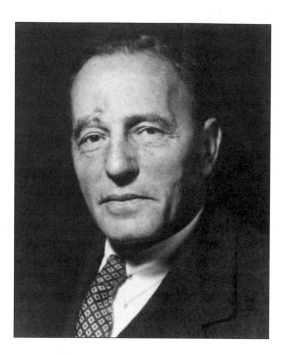

was responsible for the training of the next generation of neurosurgeons at two institutions. In addition, he left behind four major texts[16–19] and four volumes of reprints containing more than 150 publications.

When Elsberg left Mount Sinai in 1929, Harold Neuhof was appointed Chief of the Neurosurgical Service. His professional passion, however, was thoracic surgery, and in 1932 Ira Cohen became the new Chief of Neurosurgery. A member of the staff since his internship in 1911, Cohen had a distinguished career in the military during World War I. As a Major assigned to Base Hospital No. 3 (the Mount Sinai unit), he served in France. Asked to establish a new hospital at Le Braun, France, he outfitted it and ran it with distinction. While overseas, he suffered a head wound above his right brow that caused a skull fracture and a dural tear; awake and with the mirror in his hand, he instructed his colleagues as they debrided and repaired his wound.[20] The defect that remained was a distinguishing feature of every photograph of Cohen.

It was Cohen who in 1932 convinced the administration that Neurosurgery should be separated from the body of Surgery and have its own department. One year later, Cohen and Joseph Turner (then Director of the Hospital) noted, "The medical profession and the informed lay public were asking more insistently for trained specialists for these highly technical operations. . . . In no branch of surgery is it more important for the operating team to be constant. In no branch are results more dependent on attention to details, before, during, and after the operation."[21] An excellent teacher, Cohen established the formal residency in neurosurgery at Mount Sinai in 1946. Cohen was able to appoint only two Residents before his retirement in 1950. The first, Aron J. Beller, went on to become Chairman of the Department of Neurosurgery at Hadassah Hospital in Israel. The second was Leonard Malis.

Sidney W. Gross became Acting Chief upon Cohen's retirement. This appointment was short-lived, however, as Leo Davidoff was appointed Neurosurgeon to the Hospital effective February 1951. Davidoff was a brilliant individual who had received his neurosurgical training at the Peter Bent Brigham Hospital under Harvey Cushing. He had a penchant for accepting appointments at many of the hospitals in New York City and at one time or other had been the Chief at most of them. His tenure at Mount Sinai was short, and, after his resignation in June 1956, Gross was named Neurosurgeon to the Hospital and Chief of Service.

A midwesterner, Gross had trained in neurosurgery at the Neurological Institute under Elsberg. This was followed by a fellowship with Ernest Sachs in St. Louis and neuropathology training in Chicago. He was appointed to the Mount Sinai staff in 1938 and rose rapidly through the ranks of the attending staff. The first individual to use water-soluble contrast material for myelography,[22] Gross was an exceptional teacher who was revered by his Residents. In the early 1960s, the residency was expanded to include the City Hospital Center at Elmhurst, with its busy trauma service. Leonard Malis and Bruce Ralston were added to the attending staff. It was an interesting time to be a House Staff officer in neurosurgery. Anton Marti, a Resident during this period, has commented, "Because of differing personalities, backgrounds, and professional interests, the three attending neurosurgeons brought a wealth of concepts and operative approaches to the residency program. Dr. Gross drew from tried and true traditional methods. Dr. Malis brought consistent innovation to neurosurgical technique. Dr. Bruce Ralston never performed any operation the same way twice."[23] On Gross's mandatory retirement at age sixty-five, in 1969, he was appointed Director Emeritus and Consultant, and Malis was named Chief of Service.

Born in Philadelphia, Leonard I. Malis was brought up and received his early education in Atlantic City. An early bent toward technological innovation and a passion for electronics led him, as a youngster, to build a radio transmitter, boat and auto engines, and his first television set before the advent of commercial television.[24] He earned undergraduate and M.D. degrees at the University of Virginia. Following internship at the Philadelphia General Hospital, Malis served two years in the Army Medical Corps, where, without formal training, he emerged as the Chief of his hospital's Neurological Service.

Following his discharge from the military, Malis came to Mount Sinai, where he spent one year as a Neurology Resident under Israel Wechsler and then was appointed Ira Cohen's Resident in Neurosurgery. Funded by the Dazian Foundation, Malis spent a year in the laboratory of John Fulton at Yale, then a mecca for neuroscience researchers. There Malis began a number of studies that would be continued and refined throughout his professional lifetime. Recognized as a basic scientist and clinical investigator, an outstanding teacher and a superb neurosurgeon, Malis made many contributions to the field, including:

> the study of neurophysiology, creation of a true bipolar coagulator, design of a serial cassette changer for cerebral angiography, refinement of full-column myelography, understanding of spinal stenosis, introduction of the binocular microscope into the neurosurgical operating room, invention of many instruments key to neurosurgery, and perfection of microsurgical techniques to safely and completely remove tumors of the base of the skull, posterior fossa, pituitary, and spinal cord.[25]

At one point early in his tenure as Chief, Malis became concerned with a small but nevertheless serious incidence of wound infections on the Service. He instituted changes to the usual routine of antibiotic prophylaxis and added irrigation with topical antibiotic solutions. Over the subsequent five-year period, during which more than 1,700 cases were treated, the infection rate was reduced to zero, a remarkable feat.[26]

Under Malis's leadership, the Department expanded in dramatic fashion. With the opening of the surgical suite in the Annenberg building, two dedicated neurosurgical operating rooms were supported with neurosurgical specialist nurses. Malis developed, designed, and constructed a unique operating room television network that linked the operating rooms, Attending staff offices, the laboratories, and the neuroradiology suite. Laboratory space was enlarged; the residency program increased in size, attracting outstanding candidates who would receive unique training by a dedicated group of attendings. Ved Sachdev was a mainstay of the teaching program for many years until his death in 2000. Martin Camins, Allen Rothman, and Frank Moore continue their participation in all aspects of the Department's activities. Malis retired from the Chairmanship in 1991 but continued his practice for another three years. He was succeeded in the Chair by Kalmon D. Post.

Post, a native New Yorker, received his medical degree from the New York University School of Medicine, where he served his neurosurgical residency under the legendary Joseph Ransohoff. His training included a two-year appointment as a Clinical Associate in Surgical Neurology at the National Institute of Neurological Diseases and Blindness. Beginning his academic career at Tufts University, Post moved to Columbia University in 1980, rising through the ranks to become Vice Chairman of the Department of Neurological Surgery. He joined Mount Sinai in July 1991 as Chairman and Professor of the Department and Neurosurgeon to the Hospital.

Like his predecessor, Post has had a major interest in the management of acoustic and pituitary tumors. Follow-up of the patients with acoustic tumors has shown outstanding rates of hearing preservation and facial nerve function.[27] Long-term postoperative studies on a large group of patients with acromegaly have demonstrated excellent endocrine data and long-term cure rates.[28] The Department has been a beta test site for studying frameless stereotactic cranial surgery for more accurate and complete removal of primary and secondary brain tumors.[29] In the laboratory, researchers have studied the molecular biology of primary tumors, searching for a gene defect in pituitary tumors.[30–33]

The Department has extended its educational activities with a faculty that now consists of seven full-time and nine voluntary neurosurgeons and a research staff of seven. Joshua Bederson, Vice Chairman of the Department, directs the efforts in cerebrovascular surgery and is Co-Director of the Clinical Program for Cerebrovascular Disorders, a collaboration with the Department of Neurology. Isabelle Germano is Director of the Mount Sinai Medical Center Stereotactic and Functional Neurosurgery Program, an advanced multidisciplinary program that uses computer-assisted, image-guided neurosurgery to accomplish minimally invasive procedures. She is one of the pioneers of computer-assisted image-guided minimally invasive neurosurgery and an international expert in brain tumor, epilepsy, and movement disorder surgery. Subspecialization has also led to the development of expertise in endoscopic neurosurgery, microsurgery, physiologic monitoring in the operating room, and the surgery of epilepsy. The residency program is highly sought after. Collaborative programs have been initiated with the Departments of Pediatrics, Rehabilitation Medicine, and Otolaryngology. Surgical case volume has increased steadily to approximately 1,300 cases per year.

The surgeons performing neurosurgical procedures at the Mount Sinai Hospital for more than a century created an extraordinary legacy. Under the stewardship of Kalmon D. Post, the Department of Neurosurgery will further that legacy as it builds on its current excellence and formulates new initiatives in minimally invasive surgery, spinal disease, and the management of neurovascular abnormalities and tumors of the nervous system.

22

Department of Obstetrics, Gynecology, and Reproductive Sciences

ON AUGUST 10, 1856, a twenty-six-year old widow, with one healthy child, was admitted to the Jews' Hospital in her ninth month of pregnancy. Labor ensued on August 27, and at 8:34 P.M. she was "safely delivered of a fine male child,"[1] the first baby to be born at the Hospital. The postpartum course was apparently uncomplicated, although lengthy by today's standards, and, on September 22, "mother and child discharged in the enjoyment of good health."[2] This admission preceded the 1952 opening of the Obstetrical Service of the Mount Sinai Hospital by ninety-five years and eleven months.

Although obstetrical services were not offered at Mount Sinai until one hundred years after the Hospital's founding, the Gynecology Service came into early prominence. In 1877, medical and surgical services were established, with separate wards for each. In that year, Emil Noeggerath was appointed Gynecologist to the Hospital, marking an early step toward specialization in the institution.

Noeggerath was born and educated in Bonn, Germany. He subsequently emigrated to the United States, where he had expected an appointment to the medical school in St. Louis. When those plans failed to materialize, he established a highly successful practice in New York City in obstetrics and gynecology (OB/GYN). In collaboration with Abraham Jacobi, he co-authored *Contributions to Midwifery and Diseases of Women*.[3] He was also one of the founding Editors of the *American Journal of Obstetrics and Diseases of Women and Children*.

Noeggerath's research involved clinical studies on gonorrhea, including its etiology, the contagious aspects of the disease, and the fact that the disease caused sterility in women.[4] He also published on the development of carcinoma.[5] He resigned from the Hospital in 1882 over a dispute with the Trustees regarding operating privileges and returned to his native Germany, where he died of pulmonary tuberculosis in 1895.

Noeggerath was succeeded in 1882 by Paul Fortunatus Mundé, also born in Germany but brought to America at the age of four and raised in Massachusetts. His medical studies were interrupted by military service during the Civil War. After the war, he completed his studies at Harvard Medical School and spent seven years in Europe studying OB/GYN. On his return to the United States, Mundé succeeded Noeggerath as Editor of the *American Journal of Obstetrics*.

Mundé was named the first Chief of the Outpatient Gynecology Clinic in 1875: "Paul F. Mundé, with his magnificent presence and regal carriage, was affectionately admired by patients, nurses and House Staff alike."[6] Mundé's forte was gynecological surgery, a practice that in his time was approached by most surgeons and patients alike with fear and trepidation. An early disciple of aseptic and antiseptic surgery as propounded by Lord Joseph Lister, Mundé established scrupulous standards for surgery never before enforced by the Hospital.[7] He was concerned about performing extensive surgery and noted that contraindications to multiple procedures included long anesthesia time, a uterine discharge that could jeopardize a perineal repair, recent suturing in the perineum, and more than normal blood loss.[8] The results of his surgery were excellent for their time.

In dealing with cervical carcinoma, Mundé performed vaginal hysterectomies with an approximately 11 percent mortality rate. However, none of the patients was cured, and he later commented, "I have made up my mind most positively that in no case will I ever again remove the uterus for cancerous disease, whether of the cervix or the body, through the vagina or by abdominal section unless the organ is so movable that any possible extension of the disease to its surroundings can be absolutely excluded."[9]

Mundé held numerous appointments at institutions both in and out of New York City. During the mid-1880s, he was Consultant Surgeon to Mount Sinai. In 1898, he served as President of the American Gynecological Society; he was also named Honorary President of the International Congress of Obstetrics and Gynecology in 1897 and in 1899. Moreover, he was a prolific writer, authoring several books on obstetrical and gynecological management,[10] as well as a treatise on the use of electrical current as a therapeutic modality in gynecology.[11]

Under Mundé's leadership, the Gynecological Service expanded rapidly. The number of patient admissions increased from 181 in 1883 to 505 the following year. Most of the procedures were performed by Mundé himself, except during his summer vacations, when general surgeons substituted for him. In 1892, Joseph Brettauer was appointed Assistant Gynecologist to take charge of the service during the summer months. Ten years later, he succeeded Mundé as Gynecologist to the Hospital and Chief of the Gynecological Service.

Brettauer was born in the Austrian Tyrol in 1863 and received his medical degree from the University of Graz. He was well trained in general and plastic surgery, as well as in OB/GYN. He was an excellent operator in both vaginal and abdominal procedures, and he was also an exceptional organizer, whose emphasis on punctuality and esprit de corps were legacies impressed on the institution for decades to come. Brettauer served as President of both the New York Obstetrical Society and the American Gynecological Society.

Best known for his keen clinical insights and his conservative approach to therapy, Brettauer exerted wide influence, although he did little scientific writing. He was, however, one of the first to point out that prolonged postoperative ileus is almost always related to intra-abdominal infection and that an aseptic operation is the best guarantee of a good result.[12] Elevated to the rank of Consultant in 1925, Brettauer remained active in the Hospital until his death in 1941.

During Brettauer's tenure, the Gynecological Service was divided between him and Florian Krug. Trained in Germany, Krug settled in New York in 1885. Krug introduced the Trendelenberg position for gynecological surgery to America.[13] A bold surgeon and a striking personality, he wrote extensively on various subjects but never achieved the influence on the Service that Brettauer did. Krug was succeeded by Hiram Vineberg in 1916.

Vineberg was born in a small Russian town, one of twins whose mother died in childbirth. The family moved to Canada; when he decided to become a physician, he attended the McGill University School of Medicine, from which he graduated in 1878, having achieved one of the highest grades ever recorded by the school. His academic achievements were even more impressive than it would seem on the surface. Vineberg was a deeply religious man, who would not take exams on Saturdays. The authorities allowed him to be tested on Mondays, but with much more difficult questions. Upon his graduation, he received the Holmes Gold Medal for having achieved the highest marks on the final examination.

After a relatively short period of medical practice in Montreal, he became a ship's doctor, sailing to England, New Zealand, and Hawaii, where he debarked and became the physician in charge of a district on Oahu. After returning to Montreal to practice again, Vineberg decided to become a gynecologist and studied in Berlin, Danzig, Prague, and Vienna, after which he settled in New York in 1886.

Vineberg was first appointed to the outpatient Gynecology Clinic in 1890, became Chief of the Clinic three years later, and received an inpatient appointment in 1900. Rising through the ranks of the Attending Staff, he became Attending Gynecologist in 1916, and in 1921, at the age of sixty-five, he was elevated in title to Consulting Gynecologist.

A Fellow of the American College of Surgeons, Vineberg served as President of the New York Obstetrical Society and as First Vice President of the American Gynecological Society. He published nearly one hundred papers, but his most important contribution to the Hospital was his nurturing and mentoring of young physicians and gynecologists, a contribution duly noted by his colleagues in a testimonial presentation to him on his retirement from the Service in 1921. In 1936, the Hiram N. Vineberg Fellowship in Gynecology was established. In 1943, on the occasion of his eighty-fifth birthday, an anniversary issue of *The Journal of the Mount Sinai Hospital* was presented to him.[14] Active until well into his eighties, Vineberg died in 1945 at the age of eighty-seven; he had practiced medicine for sixty-five years.

When Vineberg retired, Brettauer assumed the direction of the entire Department until 1925, when Robert Tilden Frank was appointed Gynecologist to the Hospital, a position he held for twelve years. Frank was a leading gynecological scholar of his generation and one of the fathers of reproductive endocrinology.

A New Yorker, Frank began his training at Mount Sinai in 1900. Following the course of most Mount Sinai trainees interested in OB/GYN, he embarked upon further study in Europe, where Ludwig Pick, the famous German pathologist, was one of his mentors. Frank rejoined the staff and also secured an appointment at Columbia University, where his laboratory investigations produced a number of publications. "The Function of the Ovary,"[15] published in 1911, attests to his early interest in endocrinology. Four years later, he was able to demonstrate physiologically active substances in the placenta and corpus luteum.[16]

During World War I, Frank served in France as an officer with Mount Sinai's Base Hospital No. 3. He developed pulmonary tuberculosis and was sent to Colorado for recuperation. It was during his years in Colorado that he planned and began his research into the female endocrine system.

After his recovery, Frank was appointed Professor of Pathology at the State Medical School in Boulder, Colorado. In the field of obstetrics and gynecological pathology, he was a recognized master. His numerous achievements were crowned by the text he wrote, which was twice revised and which became a frequently cited standard in its field.[17] Because of the lack of laboratory facilities at Boulder, Frank moved to the National Jewish Hospital in Denver, where, at the Cooper Laboratory, he set out to isolate the female sex hormone from ovarian follicle fluid, the corpus luteum, and the placenta. He was among the first to demonstrate the female sex hormone in the follicular fluid of the ovary[18] and was the first to demonstrate circulating estrogen directly, rather than by inference.[19] He also isolated alpha-estradiol.

There are many who believe that the Nobel Prize awarded to the biochemist Edward Doisy and his colleagues from St. Louis University for their work on female hormones should rightfully have been given to Frank. Louis Lapid, a member of the Mount Sinai Department for sixty years, had access to Frank's diary and has paraphrased the acrimonious story:

> In January 1922, Frank published a summary of his previous research in the Journal Of The American Medical Association (JAMA).[20] In the Spring of 1923, Frank received a letter from an old friend, Leo Loeb, Professor of Pathology at St. Louis University. For many years, both men had engaged in ovarian endocrine research, and had communicated frequently. Loeb made inquiries about Frank's work on "female sex hormones" (a term Frank had coined), and which at the time was generally used. Loeb stated that two young investigators were starting work on this subject and were interested in Frank's research. Frank replied fully and in great detail. He was surprised, as well as devastated, when, in the September 8, 1923 issue of *JAMA*, an article entitled, "The Ovarian Hormone," appeared which described the ovarian

follicle as its source. The article referred only condescendingly to Frank's publication, which had appeared 20 months earlier, and, furthermore, misquoted him. Unfortunately, Frank did not keep any of the correspondence he had with Loeb.

However, I [Lapid] must state that Doisy's 1943 Nobel Prize Award was for determining the nature of Vitamin K, a clotting factor in blood, isolating and synthesizing pure Vitamin K1, as well as for his work on the isolation of the female sex hormone. Dr. Allen, a collaborator with Doisy and Professor of Anatomy at Yale University, apologized to Frank in private. Frank replied, "It's too private and too late." Doisy later gave Robert Frank full credit.[21]

Notwithstanding all of his Colorado accomplishments, Frank still felt the lure of Mount Sinai, and, when invited in 1925, he returned to the Hospital as Chief of the Gynecology Service, a post he held for twelve years. On assuming the position, he wrote, "It is now time to take charge of the Gynecological Service of the Mount Sinai Hospital, a proud privilege which has existed for 50 years, and has been headed by famous personages. It is now all mine to make or break."[22]

With his core staff of I. C. Rubin, a sterility expert, Samuel Geist, an endocrinologist, pathologist, and superior surgeon, and Max Mayer, a psychoanalyst turned gynecologist, Frank set out to make his Service a model for the medical community. At his instigation, an endocrinological laboratory was established, where, among others, a chick-comb test for the bio- assay of androgens and a rapid rat test for pregnancy were created. In collaboration with Morris Goldberger, Frank developed the first test to measure the levels of circulating estrogens in the blood,[23] and reported the results.[24] Frank studied hormonal factors during menopause and castration and how these factors were modified by substitutional therapy. He standardized the repairs of vaginal prolapse, vesico-vaginal fistula, and hysterectomy. With Geist, Frank originated a practical operative technique for the construction of an artificial vagina.[25]

Frank was instrumental in the organization of special clinics for the study and treatment of functional disorders and for providing contraceptive advice to all who needed it for medical reasons. For therapeutic purposes only, the first birth control clinic connected with a hospital in the United States was founded under the direction of Max Mayer in 1927. Frank stressed the importance of psychological and sociological factors as they impacted gynecological problems. In 1931, Frank described a condition manifested by change in disposition, temper, and demeanor, sometimes verging on the maniacal, in some women before the onset of menses; the condition is relieved, as though by magic, by the beginning of the menstrual flow. Frank called this condition PMS— the premenstrual syndrome.[26] Interestingly, the article was published in the *Archives of Neurology and Psychiatry*, not in an obstetrical or gynecological journal.

In 1937, Frank was elevated to Consultant, at which time Rubin and Geist were appointed Gynecologists to the Hospital. Frank died at Mount Sinai in 1949, at age seventy-four.

Isidor Clinton Rubin was a true New Yorker, who attended City College and then graduated from Columbia University's College of Physicians and Surgeons (P&S) in 1905. Accepted to Mount Sinai for his training, Rubin stayed for three years, then went abroad for several years to study in Vienna and Berlin. Returning to New York, he established a practice and was appointed to the staffs of The Mount Sinai, Beth Israel, and Montefiore hospitals. Over time, Rubin devoted more and more of his schedule and energy to Mount Sinai, rising through the ranks to become Attending Gynecologist and, eventually, Chief of Service from 1937 to 1945. He also held a faculty appointment at P&S.

In 1914, Rubin began experimental studies outlining the uterine and tubal lumens using a radio-opaque material, the goal was to identify patency of the Fallopian tubes.[27] This material, however, proved irritating to the tissues and was soon abandoned. The use of air had been suggested as early as 1849; it would be seventy years before Rubin would use it clinically with success. On November 3, 1919, Rubin performed the first tubal insufflation using oxygen.[28] As the first nonsurgical method established to test the patency of the Fallopian tubes, the achievement was monumental in the annals of OB/GYN. The chart and records of the first patient to undergo the procedure are housed in The New York Academy of Medicine library. Rubin continued his work and soon determined that carbon dioxide was superior to oxygen because of its more rapid absorption. Carbon dioxide was also less likely to cause air embolism. Rubin later developed a Kymograph that allowed for better interpretation of the results.[29]

Although tubal insufflation is considered one of the most important contributions to the study of female infertility, it was not Rubin's only

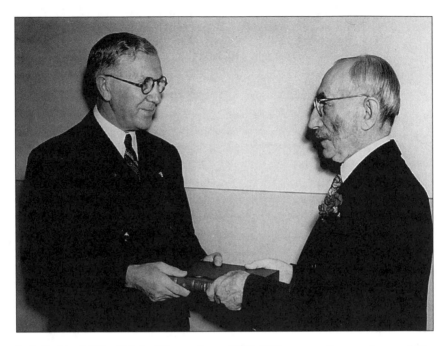

I. C. Rubin, M.D., Chief of Gynecology, 1937–1946, presenting a volume of *The Journal of the Mount Sinai Hospital* (May–June 1943) to Hiram Vineberg, M.D., Chief of Gynecology, 1915–1921. This volume was dedicated to Vineberg.

accomplishment. A man of singular vision and imagination, he was among the first to apply x-rays in the practice of gynecology, and he also wrote extensively on early carcinoma of the uterus. Rubin was the first to describe sudden shoulder pain as a symptom of a ruptured ectopic pregnancy.[30] With the development of less irritating radio-opaque solutions, Rubin was among the early advocates of their use in the radiological visualization and evaluation of the uterus and Fallopian tubes. His publications number almost one hundred and include several texts that were standards of their time.

Rubin was acclaimed throughout the world, receiving honorary degrees from the University of Athens and the Sorbonne. On the occasion of his retirement as Chief in 1947, an anniversary issue of *The Journal of the Mount Sinai Hospital* was presented to Rubin.[31] In 1954, he was accorded the rank of Chevalier in the French Legion of Honor, and in 1957 he was awarded an honorary fellowship by the Royal College of Obstetricians and Gynecologists. City College in New York honored him with its distinguished alumnus award. Ill with a heart condition for many years, Rubin succumbed to a heart attack in London on July 10, 1958, while attending an International Cancer Congress.

Samuel Geist, Rubin's Co-Director of the Gynecology Service, was born, bred, and educated in New York City. Geist joined the Mount Sinai House Staff in 1908 and after two years served a residency in obstetrics at the New York Lying-In Hospital. This was followed by a year at the University of Freiburg, where he pursued his interest in gynecological pathology.

Appointed to the staff in 1912, Geist served Mount Sinai with distinction until his untimely death in 1943. For twenty years, he was also an Associate in Surgical Pathology. A superb teacher, clinician, and mentor, Geist's door was always open to those seeking his counsel and advice. In addition to his collaboration with Frank, his early laboratory investigations dealt with the morphology of menstrual blood and its diagnostic significance. A recognized expert in the field of ovarian tumors, especially those with endocrine function, he was one of the first to study ovarian theca cell tumors. In addition, Geist made vital contributions in the field of reproductive endocrinology. He published well in excess of one hundred papers, and his text on ovarian tumors, published shortly before his death, became a classic in its time.[32]

In 1944, just prior to stepping down as Chief, Rubin had made a plea to the Trustees to develop a Maternity Service and an associated "Institute of Biogenetics."[33] The message was partially heeded, and the post–World War II years were dominated by long-range planning and fund-raising for a new building to house the Service. The last voluntary Chief of the Gynecology Service was Morris A. Goldberger, who was appointed in 1947 and served five years. A colleague and collaborator of both Frank and Rubin on numerous projects, Goldberger was also a highly successful clinician who helped shape the plans for the Department's new clinical and research facilities.

The 1952 opening of the Magdalene and Charles Klingenstein Pavilion, rising nine stories above Fifth Avenue with commanding Central Park views, provided the most modern and comprehensive obstetrical and nursery services in New York City. Mount Sinai could now expand its reputation and tradition of excellence in gynecology with a similar commitment in obstetrics. The presence of an Obstetrical Service would not only vastly improve the training program in OB/GYN but also have a salutary effect on the pediatric program by providing a newborn service.

Alan F. Guttmacher was chosen to lead this effort as the first full-time Chief of the newly named Department of Obstetrics and Gynecology. Relating to the obstetrical component of the Department, Guttmacher was fond of saying that "Mount Sinai rivaled Sarah in being the oldest primipara in history."[34] Under his leadership, the new Service would quickly achieve not only local but also regional and national attention. Born in Baltimore, Guttmacher received his undergraduate and medical education at Johns Hopkins University, where he also trained on the prestigious Obstetrical Service. During his residency, he spent one year at Mount Sinai working with Robert Frank. He then went into private practice in Baltimore, establishing a reputation for clinical excellence, personal compassion, social concern, and an extraordinary talent as an educator. For nine years prior to his coming to Mount Sinai, Guttmacher served as Chief of Obstetrics at Sinai Hospital of Baltimore and Professor at the Johns Hopkins Medical School, where he had already attained prominence in national obstetrical and family planning circles.

As a pioneer in a newly formed Department, Guttmacher moved swiftly to implement his vision for the Service, with a special focus on two areas. First, with a strongly held belief that the best obstetrical care required interaction among obstetricians and other clinicians, Guttmacher utilized the expertise of the multiple specialists at Mount Sinai readily available and desirous to serve. Pulmonologists, cardiologists, endocrinologists, diabetologists, and hematologists, among others, were recruited to form consulting services in their respective areas of proficiency. The impact of combining these talents presaged the development of perinatology as a sub-specialty of OB/GYN, specifically concerned with maternal and fetal health.

Second, Guttmacher led the difficult but essential drive for improved reproductive health, and also for reproductive freedom and choice for all women. It must be remembered that, as recently as the 1950s, contraception and abortion were not standard elements of female medical care. Most women received no direction or support for family planning or avoidance of unwanted pregnancies. Furthermore, sexually transmitted disease were misunderstood and underappreciated by practitioners, and, for the most part, physicians shared the general public view of the entire subject as carrying a social stigma. Evaluation and therapy were avoided or delayed, leading to lifelong chronic pain, disability, and, often, sterility. Guttmacher's efforts ultimately led to the availability and acceptance of contraceptive methodologies and abortion rights for all women. Outstanding obstetrical care, informed family planning, and pelvic infectious disease services became available to all women who came to Mount Sinai.

Although Guttmacher's training had been entirely in obstetrics, he saw to it that the excellence of the Hospital's gynecological services was maintained and, indeed, even improved. Joseph Gaines and Arthur Davids took over as joint Chiefs of Gynecology, alternating monthly in the capacity of Director. Both were talented surgeons who demanded excellence in patient care and who gave unstintingly of their time and wisdom in the education of the resident staff. To maintain the quality of their Service, they were most fortunate in having many extremely gifted gynecologists with them in the Department.

Louis Lapid played a meaningful role in the Department for sixty years. Born in Chicago, Lapid received his M.D. from the University of Illinois. His OB/GYN training at Mount Sinai and Boston Lying-In Hospital was interrupted by military service in World War II. A peerless clinician and an outstanding teacher, Lapid made a major contribution to Mount Sinai in 1947, when, as the Brettauer Fellow in gynecological pathology, he introduced cellular pathology to the Hospital. As he tells the story:

> I worked with Dr. George Papanicolaou. I was so enthusiastic about his work in cellular pathology that I approached Dr. Paul Klemperer, Chief of Pathology at Mount Sinai. Dr. Klemperer's mind was so open, he said he would meet with me one half hour a week for six months. If I could prove to him that a diagnosis of malignancy could be made by examination of individual cells, he would see that I got a laboratory for this study. In four months, I had the laboratory. . . . We did smears of the vagina and sputum, as well as bronchial and urine studies. I remained Director of Cellular Pathology for ten years, until it became an integral part of the Pathology Department of the Hospital and was taken over by a full time pathologist.[35]

Guttmacher's trainees would go on to distinguished careers. Joseph Rovinsky, the Co-Editor of the highly acclaimed *Complications of Pregnancy*,[36] would spend many productive years as Chief of OB/GYN at the Long Island Jewish Medical Center. The accomplishments of Nathan Kase are detailed later.

In 1962, after ten years at the helm, Guttmacher left Mount Sinai to become President of the Planned Parenthood Federation of America, a position he occupied with great distinction until his death in 1973. Guttmacher left as his legacy an exceptional staff of talented and dedicated physicians, who would form the nucleus of the Department in the Mount Sinai School of Medicine.

Succeeding Guttmacher in 1962 was Saul Gusberg, recruited from the Columbia-Presbyterian Hospital, who became the second full-time Director of the Department and Obstetrician and Gynecologist-in-Chief of the Hospital. Where Guttmacher's focus had been on obstetrics, Gusberg's area of expertise was gynecologic oncology, and he quickly established a program and fellowship in this specialty. Gusberg's work in the field extended over more than half a century. In a classic 1947 paper, Gusberg noted the association of adenomatous hyperplasia with unopposed estrogen exposure and identified the latter as a precursor to the development of endometrial cancer. This was followed by a series of papers further describing the clinical course and outcome of patients with adenomatous hyperplasia. Gusberg was also responsible for the concept of individualization in the treatment of cervical cancer. He studied the cellular nucleoprotein pattern in response to radiation in an attempt to devise a predictive test to distinguish patients who would respond to radiation therapy from those who would benefit from surgery.[37] Gusberg's third major clinical contribution was his definition of prognostic factors such as uterine size and histologic features in patients with endometrial cancer. His proposal to include them in a staging system would lead to individualized therapy based on prognosis.[38] This approach was ultimately accepted as a basis for an internationally (FIGO) accepted staging system.

As founding Chairman of the Department in the new Mount Sinai School of Medicine, Gusberg was responsible for developing the curriculum for the mandatory third-year student clerkship, for the teaching of reproductive biology, and for providing significant input to the course on human sexuality in the preclinical years. Gusberg's era was notable, not only for a marked increase in the number of women gaining admittance to the Mount Sinai Medical School but also for the beginning of the trend for more women to enter the specialty of OB/GYN.

Gusberg was active in a number of medical societies, assuming many leadership positions. He served as President of the New York Obstetrical Society, The New York Academy of Medicine, the Society of Pelvic Surgeons, the Society of Gynecologic Oncologists, and the American Cancer Society. He was also the Editor-in-Chief of the journal *Gynecologic Oncology*. After an eighteen-year tenure, Gusberg retired from the Chair in 1980. His trainees would continue in his footsteps, making far-reaching contributions to OB/GYN and gynecological oncology.

Carmel Cohen was appointed Gusberg's first Fellow in gynecologic oncology at Mount Sinai after completing his residency. Upon completion of the fellowship, he was placed in charge of the newly created Division of Gynecologic Oncology. The Division would achieve great success in many areas. A demonstration cervical cancer screening project was established in the New York City Municipal Hospital System that ultimately resulted in a significant reduction in the prevalence of the disease. Uterine aspiration sampling was shown to be possible and accurate as an outpatient procedure for endometrial cancer screening.[39] In collaboration with David Koffler of the Department of Pathology, the presence of cell-mediated immunity in patients with cervical, ovarian, and endometrial cancers was demonstrated, a finding that would establish a basis for the potential benefits of immunotherapy.[40]

In conjunction with the Department of Neoplastic Disease, the Gynecologic Oncology Group was among the first to demonstrate the utility of cisplatinum in the treatment of patients with advanced epithelial ovarian cancer[41] and also among the first to demonstrate the efficacy of the same drug in treating squamous cell carcinoma of the cervix, a malignancy thought to be completely resistant to chemotherapy.[42] An authoritative paper, describing second-look operations in ovarian cancer patients treated with platinum regimens, quantified for the first time the histologic responses to the new chemotherapy.[43]

Cohen introduced minimally invasive surgery to the Division's therapeutic armamentarium in the management of patients with gynecologic cancers and added training in laparoscopic procedures to the fellowship program.

Sheldon Cherry, recruited by Gusberg, developed a clinical and research interest in the Rh factor. Working with Richard Rosenfield,

Director of the Blood Bank, and Shaul Kochwa, they devised a biliru-bin-protein amniotic fluid index to gauge the severity of erythroblasto-sis fetalis.[44] Cherry was the first to report on Mount Sinai's use of in-trauterine transfusion in the management of erythroblastosis[45] and also was the Senior Editor of the third and fourth editions of Rovinsky and Guttmacher's text, *Complications of Pregnancy*.

Erlio Gurpide, a steroid biochemist, with a major interest in estro-gen and progesterone elaboration and metabolism, was recruited by Gusberg in 1972. His studies on estradiol and estriol in the fetal and ma-ternal circulations had important implications for the evaluation of fetal health. Through the development of tracer techniques and subsequent to multiple studies, Gurpide described the effects of estrogen stimula-tion of the human endometrium[46] and the role of hormones in the pro-duction and modulation of gynecologic cancers.[47] His notable contribu-tion to the field of gynecologic cancer was his demonstration of the mechanisms of estrogen promotion of endometrial cancer and the ra-tionale for the protective use of progesterone.[48]

In 1981, one of Mount Sinai's own returned to succeed Gusberg as Chairman of the Department. Nathan G. Kase, a graduate of P&S, was one of the last of Mount Sinai's rotating interns, completing his OB/GYN training under Alan Guttmacher and then serving a fellow-ship in the Division of Endocrinology. Moving to New Haven, Kase rose rapidly through the ranks of the faculty and served for nine years as Chairman of the Department of Obstetrics and Gynecology at the Yale University School of Medicine.

A specialist in gynecologic and reproductive endocrinology, Kase made momentous contributions to the field. In 1961, Kase and his col-leagues[49] provided the first demonstration that the human ovary could synthesize testosterone in vitro. This was followed by several papers on the subject, written by Kase with members of the endocrinology labo-ratories at Mount Sinai. In 1967, Kase published on the extraglandular production of androgens, the first documentation of the critical differ-ence between glandular secretion and total hormone production.[50] In that same year, Kase and his colleagues provided early evidence for new mechanisms of ovulation induction in previously untreatable anovulatory females.[51] This publication on the use of Clomid, and a subsequent paper on the use of Pergonal,[52] provided regimens that be-came the standard of care for the administration of these drugs. In 1973, Kase co-authored the first edition of *Clinical Gynecology, Endocrinology and Infertility.*[53] With the sixth edition appearing in 1999, the book became the largest-selling text in the specialty of OB/GYN.

Kase returned to Mount Sinai with a mandate to improve the national standing of the Department. His plans included a revitalization of obstetrical services, expansion of departmental research and education, and the modernization and consolidation of the facilities. Kase has remarked that one of the most important actions taken during his tenure was the recruitment of Richard Berkowitz from Yale to direct the Division of Perinatology and Maternal-Fetal Medicine. Under Berkowitz's leadership, plans for developing and upgrading the Obstetrical Service were immediately drawn up and implemented.

The Department's clinical research capabilities were significantly amplified by the recruitment of Trudy Berkowitz, a perinatal epidemiologist from Yale, and of Sally Faith Dorfman, of the Emory University School of Medicine, where she served as the Director of Family Planning and Adolescent Gynecology. Other major recruitments were Andrea Dunaif, trained in medical and gynecologic endocrinology at Harvard, and Marjorie Luckey, who trained in the Mount Sinai Department of Medicine's Division of Endocrinology. Dunaif, who would later become Chief of Women's Health at Harvard, achieved worldwide recognition for her pioneering studies in insulin resistance in the polycystic ovary syndrome, most of which were conducted at Mount Sinai. Luckey established a major program in menopausal medicine in the Department prior to leaving to become director of the Osteoporosis Center at St. Barnabas Health System. During the tenure of these exceptional individuals, the Department's preeminence in reproductive endocrinology, menopause, anovulation, infertility, hirsutism, and abnormalities of pubescence and contraception was dramatically enhanced.

Clinical gynecologic endocrinology and infertility services were further advanced under Victor Reyniak. Reyniak established the first gynecologic laser surgery unit in the metropolitan area. He also instituted the first New York City–based In Vitro Fertilization (IVF)program; the first Mount Sinai IVF baby was born in 1984.

Kase also stressed excellence in research, especially in developmental biology and molecular biology. The strong program in endometrial biochemistry, established by Gusberg and led by Gurpide, was further augmented by the recruitment of Jon Gordon from Yale. Gordon brought to Mount Sinai nationally acknowledged expertise in developmental biology, particularly in the areas of DNA function, re-combinant DNA technology, and, most important, the production and scientific exploitation of transgenic mice.

Kase further recognized the need for improvement and updating of the Department's educational activities. Consequently, he appointed a full-time Director of Medical Student and Resident Education. To lead the effort, Kase recruited Charles Bowers, one of the first African-American faculty members at Mount Sinai and a former student and associate of Kase at Yale.

The final area of Kase's strategy for overall improvement dealt with modernizing the Department's physical plant. The Klingenstein Pavilion was thirty years old and inadequate for the innovations in female health care and obstetrics that had become standard procedure since the building's opening in 1952. The Labor and Delivery Suites were re-designed and a contiguous Perinatology Center created. Ambulatory gynecology services were relocated to the Maternity Pavilion, creating a single patient care site for the Department's inpatient and outpatient activities.

In 1985, four years after becoming Chairman, Kase was appointed Dean of the Mount Sinai School of Medicine. By that time, the Department had undergone a major transformation, from emphasizing gyne-cologic oncology to stressing the entire spectrum of female health, with a special focus on reproductive endocrinology. In recognition of this change, the Department was officially renamed the Department of Obstetrics, Gynecology, and Reproductive Science in 1983.

After a nationwide search, Richard Berkowitz was appointed the fourth full-time Chairman of the Department. Berkowitz trained in OB/GYN at the New York Hospital; and, after obtaining a Master of Public Health degree in Population Dynamics and International Health at the Johns Hopkins School of Hygiene and Public Health, he joined the faculty of Yale and became a member of the Perinatal Unit. This unit had been a pioneer in exploring the potential of ultrasound as a diag-nostic tool for obstetrical patients and had utilized ultrasound as an in-novative therapeutic adjunct to invasive in utero therapies. Most im-portant, the Yale group developed the principle of using ultrasound as an integral part of the care provided by Maternal-Fetal Medicine spe-cialists to women who were experiencing complex medical problems during their pregnancies. This background had been a critical factor in Kase's recruitment of Berkowitz to Mount Sinai in 1982 to become Director of Obstetrics. Shortly after his arrival, Berkowitz established the Division of Maternal-Fetal Medicine and introduced the modern use of ultrasound to the practice of perinatal medicine.

Berkowitz's first fifteen years as Chairman produced many achievements. The Obstetrical Service grew from approximately 3,200 deliveries a year to a peak of 5,200 in 1997. This was attributable in large measure to the reputation of the Division of Maternal-Fetal Medicine and its Ultrasound Unit, along with the total renovation of the delivery floor. As a result of this growth, the number of residents was increased from six to seven per year in 1991, at a time when most OB/GYN residency programs around the United States were reducing their resident complements. The fellowship in Maternal-Fetal Medicine attracted outstanding individuals, many of whom are now in prestigious academic positions throughout the world. In 1986, Berkowitz and his colleagues reported the first successful intrauterine transfusion of blood given by the intravascular route directly into an umbilical vessel without the use of fetoscopy. The procedure was performed percutaneously under direct ultrasound visualization.[54] In 1991, Charles Lockwood identified fetal fibronectin as a marker for preterm birth.[55] Lockwood became Chairman of the Department of Obstetrics and Gynecology at the New York University School of Medicine.

By recruiting graduates from the residency to remain on the faculty, Berkowitz created several generalist practices that grew substantially and moved the full-time faculty away from providing only subspecialty care. As noted earlier, the Department became a center of excellence for laparoscopic gynecologic surgery. The groundbreaking efforts of Carmel Cohen and Peter Dottino to utilize minimally invasive surgery in the staging and treatment of gynecologic malignancies were further strengthened in 1997 by the recruitment of Farr Nezhat, an innovative and highly skilled gynecologic laparoscopic surgeon.

In 1994, the traditional obstetrical and gynecologic clinics were replaced by continuity clinics under the leadership of Rhoda Sperling, an OB/GYN generalist who had subspecialty training in Infectious Diseases. Sperling became a national leader in research into the epidemiology and management of HIV infection in OB/GYN patients. She was a senior author on the landmark AIDS Clinical Trials Group paper, the first to document that the use of antiviral therapy during labor and the neonatal period dramatically reduced vertical transmission of the HIV virus from pregnant women to their offspring.[56] The continuity clinics established at the Hospital became a model for outpatient OB/GYN care, and similar programs were subsequently mandated for inclusion in residency training programs by the Residency Review Committee (RRC) for OB/GYN. In 1998, leadership of these clinics was assumed by Joanna Shulman. Under her guidance, the scope of outpatient activities was broadened, necessitating an increase in clinic attending staff coverage, and a midwife service was established. As all of the Divisions of the Department grew during the late 1980s and early 1990s, so did the size of the full-time faculty.

The integrated residency at City Hospital Center at Elmhurst, directed first by Jasmin Moshirpur and later by Barry Brown, evolved into the premier unit of its type in the New York City Health and Hospital Corporation. The number of deliveries at Elmhurst rose from 3,500 in 1985 to approximately 4,700 in 1998; the majority of these pregnancies were medically complex. Despite the high-risk nature of the patients being served and the dramatic growth in volume, the perinatal morbidity and mortality statistics of this Service were the best among New York City's nineteen public hospitals. The Department was now responsible for more than 10,000 deliveries a year at Mount Sinai and at Elmhurst General Hospital. In 1993, the Department assumed responsibility for overseeing the OB/GYN program at Queens Hospital Center, replacing the Long Island Jewish Medical Center. Within a year, a new, free-standing residency was established. The departmental faculty at Queens Hospital Center grew in number and quality, and the residency program gained full accreditation in 1994.

Jon Gordon continued his highly successful laboratory program. Along with his colleagues, he had been the first to introduce recombinant DNA material into the germ line of a mammal with success;[57] he also reported the first introduction of a human gene into mice and then the transmission of that gene to two generations of offspring.[58] This work introduced the term "transgenic" into the scientific lexicon. Gordon's team also showed for the first time that the efficiency of IVF could be greatly increased if the sperm were assisted in reaching the surface of the egg using micromanipulation[59] and that this technique could be of value in treating male infertility.[60] This laboratory was also among the first to demonstrate the feasibility of genetic diagnosis by polymerase chain reaction analysis of DNA from single cells removed from the preimplantation embryo.[61] Gordon's group has expanded its horizons and, although not specifically related to the work of the Department, in 1995 reported the creation of a new transgenic mouse model for amyotrophic lateral sclerosis.[62]

As the twentieth century came to an end, Mount Sinai's Department of Obstetrics, Gynecology, and Reproductive Science had completed its transformation into a full-fledged academic and clinical enterprise, incorporating the newest branches of science and research into its curriculum and practice of medicine. The Department entered the twenty-first century fiscally stable, nationally recognized for the superiority of its postgraduate training programs, and accepted locally and nationally as a bastion of clinical excellence.

23

Department of Ophthalmology

THE FIRST RECORDED eye operation at the Jews' Hospital was performed in 1860. Seligman Teller, the House Physician and Surgeon, reported on A. L., a peddler, "who by the effect of a cold lost the sight of his right eye which was affected by cataract and glaucomatous disease. An operation was performed with success and the sight of his eye was fully restored."[1]

In 1879, Emil Gruening (1842–1914) was appointed the first Chief of a combined Eye and Ear, Nose, and Throat (EENT) Service, the first such department by two decades in a general hospital in New York. Gruening had his early education in Europe and came to the United States at age nineteen. He settled in Hoboken, New Jersey, and made a meager living tutoring. He started medical school, but, at the outbreak of the Civil War, he volunteered for the infantry, serving in Grant's command at several battles, and was present at Lee's surrender at Appomattox. He finished medical school and studied in Europe with Hermann von Helmholtz, Albrecht von Graefe, and others for three years. As was common at the time, Gruening cared for patients with disease of the eyes, ears, nose, and throat. In 1882, an Eye and Ear Department was started in the Outpatient Dispensary (OPD) of Mount Sinai. In 1883, an inpatient eye and ear ward was established, separating these patients from the general medical and surgical cases. Alice B. Brill and Edward Fridenberg were appointed to the staff to help with the increasing workload. By 1895, a spectacle and eye glass service had been added in the OPD.

The Great Blizzard of March 12, 1888, is still remembered, although many have forgotten its medical implications. The storm and the whiteness of the snow caused many cases of temporary vision problems, as well as many upper respiratory infections, many with mastoiditis. With his vast experience, Gruening became the first to perform radical mastoid drainage surgery in the United States.[2] He also designed platinum instruments for eye surgery that could withstand high temperatures for sterilization better than silver. Although aseptic surgery was introduced to Mount Sinai in the 1880s, many surgeons did not espouse the concept. Gruening, in fact, was described as holding the cataract (Graefe) knife in his mouth.[3]

One of the many bright lights in the early years of the Eye Service was William Wilmer, who was on the Mount Sinai House Staff from 1885 to 1887 and then became Gruening's assistant. Wilmer subsequently moved to Baltimore, where he founded the Wilmer Eye Institute. When Gruening died in 1914, Wilmer wrote to Emil's son, Ernest, and noted that he had no greater admiration or respect for anyone except for his own father. Ernest Gruening later became the governor of the Territory of Alaska and its first Senator when Alaska attained statehood.

Percy Fridenberg was on the Aural and Ophthalmic staff for many years. His family connections were notable. Two brothers were Mount Sinai physicians; one of his sisters, Rose, was Emil Gruening's first wife, and, after her death, another sister, Phoebe, became Gruening's second wife. Percy Fridenberg served for many years at Mount Sinai and published extensively. A 1903 case report gave a remarkable hint of the future and also an example of Fridenberg's prescience. The patient, a twenty-six-year-old physician, sustained a partial thickness laceration of the cornea, which, after healing, eliminated a previously known corneal astigmatism. Fridenberg wrote, "the prophetic eye may see, in the dim future, the operation of graduated superficial keratotomy for astigmatism."[4] And this was nearly a century ago.

Max Talmey, one of the more colorful ophthalmologists of the era, joined the staff in 1895. As a medical student in Germany, he had been introduced to a bright and personable lad of ten to whom he gave some books on science, mathematics, and philosophy. The boy was Albert Einstein, and Talmey remained in touch with him over many years. With Einstein's permission, Talmey published a popular version of the Theory of Relativity. He was also very involved in the synthetic languages Esperanto and Gloro, which were developed in that era. His critical comments about psychoanalysis published in the newspapers attracted considerable attention (including a supportive note from H. L. Mencken). He wrote on a variety of subjects: cataract, infantile paralysis, and international efforts to save energy. Talmey died in 1941.

Carl Koller (1857–1944) achieved instantaneous world renown on September 15, 1884, when he reported on the anesthetic properties of cocaine at a convention of German oculists in Heidelberg, Germany.[5]

Koller was a colleague of Sigmund Freud in the Vienna General Hospital, where Freud was studying cocaine as a possible substitution therapy for morphine addiction. Koller, in a perfect example of serendipity, noted that an animal with cocaine in its eye had no apparent sensation. He tried it in his own eye, and the rest is history. Because Koller could not afford to make the trip to Heidelberg, the report was given by Koller's friend, Joseph Brettauer, who would later become the Chief of Gynecology at Mount Sinai.

Koller left Europe and in 1888 was named the Chief of the Eye Clinic at Mount Sinai. In 1910, with Gruening's retirement, Koller and Charles H. May were named Ophthalmic Surgeons to the Hospital. Koller served until he reached retirement age in 1920. He did not rest on his early laurels but was productive in his practice and writings for many years. He was a meticulous surgeon and developed surgery for strabismus based on mathematical analysis, well ahead of his time. He also expanded the thinking in regard to eye conditions in relation to the body as a whole. He used a type of contact lens with a flat front surface that allowed a wide-field view of the fundus, a forerunner of currently used contact examination lenses and laser treatment lenses. Koller remained active, publishing on ocular tension and the intraocular circulation in 1942, during his eighty-fifth year. Koller was honored worldwide. In 1922, he was the first recipient of the Lucien Howe Gold Medal of the American Ophthalmological Society.

May (1861–1943) joined the House Staff in 1883. Three years later, he published on the experimental transplantation of rabbit eyes.[6] Shortly after the report appeared, a midwesterner with a sightless and deformed eye requested that May perform the operation on him. The procedure was successfully carried out, but the transplanted eye, which was clear at first, opacified and had to be removed on the ninth postoperative day[7] evidently one of the first cases of graft rejection ever to be reported. The patient requested a second attempt, but May demurred. *The Minneapolis Herald* reported the story, relating how May, Gruening, and Wilmer performed the operation on February 1, 1887.

May achieved international recognition for his contributions in the design of the direct ophthalmoscope[8] and for his textbook, *Manual of Diseases of the Eye*,[9] printed in more than twenty editions and in many languages. This was *the* ophthalmology textbook for decades in medical schools around the world, and the ophthalmoscope, in its more modern version, is still used everywhere. As a young man, he was a superb stu-

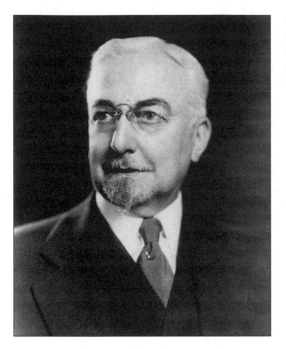

Charles May, M.D.,
developer of the May
Ophthalmoscope,
Chief of Service,
1910–1923.

dent; after completing his college courses, he was too young to be accepted into medical school. He studied pharmacy and years later published an index of *Materia Medica*. He was truly the first of the Mount Sinai ocular pharmacologists. May was also an excellent artist and did the illustrations for his own publications and for some of his colleagues. He finished the review of the eighteenth edition of his *Manual of Diseases of the Eye* two weeks before his death in 1943.

Koller and May served jointly until Koller's retirement in 1920; May was in charge of the Service until 1924 when he too reached retirement age for Chiefs and was succeeded by Julius Wolff (1870–1942). Wolff, who would be Chief for eight years, had started at Mount Sinai in 1907. He designed an instrument for iridectomy that grasped the iris and cut it simultaneously. He published on congenital defects, unilateral exophthalmos, and the use of a conjunctival flap during cataract extraction.

Every Hospital Service was impacted by World War I, and ophthalmology was no exception. Cyril Barnert, on the staff from 1906 until his death in 1930, went overseas with Base Hospital No. 3, the Mount Sinai unit. On his return, he published the history of the unit.[10]

During the 1920s and 1930s, the Department thrived. A slit lamp and a corneal microscope were acquired by the Eye Service in 1924, very advanced equipment for that time. A formal two-year residency program was started in 1927, and the following year an ophthalmic pathology laboratory opened. Photography of the back of the eye was instituted at the Hospital in 1929, and new dedicated operating rooms opened in 1933. The Resident training program increased to three years in 1938.

Isidore Goldstein (1879–1937) and Kaufman Schlivek (1881–1955) were joint Chiefs of the Service from 1932 until the untimely death of Goldstein in 1937. Goldstein wrote about optic atrophy in periarteritis and oculoplastic procedures, including the first use of a hollow gold ball, fashioned by a dental laboratory, for implant after enucleation. Most memorably, in 1935, he and Carleton Simon, a prominent criminologist, published "A New Scientific Method of Identification."[11] Based on the individuality of vascular anatomy in retinal photographs, this concept is now being embraced, not only in the movies but also in sophisticated security systems. Goldstein utilized levator recession to protect the globe in thyroid eye disease. He described reconstruction of the lids after orbital exenteration to permit the fitting of a prosthesis. He lectured and gave surgical demonstrations in Cairo, Paris, and Jerusalem, where he helped establish the ophthalmic division of Hebrew University.

Schlivek started at Mount Sinai after several years of general practice. A friend of Abraham Jacobi, he had once considered a career in pediatrics. He opted for ophthalmology, however, received excellent training with many of the outstanding ophthalmologists of the day, and became one of the finest clinicians and teachers of his time. Schlivek's opinion was widely sought throughout his career; he was consulted at his home, just two weeks before his death, about a child with only one eye.

Robert Lambert (1898–1946) became Chief of the Service in 1943 with plans for establishing an eye institute. Lambert had done research on glaucoma and designed a provocative test to diagnose the condition that was used for many years. Unfortunately, Lambert's plans never came to fruition because of his untimely death in 1946.

Lambert was succeeded by Henry Minsky (1895–1959). A creative individual, Minsky was also considered absent-minded. His training in ophthalmology started in medical school. He spent early morning hours with Oscar Diem, a pupil of the great Ernst Fuchs of Vienna. With Diem, he accompanied Fuchs on the latter's American lecture tour in 1921. Minsky's meticulous notes on the lectures were privately published. His method of a figure eight suture for repair of eyelid margin lacerations was used widely for many years.[12] His technique for trans-illumination of the anterior chamber of the eye in the operating room is still useful.[13] Minsky's interest in the changes in the retinal blood vessels in hypertension resulted in a classic 1954 paper, "Correlation of Ocular Changes in Essential Hypertension with Diastolic Blood Pressure."[14]

Interest in the embryology of the eye stimulated an organized study and collection of material at Mount Sinai in 1938. This work was done primarily by Abraham Kornzweig (1900–1982), who taught the subject at the New York University Postgraduate Medical School for many years. Kornzweig then turned his interest to geriatrics and studied retinal pathology in the aged. Considered by many to be the first geriatric ophthalmologist, he presented a monograph on the eye in the elderly at the 1971 meeting of the President's Council on Aging. With Frank A. Bassen, a Mount Sinai hematologist, Kornzweig published the classic paper defining the Bassen-Kornzweig syndrome.[15]

In 1953, Joseph Laval (1902–1992) was appointed to head the Department. He had been a Mount Sinai Intern and, as a young man, served briefly as the doctor for the Sing Sing prison in Ossining, New York. An active practitioner, Laval placed emphasis on ophthalmic surgery during his tenure. His publications include reports on cysts of the optic disc, absorption lines of the cornea, Marfan's Syndrome, vaccinia of the eyelids, the use of Gelfilm in glaucoma surgery, and steroid-induced elevation of the intraocular pressure. Laval stepped down as Chief of the Department in 1965 but remained in practice. He retired, due to failing vision, only a short time before he died unexpectedly at age ninety while walking near his home.

Frederick H. Theodore was very active at Mount Sinai during the 1940s and 1950s and did extensive research on external diseases of the eye, particularly allergy. Until the mid-twentieth century, eye medications were compounded by the local pharmacist. The highly variable concentration of medication and the far from sterile conditions that prevailed were grossly unsatisfactory. In 1950, Theodore published an early paper on the use of cortisone in the eye, and one year later he initiated a campaign that culminated in the Food and Drug Administration regulation requiring all ophthalmic solutions to be sterile. The 1958 text *Ocular Allergy*,[16] by Theodore and Abraham Schlossman, remains a useful reference work to the present day. Theodore described superior limbic keratoconjunctivitis[17] and published a number of other "firsts" in the ophthalmologic literature, especially in the area of ophthalmic infections, the complications of cataract surgery, and the "Masquerade syndrome"—carcinoma of the conjunctiva masquerading as chronic conjunctivitis.[18]

Although there were few women in medicine during the early years, the Department of Ophthalmology did include women staff, notably Alice Brill, Olga Sitchevska, Frieda Mark, and Virginia Lubkin. Lubkin was always creative with novel approaches to problems of varied nature and is still actively engaged in ophthalmic research.

Alan Barnert (1914–1979), the son of Cyril, was a member of the staff from his residency in 1940 until his death. He performed considerable research on contact lenses at a time when they were not fully accepted. A superb teacher and a provocative thinker, Barnert was highly regarded for his work in community affairs and was in charge of the clinic at the Lighthouse for the Blind. The Ophthalmology Alumni group carries Barnert's name.

In 1965, Irving H. Leopold (1915–1993) was appointed the first full-time Chairman of the Department of Ophthalmology. Recruited from Philadelphia, where he had served as Director of Research at the Wills Eye Hospital from 1949 to 1964, Leopold was responsible for developing the role of ophthalmology in the Mount Sinai School of Medicine curriculum. During his tenure, Mount Sinai affiliated with the City Hospital Center at Elmhurst and the Bronx Veterans Administration Hospital; the residency program was expanded to have five Residents in each of the three years of the program and adjusted to include the additional training sites. Leopold acquired new research facilities and recruited full-time faculty. The Department acquired its own electron microscope and also recruited Donald Wong, a full-time ophthalmic photographer. Plans were drawn up for the space in the Annenberg Building, both for the clinic and for the department offices and laboratories.

Leopold published more than two hundred papers, authored a dozen book chapters, and wrote and edited another dozen books on ocular therapeutics. He was widely recognized as an authority on ocular pharmacology and researched many compounds for their potential use in the ophthalmic armamentarium. He was honored by many ophthalmic societies and served on the scientific advisory boards of several philanthropic agencies. His skill as a speaker was vividly demonstrated when he presented a Jackson Memorial Lecture at the American Academy of Ophthalmology, a one-hour presentation given without notes and without a glance at the slides changing on the screen behind him.

Aran Safir and Andrew Ferry were major assets to the Department during Leopold's tenure. The former published on the ophthalmologic complications of juvenile diabetes; his sophisticated research on the Stiles-Crawford effect (the phenomenon by which light passing through the periphery of the eye's pupil is less efficient at stimulating vision than is light passing near the center of the pupil) was a most important contribution.[19] Safir also designed the first electronic refraction device, the Ophthalmetron, which in recent years has been followed by instruments to measure and map the cornea as well as to refract and test visual fields. In 1970, Ferry, an ophthalmic pathologist, and Barnert published their pioneering research on the use of cyanoacrylate as a tissue adhesive.[20] Beginning in 1971, and continuing for twenty years, the Department, in conjunction with the Post Graduate School, offered a course entitled "Cosmetic Surgery of the Aging Eye." This two-day seminar was created by Morris Feldstein, Virginia Lubkin, and Ira Eliasoph. With a stellar guest faculty, the course was well attended and highly acclaimed. Leopold resigned in 1974. Ferry served as the acting Chair and accomplished the move of the Department to its present location.

In 1975, Steven M. Podos was appointed Chairman of the Department of Ophthalmology. A New Yorker, whose father and grandfather were optometrists in Brooklyn, Podos trained at Washington University in St. Louis, and then remained on the faculty, rising to the rank of full Professor. His early work led to the development of the first topical nonsteroidal anti- inflammatory agent for ophthalmological use.[21] A world leader in the study and treatment of glaucoma, Podos, along with his colleagues, was the first to demonstrate that topical carbonic anhydrase inhibitors lower intraocular pressure;[22] this is now standard therapy. He and Robert Schumer developed the seminal concept of treating glaucoma as a neurodegenerative disease.[23] In the early 1990s, Podos and Myron Yanoff edited a ten-volume text.[24] Podos has served on numerous editorial boards and has held leadership positions in many ophthalmologic societies, including the Presidency of the Association of University Professors of Ophthalmology and the Association for Research in Vision and Ophthalmology.

Under Podos's leadership, the Department has achieved national and international recognition. In 2000, it ranked eighth in the United States among academic departments of ophthalmology in funding from the National Institutes of Health. Departmental scientists have been at the forefront of ophthalmological research. Thomas Mittag and his colleagues were the first to detect anti-acetylcholine receptor factors in serum and thymus from patients with myasthenia gravis.[25] Mittag later went on to elucidate the secondary messenger systems in the ciliary body of the eye. Ehud Kaplan and Robert Shapley defined the dual pathway of the visual system from retinal ganglion cells.[26] Sandra Masur and her colleagues have made fundamental contributions to the understanding of the role of the integrins in the extracellular matrix of the anterior portion of the eye[27] and have provided the first demonstration that fibroblasts' cell-cell and cell-matrix signals control phenotypic differentiation and stromal wound healing of the cornea.[28] Oscar Candia has published significant findings relating to fluid and electrolyte transport in the conjunctiva. In the clinical arena, Penny Asbell has been a leader in trials of an exciting new modality of refractive surgery utilizing plastic inserts in the cornea. Janet Serle has had a major clinical and research interest in glaucoma, and Wayne Fuchs has been a leading retinal surgeon in the Department for many years. He has also been very active in the Mount Sinai Alumni Association. The Department is one of very few to have its own pathology laboratory and pathologist. Alan Friedman has filled that role admirably for many years. Utilizing the new technology of telemedicine, Department staff carry out teaching and pathology consultations with institutions from afar.

The Resident training program, with rotations at Mount Sinai, City Hospital Center at Elmhurst, and the Bronx Veterans Administration Hospital, has been singularly successful. The program has spawned a substantial number of academic ophthalmologists who are now professors and chairmen in their own right, as well as countless ophthalmologists in private practice throughout the country. Given the Department's visionary leadership and preeminent staff, the future of ophthalmology at Mount Sinai will be bright and auspicious.

Adapted from an essay written by Ira Eliasoph, M.D., F.A.C.S.

24

Department of Orthopaedics

ALTHOUGH AN OFFICIAL Department of Orthopaedics was not established until 1909, the first orthopaedic patient (Case #9) was admitted June 14, 1855, nine days after the Jews' Hospital opened its doors. The patient was a two-year-old boy with a transverse fracture of the femur at the junction of the mid and upper third; a splint was applied, and the child was discharged "cured" after a three-week stay. Union of the bones occurred "at a slight angle but there was no perceptible shortening."[1] And this was forty-five years before Mount Sinai had an x-ray machine. A far more interesting patient (Case #25) was admitted on July 23, 1855, after having already spent six weeks at another hospital with an as yet unhealed fracture of the patella. After the patient spent another four weeks at the Jews' Hospital with no improvement, the Attending Surgeon, Alexander Mott, "ordered an apparatus by means of which the fragments could be retained in close approximation with each other."[2] Following the application of this apparatus and with "electricity pulsed through the part every other day,"[3] the patient was discharged cured on October 20.

In the nineteenth century, orthopaedics began to evolve as a specialty worldwide with the advent of institutions devoted to the care of the "crippled and deformed." At that time, the specialty dealt primarily with musculoskeletal problems in children (the word "orthopaedics" derives from the Greek ortho, meaning "straight," and pais, meaning "child"), including congenital, developmental and posttraumatic deformities of the hips, spine, and extremities, as well as infections (poliomyelitis, osteomyelitis, tuberculosis).

During the Hospital's early years, most musculoskeletal problems (i.e., arthritis) were treated on the Medical Service, while trauma, bone tumors, and infections were part of Surgery. In 1909, an Out-Patient Orthopaedic Clinic was established under the direction of Philip W. Nathan, who at the time was known primarily for his work on arthritis.[4] The recent development of the x-ray machine was a major stimulus to the understanding and treatment of bone and joint problems and fractures during this period.

In 1910, an Inpatient Service was established, and Nathan was appointed Attending Orthopaedist to the Hospital. Nathan had graduated from the New York University School of Medicine in 1893 and then spent three years studying in Berlin, during which time he also studied at the Conservatory of Music. After several years in California, he returned to New York and began to specialize in orthopaedics at both the Ruptured and Crippled and the Polyclinic hospitals. In 1903, he was elected a Fellow of the American Orthopaedic Association and joined the Mount Sinai staff in 1909.

Nathan wrote extensively; his major papers focused on bone development and its relation to bone transplants,[5] the management of poliomyelitis,[6] and tuberculous hip disease.[7] In 1932, he published a landmark work on acute infections of the hip joint, which provides a graphic description of the plight of the acute osteomyelitic orthopaedic patient in the early twentieth century and merits being quoted at length:

> the vast majority of the patients are brought to the hospital during the acute stage, the abscess is opened, the bone either drilled or curetted, and perhaps a sequestrum removed, and he is discharged after a more or less serious siege of illness, with either a draining sinus or with the disease apparently quiescent. He usually has the motion in the hip more or less completely restricted in a deformed position and in consequence is lame or must use some apparatus or crutches to be about. He may be fairly well for a while but the symptoms sooner or later return, when he is readmitted to the hospital, and the series of events of his first admittance are repeated. Again, he is discharged either quiescent or with a sinus which may drain for weeks, months, or years, when the disease again exacerbates or gives rise to metastasis. This series of events is repeated time and time again until the patient is either operated upon radically or he succumbs to a metastasis in one of the internal organs, general sepsis, or amyloidosis.[8]

Many of the cases being treated were children, and Nathan expressed his concern for these patients:

> The children cry out when anyone comes near the bed, they shriek when the dressings are changed, and are so terror- stricken when they

finally leave the hospital that sometimes months go by before they gain their mental equilibrium. I am, therefore, pleading for a more intelligent and appropriate attitude toward these patients.[9]

Percy Roberts, who joined the Department in 1914, designed a traction frame to help alleviate some of the monotony associated with being a pediatric orthopaedic patient. Unlike the devices usually employed, Roberts's frame allowed the patient to be moved about and carried out into the fresh air when so desired.[10] An imaginative and innovative man, Roberts recognized that the astragalus (heel bone) had a similar shape to the femoral head of the hip when held in a certain position, and he devised a method of using the astragalus in hip reconstruction in patients whose hip had been destroyed by tuberculosis.[11]

The initial orthopaedic staff at Mount Sinai was small, consisting of Nathan, Percy Roberts, Edgar D. Oppenheimer, and Samuel K. Kleinberg, who subsequently became Chief of Orthopaedics at the Hospital for Joint Diseases. When the Department was assigned nine hospital beds in 1923, a number of men were added to the staff, including Seth Selig, Sigmund Epstein, and Robert Lippmann. The *Annual Report* for 1924 indicates that the Department "is being organized on a firm basis and is expected to prove of great value to the other clinicians in the consultations of obscure conditions." Inpatient and outpatient treatment at the time was largely nonsurgical and consisted of bracing, manipulation of deformities, including scoliosis, and casting or traction for major fractures. Experiences in Great Britain with new surgical techniques to correct deformities, release contractures, transplant tendons, and fuse joints gained rapid acceptance in the United States. In 1934, Nathan retired at the mandated age limit, and he died the following year. For the next five years, the position of Chief of the Department remained vacant.

During the 1930s, there was growing competition between the Department of Orthopaedics and the Department of Surgery over the right to treat certain types of cases. Eventually, the Medical Board decided, in 1938, to expand the scope of the Orthopaedic Service. By the end of the decade, the Department's inpatient census had almost tripled compared to that of ten years earlier. Samuel Rupert, the first Orthopaedic Resident, graduated in 1938.

From 1939 until 1941, Robert Lippmann and Seth Selig were Co-Chiefs of the Department. In 1934, Selig was the first to report a

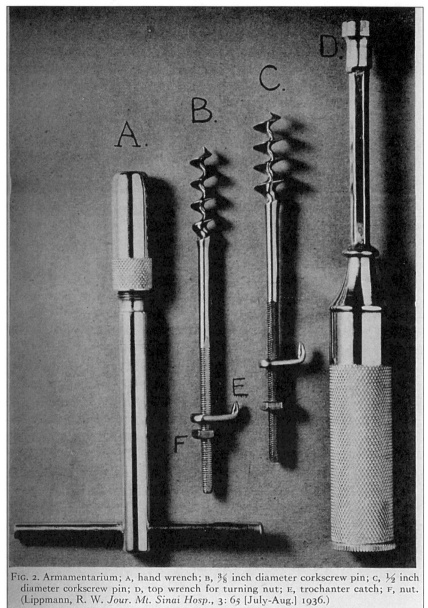

FIG. 2. Armamentarium; A, hand wrench; B, ⅜ inch diameter corkscrew pin; C, ½ inch diameter corkscrew pin; D, top wrench for turning nut; E, trochanter catch; F, nut. (Lippmann, R. W. *Jour. Mt. Sinai Hosp.*, 3: 65 [July-Aug.] 1936.)

Lippmann screw, developed by Robert Lippmann, M.D., Chief of the Orthopaedics Service, 1939–1960.

successful interinnomino-abdominal (or "hindquarter") amputation in America.[12] That same year, he was also the first to describe a safe method of operating on the obturator foramen via a perineal approach.[13] Selig also introduced the use of Kirshner wires for internal fixation in the treatment of hammertoe, allowing patients greater mobility and a shorter recovery period than did other methods in use at the time.[14] Upon Selig's death in 1941, Lippmann became the sole Chief of the Department.

Lippmann had interned at Mount Sinai from 1923 until 1925 before going to Vienna and Bologna to study bone pathology. In 1926, he was appointed Adjunct Orthopaedist and joined Nathan in practice. Lippmann was very creative in the production of new instruments. In fact, he had a workshop with power tools in his office to help in the construction and design of his inventions. His corkscrew bolt for the compression fixation of hip fractures was certainly his most famous.[15] The use of compression to stabilize fractures while at the same time stimulating early bone healing represented a great advance in internal fixation. Lippmann devised a new method of fixing depressed tibial plateau fractures without the use of metal plates and screws.[16] In addition, he was an expert on the "frozen shoulder," describing its natural history and the results of conservative and surgical treatment.[17] Lippmann also introduced "an important but unfortunately too seldom appreciated"[18] supplementary clinical method of testing for the presence of a fracture and for monitoring its healing utilizing a stethoscope (auscultatory percussion) to assess bone continuity.[19] His method was quick and painless and could be performed on the spot when an x-ray was not immediately at hand. Lippmann also described a method to measure the curve in scoliosis that was universally used. "Under Lippmann's leadership, the service grew rapidly to become a fully board approved residency training program in fractures and adult and children's orthopaedics."[20] In 1948, a pediatric orthopaedic clinic was established. The caseload at the time consisted largely of patients with osteomyelitis, tuberculosis, and poliomyelitis.

In 1949, the Department began an affiliation with the Blythedale Convalescent Home (now the Blythedale Hospital). Blythedale, located in the New York City suburb of Valhalla, in Westchester County, was a long-term care institution and provided an excellent opportunity for follow-up treatment of patients referred by other orthopaedic services in the city. The association lasted through the 1970s, by which time many of the diseases treated at Blythedale, including polio and tuber-culosis, were no longer prevalent.

Edgar Bick was the first Mount Sinai physician in charge of Blythedale. Bick came to Mount Sinai as a Clinical Assistant in the out-patient Department in 1930 and remained at the Hospital until his death in 1978, by which time he was a Consultant Orthopaedic Surgeon and Emeritus Clinical Professor of Orthopaedics. During World War II, Bick served as Chief of Orthopaedic Surgery in Mount Sinai's Third General Hospital, in North Africa, Italy, and France. Bick's early work focused on soft tissue and bone tumors[21] and on the pathology and clinical study of osteogenesis of human vertebrae.[22] Later he made notable con-tributions to the management of fractures and orthopaedic disabilities in the aged.[23,24] The departmental scholar, Bick was best known for his work on the history of orthopaedics. His definitive texts, *Source Book of Orthopaedics*[25] and *Classics of Orthopaedics*,[26] remain the standard works on the subject.

During the decade 1950–1960, the Department expanded consider-ably in activity and scope. The experience gained during World War II in trauma, fractures, and rehabilitation provided the stimulus for a sig-nificant expansion of the role of orthopaedics as a clinical specialty. Fracture management, which at Mount Sinai, as elsewhere, had been within the sphere of General Surgery, came under the domain of Or-thopaedics. With the introduction of noncorrosive metallic plates, screws, and pins, the surgical and reconstructive aspects of the specialty improved throughout the world. At Mount Sinai, Alvin Arkin, a dy-namic and imaginative orthopaedist, had a metal cup fabricated to re-place a hip socket and designed a metal cap to replace the femoral head to treat severe arthritis long before total joint replacements became a re-ality. Later, Arkin would go on to do important work on scoliosis[27] and epiphyseal growth.[28]

Throughout this period, the Department continued to embrace the concept of comprehensive and continuous care. Services were coordi-nated with the growing Departments of Physical Medicine and Social Services. Also, the Orthopaedic Out-Patient Clinic became more closely allied with the Inpatient Service. In 1954, Lippmann and Arthur Barsky, Chief of Plastic Surgery, established a hand service, which was placed under the direction of Joel Hartley, an orthopaedist, and Bernard Simon, a plastic surgeon. There, patients with deformities of the hand resulting from disease, trauma, or congenital anomaly were evaluated and treated, either on an ambulatory basis or as inpatients admitted for surgery.

Joel Hartley came to Mount Sinai in 1937 as an Assistant to Paul Klemperer in morbid anatomy. He began a residency in orthopaedic surgery in 1940 that was interrupted a year later for military service. He returned in 1946 to complete his training and then joined the staff. Hartley became Director of the Hip Clinic in 1964 and introduced cup arthroplasty of the hip to Mount Sinai. His research explored possible methods of stimulating osteogenesis by injection of chemical extracts of bone.[29] He also published *New Ways in First Aid*[30] and *First Aid Without Panic*,[31] the latter based on his personal experience surviving a plane crash in Africa and administering aid to his fellow passengers despite his own injuries. Hartley was also one of the founders of Health Insurance Plans of Greater New York, where he served as head of the Orthopaedic Department.

In 1960, Lippmann became President of the Medical Board of the Hospital, immediately before he retired from the Chair. "At the Mount Sinai Hospital, Lippmann's service and leadership over a period of forty-three years, his scientific inquiry and teaching and sense of humanity and ethical code of practice in his approach to patients, formed the foundation of the orthopaedic service and had great influence on the growth of the hospital as a whole."[32] Lippmann's sensitivity and his broad cultural background were also expressed in his excellence as a pianist, organist, and composer.

In 1960, Robert S. Siffert replaced Lippmann as Director and Orthopaedic Surgeon-in-Chief. Siffert began his residency at Mount Sinai in 1946, following service in the Air Force as a flight surgeon in India and China during World War II. Having had previous research experience, he continued investigative work throughout his career, publishing his first two of more than one hundred papers during his residency. He was a Blumenthal Fellow in pathology when he began practice. In 1949, he and Arkin introduced a new spinal biopsy needle that could obtain excellent, undistorted cores of tissue to aid in the differential diagnosis of many lesions.[33] In 1950, he used histochemical techniques to identify the role of alkaline phosphatase in matrix formation.[34]

During Siffert's early tenure, the residency program increased from three to six Residents. Siffert created subspecialty divisions and a specialty fellowship to improve the educational program. Staff participation in local and national scientific societies was also encouraged. With the advent of the Mount Sinai School of Medicine, Siffert became the first Professor and Chairman of the Department; the other staff members received faculty appointments. In 1983, Siffert was named the first Robert K. Lippmann Professor of Orthopaedics.

In the early 1960s, following study in England, Roger Levy, a recent graduate of the residency, began to perform total joint replacements at Mount Sinai. Levy was appointed Chief of Joint Replacement and over the years made fundamental contributions to the design of new prosthetic hips for total joint replacement that have stood the test of time. He has also conducted important long-term follow-up studies on the effectiveness of these devices.[35]

In 1961, Mount Sinai's affiliation with the hospitals of New York City proved a boon to the Department. The substantial increase in exposure to trauma accelerated the growth of the Department and was invaluable for House Staff training. From 1961 until 1963, Robert Hyman directed the Department's brief affiliation with Greenpoint Hospital. When that affiliation was dropped in favor of one with City Hospital Center at Elmhurst, Albert J. Schein became the first Director of Orthopaedics at that institution. Schein, trained at Mount Sinai and then a member of the Attending staff, established a reputation as a brilliant clinical orthopaedic surgeon and teacher. His pioneering clinical research with Arkin on the bone manifestations of Gaucher's disease represented a critical step forward in the understanding of the disease.[36] Following his death, Schein was succeeded by Elias Sedlin as Chief at Elmhurst. Sedlin had a strong background in research, studying the relationship of special field reactions of bone to mechanical forces and osteon formation. Most recently, Edward Yang, an expert in trauma replaced Sedlin as Director at Elmhurst and Consultant at Queens Hospital Center, another municipal hospital. Spanning the tenure of all of the Elmhurst Chiefs was Judith Levine, who has played a most important role in the teaching program for many years. Subsequent to the affiliation with Elmhurst, the residency was increased to nine positions, allowing each resident to spend one-third of his or her training in a trauma center. Integration of both staffs, common conferences, and the ability to transfer patients to receive the best care enriched both the Department and the other institutions. During this period, Resident training was also offered in associated aspects of orthopaedics at numerous facilities off campus, including New York University's Prosthetic and

Orthotic Program, Oxford University's Hemophilia Program, and a number of centers with large sports medicine programs.

In the late 1960s, the Hospital for Joint Diseases affiliated with the Mount Sinai School of Medicine, and its Director, Henry J. Mankin, became Professor of Orthopedics and soon joined Siffert as Co-Chairman of the Department at Mount Sinai. Mankin was well known for his basic research with cartilage and for the utilization of allografts in limb salvage procedures. In 1972, Mankin was recruited to Harvard, and soon thereafter the Department's affiliation with the Hospital for Joint Diseases was terminated.

Siffert's tenure was also marked by the growth of a number of specialized programs, including pediatric orthopaedics. As the Senior Orthopaedic Consultant for the New York City Department of Health (1950–1960), Siffert played a dominant role in setting the standards for quality care of the orthopaedic handicapped child throughout the City. He later established a children's orthopaedic clinic at Mount Sinai that permitted doctors from around the City to refer patients for consultation and specialized care. Jacob Katz, the pediatric orthopaedist, became the first full-time orthopaedic faculty member at the Mount Sinai campus. Katz's and Siffert's interests in pediatric orthopaedics led to a close collaboration with the Department of Pediatrics and its Chairman, Horace Hodes. Katz, a Co-Resident with Siffert, was a pioneer in the treatment of Perthes disease and other developmental disorders in children[37,38] and was Director of Orthopaedics at Blythedale from 1967 until his death in 1983. Katz's and Siffert's collaborative efforts produced both laboratory research and clinical publications. Their work encompassed microangiographic studies, the effects of trauma on growing bone, and the dynamics of the growth plate, which in turn led to the development of new operations. In association with Benjamin Nachamie, they devised a triple arthrodesis for the correction of severe cavus deformity,[39] and Siffert created an intraepiphyseal osteotomy for knee stabilization in Blount's disease.[40] The work also led to the publication of two texts[41] and a parent's guide to normal and abnormal growth.[42]

In 1969, Marvin Gilbert, the orthopaedist, and Louis Aledort, the hematologist, founded Mount Sinai's Hemophilia Center. Gilbert, internationally recognized for his work in hemophilia, was the first to report on radial head resection and synovectomy of the elbow in the hemophiliac.[43] In collaboration with George Hermann, the radiologist,

Gilbert reported on one of the largest series of hemophilic pseudo-tumors.[44] He was the first orthopaedic surgeon to become a Medical Director of the National Hemophilia Foundation in 1991 and founded that organization's Musculoskeletal Committee. He was also a founding member of the International Hemophilia Association and served as its President.

In 1972, the pediatric orthopaedist Richard Ulin joined the faculty. He contributed greatly to the expansion of the clinical program and the residency and became Chief of Pediatric Orthopaedics. Along with Siffert and Katz, Ulin was a co-founder of the Orthopaedic Club of New York. In 1975, a sports medicine program was established in conjunction with City University of New York under the directorship of Burton Berson, who introduced arthroscopy and reconstructive sports-related operations to Mount Sinai. He was also a consultant in sports medicine programs in schools throughout the City, emphasizing injury prevention.

With the Department's move to the Annenberg Building in 1974, research space and laboratory assistance became available. The basic scientists Arnold L. Oronsky and Gerald Suarez were involved in important research on cartilage metabolism and articular changes due to nonenzymatic processes. In 1982, the Department established a bioelectrochemistry laboratory with the recruitment of Arthur A. Pilla, Ph.D., and Jonathan Kaufman, Ph.D. In 1990, these researchers demonstrated that bone healing is accelerated by the application of ultrasound, which resulted in a widely used method of treatment of fractures in clinical orthopaedics.[45]

While specialized centers and programs were created and flourished, the Department never lost sight of the entire patient. A multidisciplinary team was always present at rounds and at teaching conferences. Selvan Davison, the internist, Howard Zucker or Louis Linn, the psychiatrists, and either Doris Siegel or Helen Rehr, representing Social Services, provided coordinated and integrated care. More than any other clinical service, the Department collaborated with Rehabilitation Medicine throughout the continuum of treatment and recovery.

Throughout his time as Chief, Siffert volunteered for work in CARE, the largest nongovernmental organization in the world devoted to development and emergency relief. As Chairman of the medical arm of CARE and a member of its board, Siffert served month-long tours in Tunisia, Indonesia, Afghanistan, Kenya, Peru, and Haiti, devoting his efforts to training surgeons and developing new orthopaedic programs in those countries. Despite his demanding clinical, research, and pro bono activities, Siffert was able to find the time to perfect his skills as an artist, and his woodcuts have been widely exhibited to critical acclaim. In 1986, after twenty-six years as Chairman of the Department, Siffert retired from the Chair but remained an active member of the Department as the Lasker-Siffert Distinguished Service Professor and Attending. Siffert's remarkable accomplishments in orthopaedics as a preeminent clinician, researcher, teacher, and international leader have brought him and Mount Sinai worldwide recognition.

Orthopaedics was one of the last two Departments (neurosurgery being the other) to name a full-time Chairman, and its faculty, with the exception of Katz and the Elmhurst staff, were all voluntary physicians until 1986. Nevertheless, they shouldered the entire burden of patient care, teaching, and research. In addition to day-to-day teaching at the bedside, in the operating room, and in the clinics, Ernest Barash served as Chief of Orthopedics at the Jewish Home and Hospital, Robert Zaretsky was responsible for coordinating pathology teaching, Herbert Sherry directed orthopaedic oncology and also had prime responsibility for the medical student's musculoskeletal course, and James Capozzi directed the Department's program in medical ethics.

Sheldon Lichtblau conducted the orthopaedic journal club. In addition to contributing his teaching abilities in general orthopaedics, Lichtblau maintained a special interest in clubfoot that led to the development of a new procedure for its correction.[46] Over the years, the Department received invaluable service from Michael Klein, of the Department of Pathology, in the teaching of bone pathology. Many of the graduates of the residency have remained on the faculty, while others have gone on to major academic careers at other institutions.

In 1986, the Orthopaedic Department moved from the Annenberg Building to a larger academic and practice office in the new faculty practice facility. In that same year, Michael Lewis was appointed the first full-time Chairman of the Department, which was renamed the Leni and Peter May Department of Orthopaedics. Lewis had designed the Lewis Expandable and Adjustable Lower Extremity Prosthesis (LEAP), which revolutionized the treatment of bone tumors in growing children. Instead of amputating the affected limb, surgeons removed the tumor and replaced the excised bone with a prosthesis that could be adjusted as the child grew.[47,48] In strengthening the subspecialties,

Lewis recruited full-time faculty in a number of different areas. This included Michael Hausman to direct the hand and upper extremity program, Andrew Casden in spine surgery, John Waller in foot surgery, Elton Strauss for fractures and geriatric surgery, and Thomas Einhorn as Director of Orthopaedic Research. Einhorn's elegant investigations in the field of bone metabolism[49] and in sequential enzymatic stages in bone healing[50] have broken new ground in understanding the mechanism of changes in bone metabolism and healing. Einhorn moved to become Professor and Chairman of the Department of Orthopaedics at the Boston University School of Medicine in 1997. Lewis played a primary role in attempts to integrate Orthopaedics with other Departments in the Hospital and Medical School. In 1993, Lewis left to become Medical Director of the Vanderbilt Stallworth Rehabilitation Hospital in Nashville Tennessee. Upon Lewis's resignation, Siffert, and then Ulin, served as Acting Chairmen for a combined period of three years.

In 1996, Dempsey Springfield was appointed Chair of the Department and Robert K. Lippmann Professor. An orthopaedic oncologist, Springfield occupies a prominent national and international position in the field. Drawing on his prior faculty experience at the University of Florida and at Harvard, Springfield introduced a strong educational program focusing on basic and clinically related research. Springfield has incorporated the active voluntary faculty into the program and strengthened the full-time faculty with outstanding recruitments. Timothy Radomisli, a pediatric orthopaedist, James Gladstone, who focuses on sports medicine and upper extremity surgery, and Steven Weinfeld, who specializes in foot surgery, have added strength and depth to the Department. Brian Markinson became the first full-time podiatrist on the faculty. Evan Flatow, the Bernard J. Lasker Professor of Orthopaedics, was recruited to be Chief of Shoulder Surgery. Internationally known, Flatow has done research on the physiology of soft tissue healing and ligament injury repair. The full-time and voluntary faculties have melded seamlessly to allow for rapid and innovative progress in the Department.

Mitchell Schaffler, Ph.D., an outstanding investigator in the field of bone physiology and dynamics, joined the faculty as the Director of the Orthopaedic Research Laboratory and Professor of Orthopaedics. Schaffler, assisted by Robert Majeska, Ph.D., and Carl Jepsen, M.D., has developed a team approach to musculoskeletal disease research. The program is organized into four units: a cell biology unit, which focuses on molecular mechanisms of disease; a tissue physiology unit, which examines integrated cell-tissue-organ function; a bioengineering unit, which explores biomechanical aspects of skeletal disease; and a clinical research effort, which aims to move basic research toward patient treatment. In this section of the research laboratory, Siffert and Kaufman have developed computer and simulation methods to study the dynamics of osteoporosis and the relationship between bone mass and architecture.[51] In addition to basic research, Schaffler has developed a comprehensive teaching program in anatomy.

Since the beginning of Springfield's chairmanship, the Department has grown to include twelve full-time faculty, twenty-two voluntary faculty, and three full-time research faculty. The residency is now a five-year program, with three Residents, appointed each year for a total of fifteen. As of 2000, the Department has subspecialties in hand, shoulder, spine, adult reconstruction, pediatrics, and sports medicine. More than 1,500 patients are admitted annually, more than three thousand operations are performed each year, and outpatient services have greatly increased. The Department now has five research grants funded by the National Institutes of Health.

As the Department enters the new millennium and heads towards its own centennial anniversary in 2009, it is well positioned to continue to contribute to the advancement of Orthopaedics for many years to come.

25

Department of Otolaryngology

STORIES AND ANECDOTES about the Great Blizzard of 1888 abound, and, like most hospitals in New York, Mount Sinai did not go untouched by the storm. Ironically, the blizzard provided an opportunity for an important Mount Sinai first: the first performance in America of a complete mastoidectomy, by Emil Gruening. As a result of the high incidence of influenza caused by the storm, a large number of patients with the complication of mastoiditis appeared at the Hospital. In fact, in the three years following the blizzard, more operations on the mastoid were performed at Mount Sinai than during any other previous triennial period. It was during this time that Emil Gruening perfected his technique, which included cleaning out the entire mastoid cavity and establishing a communication with the middle ear.[1,2] Earlier, incomplete procedures had led to continued drainage and the always present threat of cerebral complications. Word of Gruening's improved results became known, and physicians from outside the Hospital would frequently come to Mount Sinai to watch Gruening perform his operation.[3]

An 1862 émigré from East Prussia, Gruening served as a private in the Union Army before attending medical school in New York. In 1879, he established the Ear and Eye Service at Mount Sinai. At this point in history, otology was still in its infancy, and operations on the ear were limited. Gruening later opened the Eye and Ear Clinic for outpatients in 1884, and in 1890 he organized the Ear, Nose, and Throat Clinic. When the Hospital moved from Lexington Avenue to Fifth Avenue in 1904, the Service was assigned eighteen beds. In 1906, Gruening was elected President of the American Otological Society. In the words of Arpad Gerster, Gruening was "a well-knit man of small stature, and had a fine cut profile."[4] Others recalled his long beard, which in the early days before asepsis would occasionally touch a patient's wound during surgery. All those who remembered him agreed upon his remarkable capabilities in surgery; his hands, though large, were noted as having great lightness and deftness. According to Gerster, Gruening was able

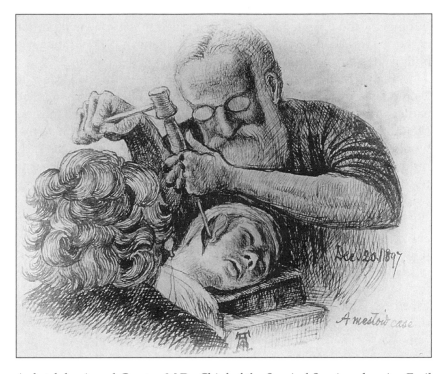

A sketch by Arpad Gerster, M.D., Chief of the Surgical Service, showing Emil Gruening, M.D., performing a mastoidectomy. Gruening was perhaps the first to do a mastoidectomy in this country. The man on the left with his back to the viewer is Abraham Jacobi, M.D., "Father of Pediatrics in America" and Mount Sinai's first pediatrician.

to raise the field of otology "from the slough of inefficiency in which he found it."[5]

In 1910, with the separation of Otology from Ophthalmology, Mount Sinai established the first independent Otology Service in any New York hospital, and Frederick Whiting was appointed Mount Sinai's first Attending Otologist and Director of Otology. Whiting had previously published the first book on ear surgery written in English, in 1905.[6] During his time as Director, Whiting introduced newly developed procedures to manage chronic ear suppuration with cholesteatoma. He was also Mount Sinai's first surgeon to perform re-section of the jugular vein for sigmoid sinus thrombosis and bulbar thrombosis and operated for abscesses located in the sphenoid portion of the temporal bone. By the time of his retirement, in 1921, Whiting had both witnessed and contributed to the birth of modern otology.

Upon Whiting's retirement, Isidore Friesner, who had come to Mount Sinai in 1920, was appointed Director of Otology. Friesner had earlier written the first book in English on the inner ear.[7] He established Mount Sinai's first residency program in otology in 1923, a move that would yield enormous benefits in the years to come. Among the early residents were men who would later make important contributions to the field, including Samuel Rosen, Irving Goldman, Harry Rosenwasser, and Joseph Goldman.

During the 1920s, research in otology at Mount Sinai focused on sinus thrombosis,[8] pathology of the labyrinth, the pathways of intracranial infection from the mastoid,[9] and tests for the early diagnosis of pontine angle tumors. Friesner established a histopathology laboratory in conjunction with Otology, and, in 1928, Joseph G. Druss established the Otopathology Laboratory. Originally located in a corner of the Pathology Museum in the basement, this laboratory eventually became part of the Eye and Ear Laboratory in the Laboratory Annex and contained one of the largest collections of sectioned temporal bones in the country. Friesner also helped establish systematic consultation between Otology and Neurology, and otologists were invited to examine all neurology cases with ear symptoms in order to rule out any otogenic central nervous system complications.

When Friesner retired in 1936, Jacob Maybaum replaced him. In 1938, shortly after the introduction of sulfonamides, the Department evaluated sulfanilamide for treatment of acute ear infections;[10] in 1939, the first audiometer was installed in the clinic. Maybaum established the field of neuro-otological diagnosis at Mount Sinai and offered postgraduate courses in the specialty. In 1940, Maybaum was the first Mount Sinai surgeon to perform fenestration procedures for otosclerosis. Five years later, Harry Rosenwasser described the first paraganglioma in the middle ear and mastoid.[11] Prior to the advent of antibiotics, ear infections were responsible for the preponderance of cases managed by otologists. Penicillin was used for the first time to treat ear infections at Mount Sinai late in 1944. By the time Maybaum retired in 1946, the emergence of sulpha drugs and penicillin had decreased the case volume of the Otology Service, and the Department of Otology merged with the Department of Laryngology to form the Department of Otolaryngology.

Like Otology, the Department of Laryngology at Mount Sinai had a distinguished early history. It began in 1903, when a separate service was created for diseases of the throat and D. Bryson Delavan was appointed the first Laryngologist to the Hospital. Already well known for his work in tumors of the ear, nose, and throat and an excellent speaker and teacher, Delavan brought a wealth of experience to Mount Sinai and added to the luster of the institution. In 1911, Emil Mayer became Director of Laryngology, a position he held for six years.

In 1917, Sidney Yankauer was appointed Director of the Laryngology Service, which was given departmental status with six allocated beds on the surgical wards. A native New Yorker, Yankauer had followed a typical path to an 1893 internship at Mount Sinai: undergraduate studies at the College of the City of New York and medical school at Columbia University's College of Physicians and Surgeons. An early appointment to the Surgery Clinic of the Outpatient Department provided the opportunity for him to develop the skills that eventually led to his appointment as Chief of Laryngology.

Yankauer's dexterity with a bronchoscope could not be matched. In 1905, he performed the first successful bronchoscopy in New York City to remove a foreign body.[12] Yankauer was also an ingenious inventor who devised many of his own instruments, including bronchoscopic tubes, irrigating tubes, tonsillectomy instruments, numerous forceps for operations on the paranasal sinuses, and a speculum for the direct examination and treatment of the Eustachian tubes.[13] Although now replaced by a disposable plastic instrument, the "Yankauer suction" tube remains an important part of the surgeon's armamentarium to this day. Yankauer also performed extensive anatomical studies of the ear, utilizing his own instruments.[14]

Yankauer's skill was legendary, and many tales of his creativity still linger today. For instance, there was the time when he and Howard Lilienthal were working together at Mount Sinai's Base Hospital No. 3 in France during World War I, and the Quartermaster accidentally locked the key inside the safe where all the men's pay was kept. Fortunately, Yankauer was able to save the day by constructing a new key out of the tools at hand, opening the safe, and thus retrieving the original key and money. Lilienthal concluded that "no wonder, with such dexterity combined with his high scientific attainments, Dr. Yankauer was recognized as one of the foremost men of his specialty."[15]

Yankauer established a special Tonsil and Adenoid ward at the Hospital in 1918. Prior to this, tonsillectomy and adenoidectomy were performed in the clinic, often without anesthesia. The Department was at the forefront in combining radiation and surgery to treat cancer of the larynx and, in 1920, reported five-year cures in two patients who underwent combination therapy.[16] In 1925, Yankauer reported having bronchscoped four hundred patients with lung abscess and treated seventy-one of them with multiple endoscopic irrigations, for a total of 3,000 procedures.[17] One year later, Yankauer proposed an improved method for the application of radium in treating cancer of the esophagus.[18] Other research studies during the Yankauer era focused on the pathology of benign tumors of the larynx,[19] the bacteriology of bronchial secretions, and the experimental production of lung abscess.

Upon Yankauer's death in 1932, Rudolph Kramer was appointed the Director of Laryngology, and in that same year he published a landmark paper with Amiel Glass describing the bronchopulmonary segments of the lung for the first time.[20] In 1939, studies were conducted of cerebrospinal fluid rhinorrhea and laryngeal lesions associated with hormone therapy. In 1942, special attention was directed toward the study of massive collapse of the lung and endoscopic treatment of esophageal varices. In 1946, with the merger of otology and laryngology, Kramer became the first Director of the new Department of Otolaryngology.

The following years were ones of great activity for the newly created Department. The ear remained a major focus of interest. In the clinic, a soundproof booth was installed for pure tone audiometry. In 1948, after performing four hundred fenestration procedures on cadavers, Samuel Rosen reported his unique experimental studies of the surgical anatomy of the ear.[21] These studies provided otologists with invaluable knowledge for avoiding errors in the fenestration procedure. Four years later, Rosen presented the first of several papers reporting a new treatment for Meniere's disease that involved electrical stimulation of the Chorda Tympani,[22] and in 1953 Rosen published his landmark paper on the success of stapes manipulation in restoring hearing in patients with otosclerosis.[23] Although the procedure had been performed earlier, results were dismal, and the practice was abandoned. Rosen is credited with its revival, and, subsequent to his success, a stapes mobilization clinic was established in 1955. Irving B. Goldman, one of Friesner's residents, pursued his singleminded interest in aesthetic surgery of the nose, which led him in 1953 to organize a two-week course in nasal plastic and reconstructive surgery at Mount Sinai.[24] The "Annual Mount Sinai Goldman Seminar on Rhinoplasty," which attracts surgeons from across the world, continues to this day under the leadership of William Lawson.

When Joseph L. Goldman was appointed Director of Otolaryngology in 1954, he was already known for having developed, in the 1930s, a successful vaccine for type III pneumococcus mastoiditis, which at that time reduced Mount Sinai's mortality rate from this disease from 24 percent to 4 percent.[25] However, with the arrival of antibiotics, the vaccine became obsolete. With the exception of four years in the Army during World War II, where he attained the rank of Colonel and received an Army Commendation Ribbon, Goldman spent his entire professional career at Mount Sinai.

As the Director, Goldman continued to make important contributions to Mount Sinai and to the specialty. In 1955, Goldman obtained approval for the Otolaryngology Service to include head and neck surgery in its program. This represented a hard-fought victory for Goldman, who would continue to spend much of his professional career advocating the right of Otolaryngology to gain control of head and neck surgery, including facial plastic surgery.[26] His position led to acrimonious debates between Otolaryngology and the Departments of Surgery and Plastic Surgery both within and outside Mount Sinai. Thanks to Goldman's forcefulness, Otolaryngology prevailed. In 1964, Goldman played a pivotal role in the formation of the American Academy of Facial Plastic and Reconstructive Surgery.[27] Irving Goldman served as its first President. Other Mount Sinai otolaryngologists who played major roles in that organization included Sidney Feuerstein and Samuel Bloom. Many of the graduates of the residency program would also go on to leadership positions in that and other organizations.

Goldman was fortunate in having Max Som, a leading head and neck surgeon, and the latter's associate, Leon Arnold, on the staff to help perform and to teach the procedures to the Otolaryngology staff and Residents. Som, an outstanding endoscopist, keenly interested in surgical research, brought many significant advances to the rapidly evolving field of laryngeal and upper esophageal surgery.[28]

Following up on the work of Yankauer in treating larynx cancer with combination radiation and surgery, Goldman, in the 1950s, introduced the concept of high-dose preoperative radiation followed by surgery in patients with advanced cancer of the larynx. A fourteen-year follow-up indicated that this combined method of therapy resulted in improved survival rates for patients with advanced cancer.[29] In 1969, the Department was awarded the Hektoen Medal of the American Medical Association for its exhibit on this management strategy.

Under Goldman's direction, members of the Department were stimulated to seek outside funding for both clinical and research activities, and their success in this endeavor is readily apparent. For example, a temporal bone bank was established in 1965 with a grant from the Deafness Research Foundation. Histopathologic studies of experimental stapes surgery in animals were conducted with support from the National Institutes of Health.

Goldman believed that, in order to have a strong department, it was of paramount importance to build a program that was centered around high-quality Residents. Thus, in 1958, he instituted a new four-year residency program in Otolaryngology. The program was immediately successful. When he became Director, there was one Resident in each year of the program; at his retirement in 1972, there were three in each of the four years. The program expanded to include City Hospital Center at Elmhurst and the Bronx Veterans Administration Medical Center. The fact that every Resident who graduated from the program during Goldman's tenure was certified by the American Board of Otolaryngology on his or her first attempt at the Board examination attests to the quality of the program, its faculty, and the House Staff. It can safely be said that the Department of Otolaryngology at Mount Sinai came of age under the stewardship of Joseph L. Goldman.

Upon Goldman's retirement in 1972, Hugh F. Biller was appointed Chairman of the Department. A superb head and neck surgeon, Biller joined the faculty of Washington University School of Medicine in St. Louis following completion of his training at the Johns Hopkins University Hospital. He was an ideal choice to further Goldman's goal of capturing all the aforementioned surgery for the Department. As noted earlier, concurrent with its drive to perform head and neck surgery, Otolaryngology made a concerted effort to become more involved in facial plastic surgery, and so in 1974 Mount Sinai offered the first facelift course in the United States given by an Otolaryngology department. The Departments's first facial plastics Fellow was appointed in 1980.

During his twenty-three-year tenure as Chairman, Biller propelled the Department to new heights. The author or co-author of three hundred clinical and research papers while at Mount Sinai, Biller, along with his faculty, made major contributions to the management of afflictions of the ear, the nose, and the throat.[30] Simon Parisier performed the first cochlear implant at Mount Sinai in 1983 and went on to become a leading proponent of the procedure as the Chief at the Manhattan Eye and Ear Hospital. Laboratory researchers investigated mechanisms of aeration of the middle ear. William Lawson would become Mount Sinai's leading sinus surgeon and publish an important text on the subject.[31] Lawson would also co-author a major work, *The Paraganglionic Chemoreceptor System*, with Frederick Zak, of the Department of Pathology.[32] Goldman, who remained active in the Department after his retirement from the Chair, would also write an authoritative text on rhinology.[33]

The advent of the laser as a therapeutic instrument led to its use in managing vocal cord paralysis and the correction of laryngeal and tracheal stenosis.[34] New procedures were developed for laryngeal reconstruction after partial laryngectomy. In 1985, Biller co-edited the definitive work *Surgery of the Larynx*.[35] The Grabscheid Clinical and Research Center for Voice Disorders was established in 1989, and Ira Sanders was appointed Research Director of the Center. Studies were conducted on larynx physiology, electromyography of the canine larynx, and the effect of laryngeal pacing in bilateral vocal cord paralysis. In 1999, scientists at the Center discovered slow tonic muscle fibers in the muscles of the human vocal cords. Because these types of muscles have not been found in the vocal cords of other mammals, the researchers postulate that they are an explanation for speech specialization in humans. These findings have created a stir among speech and language theorists, because they provide scientific support for Noam Chomsky's theory that humans have a different biology that underlies their speech ability.[36]

But the central focus of the Department continued to be in head and neck surgery. In 1981, a new surgical procedure for improved exposure of the base of the skull, nasopharynx, and cervical spine was developed by Biller.[37] Collaboration with the Department of Neurosurgery led to the creation of the multidisciplinary Division of Skull Base Surgery. In

1988, with the early collaboration of Hubert Weinberg, a plastic surgeon on the faculty of the Department of Surgery, the microvascular surgery laboratory was established. The laboratory, under the leadership of Mark Urken and housed in Department of Otolaryngology space, has been extraordinarily productive, with a focus on free-flap reconstruction of the head and neck following ablative surgery.[38] It has also proved to be invaluable in the training of the otolaryngology House Staff in microvascular surgery.

Because Biller was cognizant of the psychologic implications of ablative head and neck surgery and associated reconstruction and the problems of speech disorders, he forged strong links with the liaison service of the Department of Psychiatry. The combined rounds and consultations proved to be a boon, not only to both Departments but, most important, to the patients.[39]

The success of the residency program during the past twenty years continues to ensure the strength of the Department. In 1988, a Resident rotation in laboratory research was established, and, in 1989, the first M.D.-Ph.D. student to write a dissertation focusing on otolaryngology was accepted jointly with the Department of Anatomy and Cell Biology. By 1990, the residency program had expanded to four years of otolaryngology following one year of general surgery, and the first microvascular surgery fellow was appointed. Currently, three Residents and three subspecialty Fellows are appointed annually.

In 1995, Mark Urken was appointed Department Chairman following Biller's retirement. Urken had been Co-Director of the Microvascular Research Laboratory since 1989 and had made numerous contributions in reconstructive surgery of the oral cavity. He headed a team that was the first to report the return of sensation following reconstructive surgery using radial forearm free flaps in patients with pharyngeal defects.[40] Urken was also the first to report on a functional assessment of mastication in oral cancer patients who were rehabilitated with enosseous implants placed into mandibles that had been reconstructed with vascularized bone transferred from other parts of the body.[41]

Under Urken's dynamic leadership, the Department has evolved into multiple formal areas of subspecialization that traverse the entire scope of otolaryngology. These subspecialty areas include sleep disorders, breathing, pediatric otolaryngology, skull-based surgery, otology/neuro-otology, sinus surgery, and facial plastic surgery. Two multidisciplinary clinical teams have received national and international acclaim. The clinical voice program, headed by Peak Woo, has developed a superlative team dedicated to the diagnosis and management of the entire spectrum of voice disorders. Under the direction of Urken, the head and neck oncology program evolved into a premier center for microvascular reconstructive surgery. The clinical team includes Daniel Buchbinder, with his expertise in oral and maxillofacial surgery, and Devon Okay, whose field is maxillofacial prosthodontics. The group receives outstanding support from Peter Som (the son of Max Som), a superb head and neck radiologist, and Margaret Brandwein, who provides unique scholarship in head and neck pathology. The international acclaim accorded to the annual head and neck reconstruction course, a week-long program of lectures, workshops, and operative clinics started in 1988, serves as testimony to the success of this team. Urken's textbook, *Atlas of Regional and Free Flaps for Head and Neck Reconstruction*,[42] is one of the most authoritative texts on the subject.

As the Department of Otolaryngology makes its way into the twenty-first century, it continues to employ cutting-edge technology, now including the World Wide Web. Clinical data, including digital camera images, are posted on departmental Web sites, enabling physicians worldwide to discuss treatment options for patient care. More than one hundred years after the Department's inception, its commitment to innovative research and to high-quality patient care continues to be recognized throughout the world.

26

Department of Pathology

WHEN THE JEWS' Hospital opened its doors in 1855, pathology and laboratory services were essentially nonexistent. The need for such facilities, however, became apparent when, six months after the opening of the Hospital, Mark Blumenthal, the Resident and Attending Physician, requested permission to perform an autopsy on one of his patients to "justify himself and his reputation concerning the cause of death of the patient."[1] Permission was granted by the Directors by a single-vote margin (four to three). The following month, John Hart, the President of the Hospital, introduced a resolution "that there be no postmortems in the hospital under any circumstances whatsoever unless required by law since such examinations were entirely contrary to Jewish law."[2] This resolution passed. The Chief Rabbi of London was consulted, and, when he responded that autopsies were desecrations and could be performed only in cases of suspected murder or when the cause of death was unknown and there were other patients in the Hospital with the same disease, these very stringent regulations remained in effect. Nevertheless, when it was deemed necessary, the Directors did give their approval. These autopsies were performed by the clinicians and consisted of gross examinations only.

By the last decade of the nineteenth century, the development of research medicine made the need for laboratory services self-evident. Also, the intellectual needs of the physicians to know the cause of death and to determine where they might have made errors in diagnosis led to a gradual increase in the number of autopsies requested and permissions granted. In a move spurred by the clinicians and readily accepted by the Directors, the Hospital established a laboratory in 1893 on the second floor of the Lexington Avenue building in a small corner room. Henry N. Heineman, a member of the medical staff since 1880, was named the first Pathologist. Helping to supply the laboratory with his own funds, Heineman also appointed Frederick S. Mandlebaum his Assistant and sent the latter to Europe for further study. Shortly after Mandlebaum's return, Heineman resigned, and Mandlebaum was appointed as the first full-time Pathologist in the institution. At first, the laboratory was open only a few hours a day, and Mandlebaum's salary was five hundred dollars per year.[3]

Mandlebaum would direct pathology and laboratory services for thirty years. A meticulous and tireless worker, he not only studied all of the pathology specimens and directed research in the laboratory but also cleaned the test tubes, the instruments, and often the floor. Allergic to formalin, Mandlebaum delegated the performance of autopsies to Emanuel Libman and then to George Baehr. Mandlebaum's accomplishments were many, both as a pathologist and as an administrator. He was the first to develop the technique of identifying malignant cells in tissue fluids.[4] His studies on Gaucher's disease over a period of many years, often in collaboration with Nathan Brill, paved the way for a century of interest in this genetic disorder on the part of many of Mount Sinai's staff.

Mandlebaum appointed Charles A. Elsberg his first Assistant in Pathology in 1896. Elsberg published his first paper on the serum diagnosis of typhoid fever one year later.[5] This seminal study on the Widal reaction later allowed the Hospital to trace an epidemic of typhoid in the Nurses Training School to an employee who was probably a typhoid carrier. Elsberg also published the results of the first animal experimental study performed in the laboratory on the repair of wounds of the heart.[6] Elsberg's paper was the first of thousands of publications to result from experimental work at the laboratories of The Mount Sinai Hospital. As with so many of the physicians who were Assistants or Volunteers in pathology, Elsberg would go on to great fame in his chosen field, in his case neurosurgery.[7] In 1910, Elsberg would also be responsible for the introduction of intratracheal anesthesia.[8] Elsberg tells a delightful story about the early days of the laboratory:

> White mice, rabbits and guinea-pigs were kept in a cage in the subbasement of the hospital. In the daytime the cage was rolled out into the hospital yard and at night was kept in one of the corridors. If one can apply the term to an animal cage, this cage had a checkered career. One day a grocery wagon upset the cage and the guinea-pigs and mice escaped and frightened convalescent patients who were sitting in the yard. As a result, considerable diplomacy was required before permission could be obtained to continue to keep the animals.[9]

The move of the Hospital to the 100th Street site provided the Department with its own laboratory building and allowed for expansion in both numbers of staff and scope of work. Mandlebaum created divisions within pathology and established dedicated laboratories for chemistry and bacteriology. In 1902, the first Chemistry Department in any New York hospital was instituted, directed by Samuel Bookman. The Pathology Department expanded slowly at first. By 1907, there were fifteen staff members, all of whom not only were involved in clinical work but also were encouraged from the outset to become involved in research endeavors. In that year, approximately two thousand tests were performed in total by all of the laboratories. By 1923, the staff numbered twenty-three professionals, twenty-two of them physicians. At that time, the Department had Divisions of Clinical Pathology, Neuropathology, Serology, Surgical Pathology, Bacteriology, and Physiological Chemistry. In the twelve-month period from July 1, 1922, to June 30, 1923, 15,386 tests were recorded, a dramatic contrast to the year 2000, when more than 925,000 tests were performed in the combined laboratory programs.

The pathology staff was joined by many of the Hospital's physicians, who would devote many hours to work, study, and research in the laboratories, often at night, after the day's other work was done.[10] In 1908, as a result of his laboratory and clinical experiences as a young surgeon, Leo Buerger described "thromboangiitis obliterans," to be known forever after as "Buerger's disease."[11]

A major participant in the studies conducted in the pathology laboratory was Nathan Brill. Based upon a study of two hundred twenty-one cases collected over many years, he described a form of endemic typhus that became known as Brill's disease.[12] In 1901, Brill described the clinical features of Gaucher's disease in three cases occurring in the same family.[13] Mandlebaum provided an extensive description of the pathology of the disease in 1912.[14] The patient whose autopsy was reported was a four-year-old child. One year later, Brill and Mandlebaum described the pathologic features of the disease and introduced the eponym of Gaucher.[15] As it turned out, Gaucher had misinterpreted the disease in his 1882 description. Believing erroneously that the cause of the splenic enlargement was a tumor, he used the term "primary epithelioma of the spleen."[16] Therefore, some felt that this illness, too, should rightfully be known as Brill's disease. And then, in 1925, in another study, Brill, in collaboration with George Baehr and Nathan

Rosenthal, described a form of lymphoma that became known as Brill-Symmers disease.[17]

Emanuel Libman, after serving as a member of the House Staff and after studying in Europe, was appointed Assistant Pathologist and devoted part of his early career to developing the techniques and application of blood culture. His 1906 publication, "Experience with Blood Cultures in the Study of Bacterial Infections,"[18] was an important contribution to this field. Out of this grew his interest in bacterial endocarditis, of which he was a lifelong student. A 1910 paper introduced the terms "acute" and "subacute" and called attention to the café-au-lait color of the skin and many other clinical features of bacterial endocarditis.[19] In 1924, Libman and Sacks described the abacterial "atypical verrucous endocarditis" lesions associated with lupus erythematosus (Libman-Sacks disease).[20] It is alleged that, while in charge of the autopsy service, Libman was not reluctant to employ a technique often used at the time to obtain organs in an interesting case when permission for autopsy was not forthcoming: the physician wore a shoulder-length rubber glove while retrieving organs either transvaginally or transrectally.[21]

In 1919, George Baehr returned to Mount Sinai following his service overseas as the Commanding Officer of the Hospital's World War I Unit Base Hospital No. 3. At that time, he took over Pathology's Morbid Anatomy and Autopsy Service, a position he held until 1926. Although, like Libman, Baehr was best known for his prowess as an internist, many of his most important achievements were in the realm of pathology. He provided the first description of the renal lesions in subacute bacterial endocarditis.[22] In 1935, Baehr, in association with Paul Klemperer and Arthur Schifrin, published "A Diffuse Disease of the Peripheral Circulation (Usually Associated with Lupus Erythematosus and Endocarditis)."[23] This paper represented an important step in stimulating the interest of Mount Sinai physicians in lupus. One year later, the same authors published the definitive description of the pathology of thrombotic thrombocytopenic purpura.[24] In 1940 Baehr and Klemperer described giant follicle lymphoblastoma, considered at that time to be a benign form of lymphoma.[25]

Eli Moschcowitz, trained in pathology and medicine, with appointments on both services at Mount Sinai and at Beth Israel Hospital, made landmark contributions to medicine. He was the first to describe the eosinophilia that accompanies the allergic response.[26] And, with

Abraham Wilensky, he delineated granulomatous lesions of the small intestine in 1923,[27] nine years before Burrill Crohn, Leon Ginzburg, and Gordon Oppenheimer elucidated regional ileitis,[28] work that also had its origins in the pathology laboratory. Moschcowitz also was the first to describe both thrombotic thrombocytopenic purpura (Moschcowitz's Disease)[29] and pulmonary hypertension.[30]

Since its inception, the neuropathology laboratory has been directed by individuals who have contributed in a meaningful way to the field. Joseph Globus, Mount Sinai's first neuropathologist, in collaboration with Israel Strauss, the Chief of Neurology, characterized the clinical and pathological features of the malignant brain tumor spongioblastoma.[31] In addition, Globus will always be remembered as the founding Editor-in-Chief of The Journal of the Mount Sinai Hospital, a position he held for eighteen years.

Louis Gross, a graduate of McGill University School of Medicine (1916), was appointed Associate Pathologist in 1925. A highly skilled musician who played several instruments and already established as a leading research scientist in the anatomy and pathology of the heart,[32] Gross was appointed Acting Chief of Pathology when Mandlebaum developed subacute bacterial endocarditis, which caused his death in 1926. After Paul Klemperer's arrival, Gross was appointed Director of the Pathology, Chemistry, and Bacteriology Laboratories, a position he held until his untimely and tragic death in a plane crash in 1937. A major work that proved that Libman-Sacks disease was, in fact, associated with lupus erythematosus and not related to either rheumatic fever or subacute bacterial endocarditis had been completed by Gross in 1936 and was published posthumously in 1940.[33]

In 1926, Paul Klemperer was appointed Director of Pathology and Pathologist to the Hospital. Born and trained in Vienna, Klemperer emigrated to America in 1921 "because he felt that as a Jew his future in Vienna was limited."[34] After two years at Loyola University in Chicago, he became an assistant professor of pathology in the New York Post-Graduate Medical School. It was here that Klemperer met and established his relationship with Sadao Otani, who would join Klemperer at Mount Sinai immediately after the latter's recruitment. "The bond of personal loyalty and professional collaboration that was forged between them at the Post-Graduate Hospital in 1925 was never broken."[35]

A superb teacher, whose clinical pathological conferences attracted audiences far wider than the members of his own department, Klem-

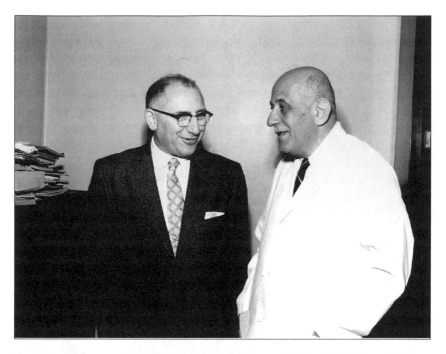

Paul Klemperer, M.D. (right), Chief of Pathology (1926–1955) talks with Hans Popper, M.D., Ph.D. Popper succeeded Klemperer as Chief of Pathology, serving as Chairman and Professor until 1972.

perer was the epitome of the compassionate, humane physician, with a soft voice, childlike humor, and a twinkle in his eye. Responding his continual emphasis on pathological anatomy as the mainspring of clinical investigation, the Hospital staff achieved autopsy rates of 80 percent within a few years of his arrival. Klemperer was the author or coauthor of almost eighty publications, a number of which were milestones in the field. In addition to those already cited, he was responsible for clarifying the relationship between cavernomatous transformation of the portal vein and Banti's disease,[36] and, with Otani, he described the changes in malignant nephrosclerosis.[37] The description by Klemperer, Abou Pollack, and Baehr, in 1941, of the pathology of disseminated lupus erythematosus[38] was a key publication in the evolution of the concept of collagen disease.[39]

As important as Klemperer's own contributions to pathology were, it was his forging of the Department that would be his legacy to

Sadao Otani, M.D.,
Pathologist.

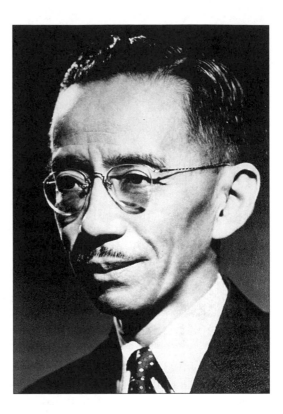

Mount Sinai. His first recruitment, Sadao Otani, would provide Mount Sinai with outstanding surgical pathology services for four decades. Otani, trained in Japan and Germany, "was a man of few words. He spoke sparingly, wrote little, and published less. This verbal frugality was backed by a powerhouse of intellect, talent, and experience in a tiny (5 ft 2 in, 100 lbs) frame. His sprightly, shy figure was a commanding presence . . . for 42 years."[40] Although Otani published fewer than a dozen papers, he was responsible for defining eosinophilic granuloma of bone.[41] In Harry Rosenwasser's delineation of a carotid body tumor of the middle ear and mastoid (later to be renamed glomus jugulare tumor), credit for the pathologic description is given to Otani.[42]

But publications were not what Otani was about. Surgeons called him to the operating room to perform a frozen section for diagnosis or went to his office with microscopic slides of a difficult case to obtain the correct diagnosis about a given lesion. And they were rarely disappointed. Not only would he review the case at hand, but also his prodigious memory would lead him to exactly the right slide of a previous, similar, difficult case, kept in a huge pile of slide trays on his desk. Unfortunately, on his desk was also a huge ashtray; Otani was a constant smoker, and this would eventually lead to his disabling emphysema, the cause of his death in 1969.

Although the majority of the staff recruited by Klemperer were either general or surgical pathologists, specialization became the order of the day, as it did in the clinical arenas. Alice Bernheim, a surgical pathologist, in collaboration with her husband, the gastroenterologist Abraham Penner, described the visceral changes in shock (Penner-Bernheim syndrome).[43] They then conducted an elegant series of experiments to establish the etiology of the condition as being due to diminished blood flow to the viscera.[44]

A native of Poland, where he received his medical degree and early pathology training, Jacob Churg completed his training at Mount Sinai in 1943. Called into the service almost immediately thereafter, he returned in 1946 to spend more than fifty years at Mount Sinai, as well as at other hospitals in the metropolitan area. With more than three hundred publications, Churg is best known for his studies on allergic granulomatosis in collaboration with Lotte Strauss (Churg-Strauss syndrome).[45] Churg also made significant contributions to the understanding of renal pathology. He introduced thin sectioning of renal specimens and special stains to study the intricate alterations of the diseased glomerulus and applied new techniques for the preparation and examination of renal biopsy tissue for electron microscopy when that modality was in its infancy.[46] The renal pathology group that included Strauss and Edith Grishman was most productive for many years. Collaborating with Irving Selikoff and E. Cuyler Hammond, Churg performed the pathological studies on asbestos-related diseases that linked asbestos exposure and smoking to lung neoplasia and the development of mesothelioma.[47] Lotte Strauss became the Department's first pediatric pathologist and made valuable contributions to fetal and developmental pathology.

Paul Klemperer retired in 1955 but continued working. He established a cell research laboratory, helped young investigators with their work, and took up the study of medical history. A myocardial infarct in August 1963 proved progressively disabling, and he died March 3,

1964. Otani became Acting Chief upon Klemperer's retirement, a position he would hold for two years.

In 1957, Hans Popper was recruited from Chicago as Pathologist-in-Chief to The Mount Sinai Hospital. Born and trained in Vienna, where his early work was in biochemistry, he fled Austria in 1938 to escape an imminent arrest, just as his predecessor Klemperer had done seventeen years earlier. And, also like Klemperer, he settled in Chicago, eventually becoming Director of Pathology at Cook County Hospital. It was here that he established his national and international reputation and became known as "the Father of Modern Hepatology." In collaboration with his long-time associate Fenton Schaffner, he published the first modern English-language textbook on the pathology of the liver.[48] Popper was the principal force behind the creation of the Hektoen Institute for Medical Research and the founding of the American Association for the Study of Liver Disease and the International Association for the Study of the Liver.

Unarguably, Hans Popper had the greatest impact on Mount Sinai of any physician associated with the institution during the second half of the twentieth century. Not only did he take an already outstanding Department of Pathology to new heights; he also recognized that, in order to maintain its preeminence as a leading academically oriented hospital, The Mount Sinai Hospital required its own medical school. He then became the driving force in persuading the Trustees, the Administration, and the medical staff to proceed. The idea of a medical school associated with the Hospital was not new; it had been broached as early as 1873, when Samuel Percy asked the Directors whether they would consider opening a medical college, but the Board members responded that they deemed the suggestion not "expedient."[49] Once the idea was agreed upon, Popper established the philosophical basis for the school, served as the first Dean for Academic Affairs, and can rightfully claim the accolade of being the "Father of the Mount Sinai School of Medicine."[50] In 1972, upon the unexpected death of George James, who was then President and Dean of the School, Popper gave up the Chair in Pathology to become acting President and Dean until Thomas Chalmers took over in September 1973. Popper continued his studies of the liver and remained active until just a few weeks before his death on May 5, 1988, due to pancreatic cancer.

As a hepatopathologist, Popper was a world leader and had no peer. With almost eight hundred publications and as the author or editor of twenty-eight books,[51] he studied every aspect of liver pathology and pathophysiology and was in large part responsible for modern concepts regarding the organ. Additionally, Popper was responsible for the training of many of the Chairs of Departments of Pathology, not only in America but around the world, and was also a superb mentor to investigators at the National Institutes of Health who were interested in liver disease.

A full discussion of Popper's achievements is beyond the scope of this work,[52] and many have said that a Popper biography would be an international best-seller. The *Lancet* capsulized Hans Popper's career as follows:

> Dr. Popper's researches concerned almost all aspects of liver function and structure. He embraced molecular biology. . . . He regularly addressed large medical audiences all over the world but was just as happy sitting with one or two junior doctors around a microscope. His charisma and reputation enabled him to advance the careers of his students, stimulate his associates, and transform a dull medical meeting into a happening. His enthusiasm and energy were boundless.
>
> His literary output . . . was enormous. The series "Progress in Liver Disease," co-edited with his friend and pupil Fenton Shaffner has appeared regularly since 1961. Honorary degrees (14), prizes, and medals were awarded to Popper by universities and governments all over the world. . . . Throughout his life he spanned European and New World medicine. His influence on colleagues was immeasurable. He was a congenial companion and everyone's friend.[53]

As noted by Schmid and Schenker, there was no greater tribute to this outstanding scientist, teacher, and academic leader than that paid to Popper by the students of the Class of 1974 of the Mount Sinai School of Medicine:

> Few times in life is one fortunate enough to come to know a man as rare as Dr. Popper. He is a kind and gentle individual, a scholar and teacher who loves learning and who delights in sharing his knowledge with others. He loves life with an exuberance which he joyously imparts to those around him. We feel privileged to dedicate the 1974 yearbook to Dr. Hans Popper.[54]

Many of Popper's recruits to the Pathology Department would go on to leadership positions in the discipline in hospitals and schools throughout the world. Fiorenzo Paronetto, Frederick Zak, Stephen Geller, and Emanuel Rubin would chair their own departments in major academic centers. Those who remained at Mount Sinai would help Popper's successors take the Department to ever greater heights in service, teaching, and research. Swan Thung, for example, who is now also involved in gene therapy research, is readily acknowledged as one the world's premier hepatic surgical pathologists.

Emanuel Rubin, a long-time member of the faculty, succeeded Popper as Chairman in 1972. Rubin served for four years, then left to become Chairman of the Department of Pathology, Anatomy, and Cell Biology at Thomas Jefferson University School of Medicine. Steven Geller, now the Chairman of Pathology at Cedar-Sinai Medical Center in Los Angeles, was Acting Director of the Department until 1978. True to their mentor, both Rubin and Geller have a major interest in liver pathology and have made many contributions to the field.

Jerome Kleinerman was recruited from Case Western Reserve University in 1978 to take over the Department. Kleinerman was internationally recognized for his accomplishments in the pathology of environmental lung disease and chaired the Department until 1986, when he left to return to his native Cleveland.

In 1988, Alan Schiller was appointed the third Irene Heinz Given and John LaPorte Professor of Pathology and Chair of the Department. World renowned for his work in bone pathology and his expertise in the effects of space and weightlessness on bone structure, Schiller has served on the Space Science Board of the Committee on Space Biology and Medicine of the National Academy of Sciences and as a member of the Life and Microgravity Sciences and Applications Advisory Committee of NASA. He was recently appointed to the Board of Directors of the National Space Biomedical Research Institute. A superb teacher and blessed with an ebullient personality, Schiller has taken the Department to new heights in clinical pathology and research.[55]

Building upon the earlier asbestos research of Churg and Selikoff, Thomas M. Fasy and Edward M. Johnson and their colleagues have helped elucidate the molecular mechanism of asbestos carcinogenesis. Their discovery that chrysotile asbestos fibers can transfer DNA molecules into cells or from one cell to another has led to further investigation on how this mechanism, now known as transfection, can cause cancer. This mechanism, coupled with their discovery that asbestos enhances DNA recombination, helps explain both the sensitivity of mesothelial cells to carcinogenesis and the long latency period for the development of mesothelioma.[56]

Daniel Perl's laboratory has explored the relationship between ingestion of aluminum and the development of Alzheimer's disease. These studies have been carried out partly in the Trobriand Islands and Guam, where Alzheimer's is rampant. They have found that the extremely high concentrations of aluminum in the drinking water of these islands has resulted in the presence of the metal in the tangled neurofibrils characteristic of Alzheimer's. Further recent work by Paul Good, David Burstein, and Donald S. Kohtz has discovered a pathway leading to Alzheimer's disease that involves the protein semaphorin.

In the 1990s, several new disease-related genes have been identified by Andrew D. Bergemann and Johnson, who have discovered the Pur family of proteins and their respective genes. These proteins are both DNA- and RNA-binding factors and are involved in multiple processes, including DNA replication, gene transcription, and RNA translation. One of these proteins, Pur-alpha, is essentially commandeered by the HIV virus upon infection. This protein is essential for efficient HIV virus replication, as well as for the ability of HIV to induce certain opportunistic viral infections. Much of this work on AIDS is stimulated by the existence of the Manhattan HIV Brain Bank, directed by the neuropathologist Susan Morgello. This facility performs rapid autopsies on AIDS patients that provide fresh central nervous system tissue suitable for molecular studies.

Sadly, the Viennese connection to research in the Department has recently come to an end with the death of the pediatric pathologist M. Renate Dische, in January 2002. In addition to her own work in pediatric cardiovascular pathology, she was the wife of Zacharias Dische, of Columbia University, the developer of the Dische diphenylamine test, an assay for DNA, without which much of the seminal work in twentieth-century molecular biology would have been impossible.

In addition to providing clinical excellence and performing outstanding research, Department faculty play a critical role in Medical Center teaching activities. Faculty contributions to the educational activities of all the other departments bear mention. Michael Klein, the bone pathologist, has won numerous teaching awards from the student body. Steven Dikman's expertise in renal pathology has been vital to the nephrologists and to the kidney transplant team. Margaret Magid's interactions with the pediatricians and pediatric surgeons cannot be overestimated, and the Department of Surgery benefits daily from the wisdom of Noam Harpaz, the gastrointestinal pathologist. The contributions of Ira Bleiweiss to the Breast Service and James Strauchen in lymphatic pathology have been invaluable. Recognition is due to Mamoru Kaneko, who for more than three decades has been the senior surgical pathologist and a most noteworthy successor to his mentor, Otani.

The Department has become a leader in clinical pathology, as well. It has built the largest robotic laboratory in the world, with a reputation that attracts visits from clinical pathologists worldwide.

From the first small, one-room laboratory in a corner of the second floor of the Lexington Avenue hospital building, the Department has evolved into an outstanding academic Department of Pathology. It can point with pride to its greatest legacy—its many graduates who occupy senior positions and Department Chairs in pathology throughout the world.

27

Department of Pediatrics

WHEN THE JEWS' HOSPITAL first opened, children were admitted to the Hospital and placed on adult wards. The development of a separate pediatric service had to wait for the rise of pediatrics as a specialty. The emerging field owed much to the efforts of one man, Abraham Jacobi.

Shortly after graduating in medicine from Bonn University, in 1851, Jacobi was jailed in Germany for high treason for his membership in the underground Communist League in the Democratic Revolution. After two years, he was able to escape to England, where he stayed briefly with Karl Marx and Friedrich Engels and from which he eventually emigrated to the United States, late in 1853.[1] Settling on the Lower East Side, he began a private practice. Jacobi stated:

> The first of my professional successes was the fact that it took my first patient only a fortnight after my new shingle began to ornament No. 20 Howard Street, to call on me with his twenty-five cent fee. . . . His only excuse for coming at all was that he had heard of me. I think that I must have gathered many more such fees, for after less than four years I was the founder of the German Dispensary, in which treatment was strictly gratuitous.[2]

In 1859, Jacobi and the obstetrician Emil Noeggerath published *Contributions to Midwifery and Diseases of Women and Children*.[3] Jacobi was appointed Attending Physician at the Jews' Hospital in 1860. In that same year, he was also appointed to the first pediatric professorship in this country, the Special Chair of Diseases of Children, at the New York Medical College.[4] Two years later, he established the first pediatric clinic in the United States at that institution, where he set the precedent for pediatric teaching across the United States. Jacobi suggested that pediatrics was a scientific as well as a clinical specialty. In the ensuing years, he accepted two other appointments, one at the

Abraham Jacobi, M.D.,
Chief of the Pediatrics
Service, 1878–1883.

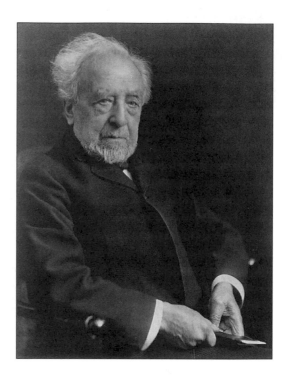

University of New York in 1865 as Clinical Chair and Professor of Pediatrics and the other at the College of Physicians and Surgeons in 1870, first as Clinical Professor of Pediatrics and later as Professor and Chair. He served in these capacities at that institution for twenty-nine years. All of these appointments were concurrent with his service at the Jews' Hospital, later Mount Sinai.

In 1875, a Children's Department in the Dispensary at Mount Sinai was organized to resemble the one at New York Medical College. Since the Trustees did not want the same person in charge of both inpatient and outpatient services, they appointed Mary Putnam Jacobi to head the Out-Patient Service. She had earlier gone to the Female Medical College in Pennsylvania and was the sixth woman to graduate from any medical school in the United States. She sought additional training and was the first woman graduate of l'Ecole de Medecine in Paris, returning to the United States in 1871. She and Jacobi married in 1875. Together they published *Infant Diet*,[5] which was adapted to public use and became the "Spock" of those days.

Because the Children's Department facilities in the Dispensary were not sufficient to care for the great number of children referred to the Hospital, a formal Pediatric Service was established within The Mount Sinai Hospital in 1878. This was the first pediatric service in New York City in a general hospital and one of the first in the United States. Abraham Jacobi was appointed Hospital Pediatrician in 1879 and served as Chief of Service until 1883. He remained a Consulting Pediatrician until his death in 1919 and served as President of the Mount Sinai Medical Board for many years.

In addition to his busy clinical and teaching activities, Jacobi was very active in organized medicine. He was a prolific writer whose works were published in a collection of eight volumes.[6] In 1981, Lewis Thomas stated, "Dr. Jacobi was obviously one of the major thinkers of his time in academic medicine. He wrote with intelligence and clarity."[7] Jacobi played an integral role in securing congressional funding for the *Index Medicus* and was a founding Editor of the *American Journal of Obstetrics*. He was the first President of the American Pediatric Society and also served as President of the New York Medical Society, The New York Academy of Medicine, and the American Medical Association. Jacobi was an indefatigable children's advocate, who repeatedly spoke out against child labor and strongly supported the establishment of milk stations. In 1910, the library of The Mount Sinai Hospital was named for Jacobi. To further honor his name, in 1952, at the one hundredth anniversary of the founding of the Hospital, the Jacobi Medallion was established by the Associated Alumni of Mount Sinai.[8] Jacobi is recognized to this day as "the Father of Pediatrics" in the United States.

Barnim Scharlau was appointed to succeed Jacobi as Chief of the Service in 1883 at the latter's suggestion. Arpad Gerster, the surgeon, commented on Scharlau's performance: "He attended to his duties with exemplary diligence, but on account of his intolerant and irritable disposition, was constantly at war with the house staff and the authorities of the training school for nurses."[9] Scharlau served until 1900, when Henry Koplik, who had been Adjunct Visiting Physician to the Children's Service since 1891, was appointed Attending Pediatrician and Chief.

In 1889, Koplik founded the first station for the distribution of sterilized milk in New York City at the Good Samaritan Dispensary in lower Manhattan, where he served as Director.[10] In 1896, Koplik described the diagnostic spots of measles in the buccal mucous membranes, which to this day bear the name "Koplik spots."[11] He was one of the first pediatricians to take an interest in bacteriology and conducted fundamental studies on diphtheria and pertussis organisms. He was an outstanding clinician, strict and demanding of his trainees. With Jacobi, he was a founder of the American Pediatric Society and served as its President. Koplik's skill as a pediatrician was renowned throughout New York City, in part because of the great number of children he saw in his practice, often treating up to fifty patients on a single Saturday. As one story goes, a woman once brought her child to see Koplik despite the fact that she knew the child to be perfectly healthy, because her mother told her that "every New York child should be seen by Dr. Koplik at least once."[12] Koplik retired from his hospital duties in 1925, having served with distinction for thirty-four years. He died two years later.

When The Mount Sinai Hospital moved to its third home, on Fifth Avenue, in 1904, a Children's Pavilion, funded by Henry Einstein in memory of his son Lewis, was built. This building, on the south side of 101st Street, included cheerful wards, play spaces, a solarium on the roof, and a view of Central Park. In 1922, the new Einstein-Falk Children's Pavilion was opened on the south side of 100th Street, opposite the Administration Building. At this time, a new pediatric outpatient facility, the Walter Children's Clinic, also opened next door. These buildings served the Department until they were taken down, in 1969, to make way for the Medical School's Annenberg Building.

A number of Mount Sinai physicians who were not pediatricians have made major contributions to the diagnosis and management of diseases of children. In 1887, Bernard Sachs described the clinical features of what is now known as Tay-Sachs disease.[13] The second disease to bear the eponym of a Mount Sinai physician was nephrosis (Epstein's disease), described by Albert A. Epstein.[14] The growth of pediatric urology as a specialty received a major impetus when Edwin Beer, Chief of the Urology Service, devised the first pediatric cystoscope in 1911. Beer and Abraham Hyman, the former's successor as Chief of Urology, collaborated to publish the first American text on pediatric urology, entitled *Diseases of the Urinary Tract in Children* in 1930.[15]

Ira Wile, who joined the Pediatric staff in 1904, developed an early interest in child psychiatry, behavioral and social problems of children, and child education. In 1919, he opened the first child guidance clinic in the United States. Named the Children's Health Class, it became the first vehicle through which preventive medicine was integrated on an equal footing with the rest of the pediatric activities of the Hospital. Wile stated that "the class is founded on the positive idea of health rather than the negative idea of disease."[16] He further stated, prophetically, that "the attention of the clinic is directed chiefly to the periodic examination of children between infancy and school age. This is a period during which the health of poorer children is commonly neglected, and when physical and psychological mismanagement may readily implant the seeds of disease against which the Department of Health and other agencies subsequently struggle in vain."[17] These seminal ideas were further publicized in subsequent papers and writings.

In 1923, the Hospital invited Bela Schick, a pediatrician of renown in Europe, to come to Mount Sinai and serve as Pediatrician to the Hospital. In collaboration with Clemens von Pirquet, Schick had already conducted his groundbreaking work on antigen/antibody reactions, which laid the foundation for immunity and hypersensitivity.[18] It was they who introduced the term "allergy." Schick also had done his pioneering studies on diphtheria, developing a skin test with toxin from diphtheria organisms.[19] The "Schick Test" was the first of many skin tests used to determine whether a child was immune or susceptible. The Schick Test was part of an early public health campaign, with newspapers and radios asking, "Have you been Schicked?"

These contributions rank among the great achievements in medicine. In the preface of the biography *Bela Schick: The World of Children*, Rene Dubos observes:

> The history of medicine can boast of many physicians who achieved fame by contributing discoveries to the fabric of theoretical science; of others who became known because of their art as clinicians; of still others who organized the policies of public health under which we function today. But few are those, who like Bela Schick, have operated successfully in all three fields of medicine, and who have succeeded in translating their own theoretical scientific studies into clinical skill and social action.[20]

When Schick arrived at Mount Sinai, he found M. Murray Peshkin at work in the fledgling Pediatric Allergy Clinic and encouraged him in his efforts to study and treat asthma and allergy in children. Peshkin ultimately published more than one hundred articles in the field. He was best known for his work on the impact of psychological factors on asthma. He advocated removing asthmatic children from their homes, a "parentectomy," so that they could be placed in better climates, as well as away from the pressures of family. He established the Children's Asthma Research Institute in Denver, Colorado, which was later absorbed by the National Jewish Hospital, the latter initially founded for the treatment of tuberculosis. Peshkin reached retirement age in 1952 but continued his efforts. He was chosen as the first presenter of the Bela Schick Memorial Lecture of the American College of Allergists in 1968, and in 1980 he died.

Schick would serve Mount Sinai as Chief for nearly two decades. An inspiring teacher, Schick led rounds characterized by continuous stimulation of his younger colleagues, such as Peshkin; a searching approach to problems at the bedside; and his exemplary behavior to the infants and their parents. During Schick's tenure, a residency program was created, with the first two physicians graduating in 1924. As noted by Peshkin, "By word of mouth the opportunities that existed for those interested in pediatric training became widely known, and doctors of both sexes competed for the privilege of obtaining staff appointments. Dr. Schick's innovation was to give competent female doctors an equal opportunity with men to compete for positions on his staff."[21]

By 1939, Schick felt compelled to complain about the lack of an Obstetrics Service in the training of young pediatricians. In a report on the "Needs of the Children's Service," Schick listed as his primary "need":

> First: A ward for newborn infants. It is impossible to educate physicians in the treatment of infants without having the opportunity of observing newborn children. Such a department necessitates the establishment of a maternity ward, which is also an urgent need of the hospital. . . . The inclusion of a ward for newborn children is also necessary to afford a physician the experience needed for certification by the Board of Pediatrics.[22]

Unfortunately for Schick and his successors, the Maternity Service at the Mount Sinai Hospital would not be established until 1952.

Schick was recognized often for his contributions to Mount Sinai, to his profession, and to the health of children. He received the John Howland Award, the highest award in pediatrics, and the Gold Medal of The

New York Academy of Medicine. Schick remained Chief of Pediatrics at The Mount Sinai Hospital until 1942, when he was named a Consultant.

Although Schick made great progress in encouraging women to enter the field in the 1920s and 1930s, Sara Welt, in 1887, was, in fact, the first woman to be appointed an Adjunct Pediatrician at Mount Sinai. She remained closely affiliated with the Pediatrics Department until her death in 1943, at which time she bequeathed nearly $1 million to establish the Sara Welt Fellowship in Research Medicine, a loan fund for young physicians who needed financial help and for support of the Pediatric Clinic.

One of the women trainees in Pediatrics at Mount Sinai during Schick's tenure was Jean Pakter, who would devote more than half a century to serving the City of New York and the nation as an advocate for maternal and child health. Her many noteworthy studies of maternal and fetal mortality, prematurity, sudden infant death syndrome[23] and her promotion of breast feeding led deservedly to numerous honors and awards.

After Schick's retirement in 1942, Murray Bass, one of Mount Sinai's most respected clinicians, served as Acting Chief. Bass was a pediatrician beloved by his patients and their families. At ward rounds, he was stimulating, inspiring, and instructive. His publications on lead poisoning from neonatal nipple shields, vitamin A deficiency in infants, and periorbital edema in infectious mononucleosis, among others, characterized his concern for urgent practical problems in children.[24] He retired as Director of Service in 1948 but remained in private practice until 1960.

Samuel Karelitz, trained by and an early associate of Schick, made a singular contribution to infant care as the first to advocate continuous intravenous fluid administration to combat infant dehydration.[25] By switching from intermittent to continuous infusion, physicians were able to reduce mortality rates by 75 percent. Karelitz and Schick also introduced isolation cubicles for infants into the Department. Originally conceived by Schick and von Pirquet, these glass-enclosed cubes were the precursors of the current isolettes. Karelitz served as an enlisted man in World War I, but in World War II he was a Lieutenant Colonel in the Medical Corps and the Chief of Medicine of Mount Sinai's Third General Hospital.

Bass and Karelitz developed a cadre of clinicians that included Jerome Kohn, Alfred Fischer, George Ginandes, Samuel Delange, Sidney

Blumenthal, and Ralph Moloshok, among others. These experienced pediatricians and the younger colleagues whom they nurtured made the Pediatric Department an outstanding clinical group and a haven for consultation referrals from the region. Karelitz, in addition, was very active in the American Academy of Pediatrics. He stimulated the development of standards to guide pediatricians and prospective adoptive parents and was awarded the Clifford Grulee Award, the highest award of the Academy. Karelitz left Mount Sinai in 1953 to become the founding Chairman of the Department of Pediatrics at the Long Island Jewish Medical Center.

The arrival of Horace Hodes in 1949 as the first full-time Chief of Pediatrics ushered in a new era for the Department. Hodes had served as the Physician in Charge of the Sydenham Hospital for Infectious Diseases, in Baltimore. While there, he reported his work on the virus of diarrhea, the first such agent to be identified as a cause of diarrhea in humans.[26] For this seminal work, he received the prestigious Mead Johnson Award for Research in Pediatrics in 1946.

Hodes was the consummate academic pediatrician, who combined excellence in research, teaching, and clinical skills. His own continuing research at Mount Sinai involved further identification of the poliovirus, the nature of poliovirus in breast milk, and the characteristics of endotoxin. In addition to performing important laboratory work, he was an outstanding teacher and a superb clinician, always interested in the challenging case. When he was called about a child with an unusual rash, his answer was, "I'll be in your office in five minutes."[27]

The pace of both laboratory and clinical departmental research intensified and flourished under Hodes. Upon his arrival, a new laboratory was built on the roof of the Walter Children's Clinic building with funds donated by the Dorothy H. and Lewis Rosenstiel Foundation. Alex Steigman and Edward Bottone pioneered the administration of penicillin to all newborns in the delivery room to prevent their contracting Group B streptococcus infection from infected mothers.[28] The policy was soon adopted nationwide. Hodes invited Richard Day, who was retiring from the Columbia University College of Physicians and Surgeons, to join the service and to establish a modern newborn nursery. Both Hodes and Day served as President of the Society of Pediatric Research and the American Pediatric Society, and both received the John Howland Award of the American Pediatric Society.

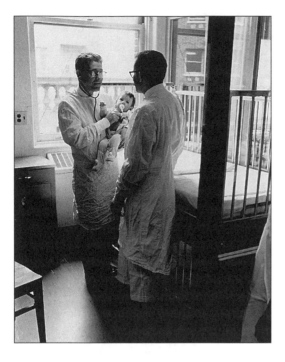

Horace Hodes, M.D. (facing, with baby), Chairman and Professor of Pediatrics, 1949–1976.

Hodes was heavily involved with the educational mission of both the Department of Pediatrics and the Hospital. He was instrumental in developing, organizing, and preparing for the Mount Sinai School of Medicine. He made major improvements in the Department's educational efforts. Bedside rounds became a daily event. They were attended and prepared by the Interns and Residents and led by the Attending Pediatricians. Formal Grand Rounds were held weekly, and a monthly Schick Lecture was held in the evening. Given by a leading pediatric personality, the lecture attracted pediatricians from across the region. For those who worked with Hodes, going on rounds each morning and hearing him describe measles, meningitis, and scarlet fever was an unforgettable experience. Hodes's charisma attracted an outstanding group of Residents, Fellows and Attendings, all of whom helped create a leading Department of Pediatrics. Donald Gribetz, who first met Hodes in Baltimore, joined the staff shortly after Hodes's arrival and practiced at Mount Sinai for more than half a century. A preeminent clinician, Gribetz published widely on renal disease in the pediatric population. Later joined by his brother, Irwin Gribetz, the two cared for the children of a significant proportion of the staff.

Hodes was given what his predecessors had been denied: a Maternity Service at the Hospital. No longer would the Residents be sent elsewhere for their instruction in newborn care. In 1952, the Maternity Pavilion opened, with a Newborn Nursery planned and staffed by the Department of Pediatrics. The following year, a Premature Nursery was opened with forty-four beds. Other subspecialty divisions expanded or created under Hodes were Pediatric Orthopaedics (1949); Pediatric Cardiology (1963); the Adolescent Health Center (1968); and a Neonatal Intensive Care Unit (1969). Hodes showed great institutional leadership as he established a number of new programs. In 1953, he opened a respirator center for both adults and children with poliomyelitis. A daily census of ten to fifteen paralyzed patients in iron lungs was seen personally by Hodes almost daily. To watch him perform a tracheostomy on a patient with polio in an iron lung was an eye-opener.[29]

In 1966, with the advent of the Medical School, a laboratory in human genetics was deemed necessary. Interested in the specialty, Hodes created space in the Department of Pediatrics for the new Division. Kurt Hirschhorn, an internist by training and well recognized for his research in the field of genetics, was recruited from New York University and brought his genetics laboratory to Mount Sinai.

When Hodes retired in 1977, he was succeeded by Hirschhorn, who moved from his position as Professor and Chief of the Division of Genetics. Hirschhorn quickly appointed Hodes Chief of the Division of Infectious Diseases, where the latter remained extremely active and productive in research, patient care, and teaching until shortly before his death in 1989. Two years later, the library of the Department of Pediatrics was named for Horace Hodes.

In 1967, Hirschhorn received a National Institutes of Health training grant to support a Ph.D. program in human genetics. This program continues today under the direction of Robert Desnick, who replaced Hirschhorn as Chief of the Division of Genetics. In 1992, Human Genetics became a separate department.

Hirschhorn enlarged the Department, adding new clinical and research divisions and increasing the number of full-time faculty. In 1977, the Department received a federal designation as a Pediatric Pulmonary Center. Under the current leadership of Meyer Kattan, the Division has conducted major studies in the management of asthma and the pulmonary effects of HIV infection. A Division of Pediatric Rheumatology was established in 1989. From its inception in 1969, the Division of Neonatology, currently directed by Ian Holzman, has been a tower of strength within the Department. Necrotizing enterocolitis, as a major problem of the premature newborn, has been studied extensively both at the bedside[30] and in the laboratory.[31] In collaboration with the Department of Obstetrics, Gynecology, and Reproductive Science, the Neonatology group also reported the first successful attempt at fetal surgery after Caesarean delivery but prior to the clamping of the umbilical cord, thereby permitting fetal oxygenation without the need for intubation.[32]

Hirschhorn is a world-renowned authority on biochemical and molecular genetics and cytogenetics, having published more than three hundred papers. In cytogenetics, his name has been attached to the Hirschhorn-Wolf syndrome, which he was instrumental in describing.[33] His work in genetics began with studies of the genetics of hypercholesterolemia and other lipid disorders. In the early 1960s, he discovered the mixed lymphocyte reaction that was one of the major starting points of the field of cellular immunology and immunogenetics.[34] His investigations have been fundamental in the understanding of a number of inborn errors, including several lysosomal enzyme defects, Menkes Syndrome, and Fanconi Anemia.[35]

Hirschhorn has been President of the American Society of Human Genetics and the Harvey Society and is a member of the Institute of Medicine of the National Academy of Sciences, as well as a number of other prestigious societies. Among other awards, he received the William Allan Award from the American Society of Human Genetics in 1995, the top prize in the field.

In addition, Hirschhorn has made other contributions to the Department and the institution. During his tenure, the Children's Center Foundation was established to support child-centered programs. He was also instrumental in developing an ethics program at Mount Sinai and was one of the founders of the Hastings Institute for Biomedical Ethics, where he continues to be an active member.

When Hirschhorn retired from the Chairmanship in 1995, Neil Leleiko, Chief of Pediatric Gastroenterology, was named the Acting Chair, a position he held until Frederick J. Suchy assumed the leadership of the Department in 1996. An internationally recognized pediatric gastroenterologist and hepatologist, Suchy edited the definitive text on liver diseases in children.[36] His several prestigious research awards include the American Liver Foundation Pediatric Research Prize and the Excellence in Research Award from the American Academy of Pediatrics.

Under Suchy's leadership, the many departmental Divisions continue to expand their activities in both patient care and research.[37] With the support of the Jaffe Family Foundation, the Division of Pediatric Allergy and Immunology is one of only three in the country to offer a comprehensive program for the diagnosis and treatment of disorders related to food allergy. In collaboration with its counterpart in the Department of Medicine and the support of the Jeffrey Modell Foundation, the Division has created a national resource center for patients with primary immunodeficiency.

Investigators in the Division of Gastroenterology, Hepatology, and Nutrition continue to seek an understanding of the mechanisms that underlie gene transcription in the intestine and on the developmental regulation of bile acid transporters in the liver. Sophisticated molecular and cellular biological techniques are being used to study the mechanisms that underlie liver development and cholestatic liver disease. Continuous care is also provided to more than five hundred patients with inflammatory bowel disease.

In addition to being a national leader in the management of sickle cell disease, the Hematology/Oncology Division has an extensive research program in place for studying the clinical and basic science aspects of hemophilia and other clotting disorders, as well as for performing basic research on the genetic aspects of embryonal rhabdomyosarcoma. The Nephrology group continues its efforts to originate a noninvasive rapid detection method for early graft rejection among organ transplant recipients. Host immune system cells have been identified in urine and bile from kidney and liver transplant recipients, respectively, many days before clinical signs of rejection appear, permitting earlier and more effective treatment.

The Pulmonary Division continues its asthma studies and is one of seven centers funded to formulate an intervention strategy for reducing asthma morbidity by educating physicians and patients about environmental factors responsible for inducing asthma. A major focus of research for the infectious disease group is the prevention of Epstein-Barr virus infection in transplant recipients. In the laboratory, researchers are investigating aspects of the host's defense against infectious disease.

One hundred fifty years after the founding of the Jews' Hospital, the Pediatric Service consists of seventy-five ward beds, fifty-five healthy newborn bassinets, eight intensive care beds, and thirty-five neonatal intensive care beds. There are seventeen subspecialty divisions engaged in patient care, teaching, and clinical and laboratory research activities. The seventy-one full-time and forty voluntary faculty are entrusted with the education of fifty pediatric house officers, twenty-five Fellows, and 110 medical students. If he were here today, Abraham Jacobi would surely take great pride in the efforts of the Department of Pediatrics in acquitting its responsibility for the continuing care, well-being, and development of children.

Adapted from an article by Donald Gribetz, M.D., published in *The Mount Sinai Journal of Medicine* 64 (1997): 392–398.

28

Department of Physics

IN THE 1920 Annual Report, Leopold Jaches, Radiographer to the Hospital, expressed the need for "the employment of a trained physicist to obtain and measure the emanations and do much of the technical work connected with the use of radium."[1] However, it was not until 1929 that the physicist Carl Braestrup was appointed on a part-time basis to the Department of Roentgenology and Radiotherapy. Radiology and Radiotherapy became separate departments in 1939; a formal physics laboratory was established three years later during a reorganization of the laboratories. The "main activities of the Physicist were directed towards establishment of cooperation with the other clinical and laboratory departments."[2] Thus, the tasks of monitoring the radiation exposure of employees and of ensuring that the equipment was properly calibrated fell to the physics laboratory. The linkage of the laboratory and the clinical departments led to a number of improvements in equipment safety and standardization. All radiation-emitting devices were standardized at regular intervals; a targeting device was constructed to direct x-ray beams to the center of the area being treated; an alignment chart was designed for measuring x-ray dosage at different distances and for calculating exposure time; and a portable, lightweight Geiger-Mueller counter was built for locating radium to guard against possible loss or misplacement.

Sergei Feitelberg was the physicist who made it all possible. Feitelberg first came to Mount Sinai in 1939 in the newly formed laboratory Department of Pharmacology and was appointed Physicist to the Hospital in 1941. Following two years in the Army Signal Corps during World War II, Feitelberg returned to the physics laboratory. It was an especially exciting and fruitful time to be there. "The disclosure of spectacular war work on nuclear fission acted as a stimulus to plans and discussions of research with radioactive tracers. A substantial grant was received from the Hospital for this type of research and will permit the realization of some of these plans in collaboration with other departments of the hospital."[3]

Radioactive isotopes would become Feitelberg's life work. With materials provided by the Atomic Energy Commission, the Physics Laboratory began experiments with the use of radioactive iodine for hyperthyroidism. The new research activity necessitated the expansion of the Department's personnel. Whereas in the prewar years Feitelberg was the only physicist working in the laboratory, by 1947 there were six full-time and two part-time physicists in the lab, with one assistant physicist assigned solely to the Radiotherapy Department.

In 1948, a multidisciplinary Radioisotope Group, consisting of the physicists and clinicians, was established to investigate the diagnostic and therapeutic use of radioactive isotopes. A major publication of the group in that same year on the use of radioactive iodine in the diagnosis of thyroid disease laid the foundation for the technique of scanning.[4] In the early years of radioisotope use, the availability of the isotopes was limited to hospitals. As a result, the number of doses of radioactive iodine given increased significantly from 1950 to 1952. In 1953, the Atomic Energy Commission began to release a limited number of radioactive isotopes for use in the private offices of qualified physicians. Consequently, hospital usage leveled off. Research activities however, continued to expand.

In 1954, the Department was officially dedicated as the André Meyer Department of Physics, with Feitelberg as Director. A subsequent move into the newly built Atran Laboratory building resulted in the consolidation of departmental activities. Although day-to-day activities continued to involve radiation equipment maintenance, collaborative research remained paramount. During the 1950s, therapy of hyperthyroidism was moving rapidly from surgery to control by drugs and radioactive iodine. The leader of this movement at Mount Sinai was Solomon Silver, the endocrinologist.[5] His early research in the use of radioactive I^{131} would make him preeminent in the field.[6-8] In 1958, Feitelberg and Silver would collaborate with Edith Quimby, a physicist at Columbia University, to publish a landmark book summarizing the work to date on the clinical and research use of radionuclides in multiple areas.[9] One year later, after ten years of experience using radioactive isotopes, the Physics Department would report the largest group of patients ever treated with radioactive iodine for hyperthyroidism.[10]

With the advent of the Medical School in the mid-1960s, Feitelberg became intimately involved in the development of the basic sciences curriculum. As a member of the National Committee on Radiation Protection and of the Human Applications Advisory Subcommittee of the Atomic Energy Commission, Feitelberg had influence far beyond Mount Sinai. He would remain active until his death in 1967, having "equally influenced the scientific growth, the pioneering in new areas, and the development of the spirit of Mount Sinai."[11]

Silver served briefly as Acting Director until 1968, when the integration of Physics, Nuclear Medicine, and Biomedical Engineering created a renamed André Meyer Department of Biophysics and Biomedical Engineering of the Mount Sinai School of Medicine, with Jay H. Katz as Director.

In 1973, Stanley Goldsmith was appointed the Director of a once again renamed André Meyer Department of Physics and Nuclear Medicine, now within the Hospital's table of organization. Goldsmith established a Nuclear Medicine Fellowship Training Program; many of the trainees would go on to head departments of nuclear medicine across the country. During Goldsmith's tenure, the Department was actively involved in nuclear cardiology, performing the first thallium stress myocardial perfusion imaging in New York City.[12] Goldsmith was at the forefront in the development of combined WBC and bone marrow imaging for the diagnosis of peri-prosthetic osteomyelitis and vertebral osteomyelitis, now standard procedures.[13,14] The Department also established the first bone mineral absorptiometry clinical service in New York.

In 1991, the Physics Department returned to its roots and was incorporated as a Division within the Department of Radiology. Two years later, Josef Machac, the former head of nuclear cardiology, was named Director of Nuclear Medicine. Dedicated to bringing the latest innovations in nuclear medicine to Mount Sinai and to strengthening the training program, Machac recruited additional faculty, including Chun Kim, a former member of the Division, and Boris Krynycki. New staff members were added in nuclear cardiology, physics, and radiochemistry. The efforts of Shlomo Hoore, as the head of a new radiation safety team, and Machac, who chaired a new human use radiation safety committee, made it possible for Mount Sinai to obtain a Broad License, allowing the institution to use new diagnostic and therapeutic modalities even before Federal Drug Administration approval.

During Machac's tenure since 1993, the practice of nuclear medicine has changed dramatically. Imaging of colorectal and prostate cancer with labeled antibodies, neuroendocrine tumors with Indium-111 Octreotide, and brain tumors with thallium-201 SPECT and the detection and localization of parathyroid tumors with combined I-123 and technesium-99m Sestamibi are now routine. Lymphoscintigraphy and sentinel node identification have revolutionized the management of breast cancer. The therapy of thyroid cancer with radioiodine and whole-body thyroid imaging has become more sophisticated, and palliation of pain from bone metastases in breast, prostate, and lung cancer has been improved with Strontium-89 and Samarium-153. With the acquisition of a whole-body PET scanner, imaging with F-18 fluorodeoxyglucose has markedly improved the diagnosis and staging of many tumors. New isotopes have enhanced the diagnosis of ischemic heart disease and the identification of viable myocardium in the presence of severe ventricular dysfunction.

In spite of the formidable challenges posed by the changes in healthcare financing and modes of medical practice, the Division of Nuclear Medicine has flourished by providing efficient, quality service to patients and referring physicians, while at the same time pursuing innovation and research.

29

Department of Psychiatry

THE CARE OF the mentally ill has been part of the tradition of The Mount Sinai Hospital since it opened in 1855. From the very first, the Jews' Hospital was one of only a few general hospitals in this country that admitted mentally ill patients. This was in contrast to the practice at the time of sending patients with mental illnesses to "insane asylums" or jail. Examination of histories from the first Case Book of the Hospital reveals that mentally ill patients admitted to the Jews' Hospital were treated by general physicians and were often discharged not improved, and some were transferred to the "Lunatic Asylum."[1] Nevertheless, despite this history of providing care for the mentally ill, it would be almost a century before the Department of Psychiatry was established.

The opening of a neurology clinic (1890) and then an inpatient Department of Neurology at Mount Sinai (1900), with Bernard Sachs as its Chief, occurred at an interesting time in the history of psychiatry. Sachs did evaluate patients with psychiatric disorders in the Hospital and considered himself a neuropsychiatrist. He believed that the anatomy and physiology of the nervous system played a fundamental role in psychiatric disorders. During the early years of the twentieth century, open warfare developed between neurologists and psychiatrists over scientific issues regarding the etiology and treatment of psychiatric disorders. Sachs, as a leader in the field and as the editor of the *Journal of Nervous and Mental Diseases,* attempted to function as a mediator and to reduce the friction between neurology and psychiatry.[2] The net result led to the establishment of psychiatry as a specialty.

In 1913, Clarence P. Oberndorf (1882–1954) was appointed Clinical Assistant in Neurology and established the first psychiatric clinic in a general hospital in New York within the Neurological Department in the Dispensary, thereby providing the setting for the beginning of psychiatry as a medical specialty at The Mount Sinai Hospital.[3] Oberndorf was deeply committed to psychoanalysis and was one of the charter members of the New York Psychoanalytic Society, founded in 1911.

In June 1919, as part of the Hospital's commitment to the advancement of preventive medicine, Ira Wile established a Children's Health Class in the children's dispensary. This was the first child guidance clinic in the United States to function as an integral part of a hospital's pediatric service. Wile and the Children's Health Class played an important role in the development of the child guidance and child psychiatry programs at Mount Sinai and in New York.[4]

The post–World War I years saw a reorganization of the medical staff, and the inpatient and outpatient staffs were merged. In psychiatry, however, Oberndorf, although Chief of the Mental Hygiene Clinic, had no inpatient responsibilities. Nevertheless, progress was being made in establishing psychiatry within the institution, even though it was only on an outpatient basis.

By the 1920s, Sigmund Freud's reputation in analysis had grown considerably. Younger neurologists were becoming increasingly interested in psychodynamic concepts, and psychotherapy became a large part of their practice. One of them, Adolph Stern, a Clinical Assistant in the Neurological Clinic under Sachs, not Oberndorf, was utilizing psychoanalytic concepts in treating children in the Clinic as early as 1915.[5] Sachs was increasingly incensed at the escalating interest in psychoanalysis among young neurologists on his service. During these years, Freud had analyzed a sizable number of the staff of the Neurology Service at Mount Sinai, including Adolph Stern, who was the first American to be analyzed by Freud.

Oberndorf also decided, in 1921, to have a personal analysis with Freud. Sachs's antipathy towards psychoanalysis had increased steadily, and he reluctantly signed Oberndorf's leave of absence. Oberndorf returned after a year of analysis in Vienna; the interest in psychoanalysis was clearly evident in the Clinic, as was the need for caring for milder cases of mental illness without hospitalization.

In spite of Bernard Sachs's strong views about analysis, Oberndorf and his colleagues were able to achieve significant growth in the psychiatry program in the outpatient setting. Sachs, however, repeatedly refused Oberndorf's requests that psychiatry be an independent department.[6] By 1924, the year of Sachs's retirement as Chief, the Mental Health Clinic had a marked increase in activity, with 350 new cases.

The appointment of Israel Strauss in 1924 to succeed Sachs brought a new view of the relationship between neurology and psychiatry to the Neurology Department. Strauss had trained at Mount Sinai and in

Vienna in both neurology and psychiatry and preferred to be known as a neuropsychiatrist, rather than as a neurologist. He emphasized the importance of psychodynamic psychiatry and psychoanalysis in the understanding and treatment of mental disorders. Furthermore, he believed that the psychiatry program at Mount Sinai was not sufficient to meet the treatment needs of the Jewish population in New York, and specifically, that it was inadequate to treat patients who were not strictly ambulatory but who were not ill enough to require state hospital care. In 1919, he assembled a group of distinguished neurologists and psychiatrists at The Mount Sinai Hospital to discuss and study this issue. The following year, he organized the Committee for Mental Hygiene among Jews, an effort that eventually led to the establishment of Hillside Hospital.[7]

The Mental Hygiene Clinic at Mount Sinai had become known as a major mental hygiene facility in New York by the late 1920s. Social workers were added to the program, as were occupational and recreational therapists. The medical staff grew and included leaders in the psychoanalytic movement in New York. For example, Sandor Lorand, who was among the first group of emigré European analysts, played an influential role in the growth and development of analysis in America and was actively involved in the psychiatry program at Mount Sinai. In addition to the treatment and care of patients, the Clinic offered lectures and clinical demonstrations and taught psychoanalytically oriented psychotherapy to physicians at the postgraduate level.

Oberndorf and other members of the clinic at Mount Sinai participated vigorously and directly in the growth and organization of the New York Psychoanalytic Society and Institute and the American Psychoanalytic Association. Oberndorf held offices in both organizations and was President of the American Psychoanalytic Association in 1924.

Throughout the 1930s, the Psychiatry Section of the Department of Neurology, now numbering a dozen physicians and a clinical psychologist, continued to grow. The Mental Health Clinic treated large numbers of patients, with increased interactions between the psychiatrists and referring doctors from other clinics. Several psychiatrists were also beginning to consult on the wards, and, in 1934, George Baehr, Chief of one of the two Medicine Services, invited Lorand to participate in weekly rounds on his service. This was the first time that a psychiatrist had taken part in medical rounds and marked the beginning of a psychiatric liaison program in medicine.[8] Lorand was also beginning psychosomatic studies on hypertension with Eli Moschcowitz, an Associate Physician on the Medical Service, and on spastic colitis with Bernard Oppenheimer, Chief of one of the Medical Services.[9]

The appointment of Israel Wechsler in 1938 to succeed Strauss brought to the Department of Neurology an individual kindly disposed to psychiatry and very encouraging about its future at Mount Sinai. But Wechsler was also acutely aware of the interactions between the two disciplines and was of the view that "It is no exaggeration of fact to say that there can be no psychiatry or understanding of mental disease without knowledge of the nervous system and its disorders."[10] Like his predecessors, Sachs and Strauss, Wechsler steadfastly refused requests from the psychiatrists for a separate department, and tensions rose. In 1939, a committee appointed by the Joint Conference Committee of the Hospital (probably at Wechsler's request) recommended a reorganization of the Psychiatry Division, noting that "this Division has been working unsatisfactorily for some time past due in large part, to questions of personalities."[11] Oberndorf and Lorand resigned, and Lawrence S. Kubie, a leader of the psychoanalytic movement and a faculty member of Columbia University's Neurological Institute, was appointed as the new Director of the Psychiatric Division. Kubie came to Mount Sinai with elite medical, scientific, and psychoanalytic training and experience. Furthermore, his family involvement with The Mount Sinai Hospital dated back to 1855, when the Hospital opened, and his great-uncle, Mark Blumenthal, was the first Resident and Attending Physician.

At the time of Kubie's appointment, he was President of the New York Psychoanalytic Society and Secretary of the American Psychoanalytic Association. He was also on the Advisory Board of a group of influential scientists and clinicians who established the journal *Psychosomatic Medicine*. This was the heyday of the psychosomatic movement, and the appointment gave Kubie the opportunity to bring psychoanalysis closer to medicine by applying psychoanalytic concepts to the understanding of medical illness.

In 1939, Kubie began to develop his innovative psychosomatic program, but it would require a much larger staff of psychiatrists willing to devote time to both the clinical and the research aspects of the program with its multidisciplinary interactions. By a horrific turn in world events, a pool of psychoanalysts became available to staff Kubie's blueprint for psychiatry at Mount Sinai. Hitler's anti-Semitism had driven many European physicians to America, and, from 1933 on, Mount Sinai welcomed large numbers of them with open arms. In 1938, Kubie became Chairman of the Emergency Committee on Relief and Immigration of the American Psychoanalytic Association, which was involved in all matters related to refugee analysts. It is not surprising that Kubie began to utilize this group of refugee analysts, all of them eager to participate in clinical programs, as a means of expanding his much-needed staff. Among the group of refugee analysts working at Mount Sinai were many who became distinguished leaders and teachers of psychoanalysis in this country. These included Rene Spitz, Margaret Mahler, Annie Reich, Heinrich and Olga Lowenfeld, and Melitta and Otto Sperling, among others.

The Hospital's Annual Report for 1939 noted:

> The psychiatric division has been entirely reorganized during the past year. Most expert psychiatric service is now available on the medical and some surgical wards and in medical clinics of the Out-Patient Department. The psychiatrists are now working shoulder to shoulder with the internists and surgeons and giving immeasurable assistance in the understanding and relief of many psychosomatic disorders. The reorganization of the psychiatry service constitutes an important change in the clinical services of the Hospital.[12]

In less than a year, the expanded staff provided consultation to all Hospital departments and initiated a number of clinical research studies. Wechsler and Kubie worked well together, and psychiatry was making its presence felt in all areas of the institution. Kubie published a widely quoted paper describing the psychiatry program at Mount Sinai that served as a blueprint for psychiatry in a general hospital.[13] Kubie was highly praised for his efforts by Wechsler and the Hospital administration.

Within very short order, however, the harmony began to disintegrate as Kubie pressed for still more staff, and Wechsler began to lose more of his neurologists to the war effort. In January 1943, Kubie and most of his staff, including the refugee analysts, resigned. A few months later, Kubie sent a letter to the President of the Board of Trustees, with copies to every member of the Board and every member of the Medical Staff, to clarify what had taken place from his perspective. Kubie suggested that, in the future, psychiatry must be an independent service on an equal basis with medicine and surgery in order

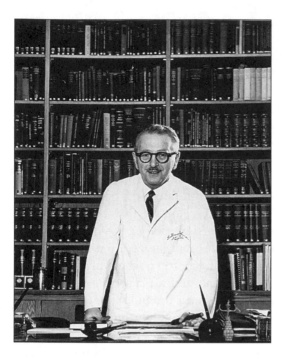

M. Ralph Kaufman, M.D., first Chairman and Professor of Psychiatry at Mount Sinai Hospital, 1945–1971.

to prevent these difficulties.[14] Other senior members of the psychiatry program concurred.

Following Kubie's resignation, Sol Ginsburg was placed in charge of the Psychiatry Section. Ginsburg had trained in neurology at Mount Sinai and then shifted his interests to psychiatry. He was not a psychoanalyst and was primarily interested in psychiatric rehabilitation and in his subsequent career was a leader in this area. For the duration of the war, the Psychiatry Section carried on with a depleted staff and provided the needed services to the Hospital.

In May 1945, after a year of study, a Board of Trustees' Special Committee on Psychiatry recommended that an independent Psychiatry Department be established with a full Attending in charge, thereby giving it the same status as other Hospital departments. Seven months later, with World War II now over, the Board appointed M. Ralph Kaufman Psychiatrist to the Hospital. The Department was launched in January 1946.

Much of Kaufman's early career had been spent in Boston. He had been Clinical Director of the McLean Hospital and one of the founding members of the Boston Psychoanalytic Society. As an attending at the Boston Beth Israel Hospital, he initiated a consultation-liaison program and laid the groundwork for the development of psychiatry in a general hospital. During World War II, Kaufman volunteered for service in the Army and served as the Executive Officer of the Army School of Psychiatry and also as Consultant in Neuropsychiatry in the Pacific. He participated in five campaigns and demonstrated the therapeutic effectiveness of psychiatry in front-line rehabilitation. Kaufman received numerous citations and medals and was discharged as a Colonel.

Originally appointed on a geographic full-time basis, Kaufman soon requested a status change to full time, since the pressure of seeing patients detracted from his ability to develop the Department. Because of limited funding, a large number of voluntary physicians were appointed, and the Psychiatric Clinic was reorganized to provide a more appropriate atmosphere for treatment. Kaufman set about structuring a liaison program, and within a year he had a Liaison Psychiatrist appointed to each of the major services and the outpatient clinics. This program became a major component of the Department and served as a model throughout the country.

Ground floor units of the Hospital were rearranged for a psychiatric inpatient service, and on March 10, 1947, Ward A, a psychiatric ward of twenty-one beds, was opened. Admissions were limited to outpatient or hospital patients who required psychiatric care, thereby creating a psychosomatic service with many extremely sick patients. In the absence of psychotropic drugs, therapy was mainly psychoanalytically oriented.

Prior to the opening of the unit, Kaufman appointed Fred Brown, Ph.D., to establish a Division of Psychology. Brown saw the main role of the psychologist as contributing to diagnosis and clarifying problems of psychodynamics and prognosis of patients. The Division grew rapidly and was involved in many research projects. Brown received a psychology training grant and designed a very popular program, publishing a number of papers concerned with psychosomatic medicine. He retired after more than twenty-five years as Director of the Division, having played an important role in clinical services, training, and research.

In January 1948, Edward Joseph and Oscar Sachs were appointed as the first Psychiatric Residents at The Mount Sinai Hospital, and both remained members of the Department of Psychiatry for most of their careers. Joseph was active in the clinical and teaching activities of the Department and served as the Acting Director in 1970–1971. Well known for his psychoanalytic research on twins, Joseph played a major role in the psychoanalytic movement in New York and nationally and was President of both the American Psychoanalytic Association and the International Psychoanalytic Association.

Psychiatric services for children were included in the new Department, and the Pediatric Child Guidance Clinic became part of the Department in 1945 under the direction of Abram Blau, an experienced child psychiatrist. The Division grew over time and included pediatric inpatient and outpatient liaison services and child psychiatry outpatient clinics. Two beds for child psychosomatic problems in the Pediatric Pavilion were made available in 1951 and were the beginning of inpatient child psychiatry in the Hospital. Shortly thereafter, the Division was approved for training, and Elizabeth Kleinberger was appointed the first Fellow in child psychiatry. She remained on the staff and was in charge of the inpatient child psychiatry unit for many years.

With a lack of space and a staff of voluntary physicians with limited time commitments, the Department was able to undertake little research. However, several notable contributions had an important influence on the development of psychiatry as a clinical discipline.[15] Papers describing the Mount Sinai Service served as primers for establishing psychiatry in the general hospital, using a psychosomatic frame of reference. Drawing on his experiences in liaison psychiatry, Louis Linn, a senior member of the Department and a well-known psychiatrist and psychoanalyst, published the classic book *A Handbook of Hospital Psychiatry*.[16] Laboratory investigation, however, was not altogether neglected. Sidney Margolin, who joined the staff in 1946, collaborated with Kaufman and members of the Gastroenterology Division in measurements of gastric function during psychoanalysis.

Charles Fisher, known for his earlier work, which demonstrated that hypothalamic lesions cause diabetes insipidus, joined the Department in its early days and would serve for more than forty years as an active and productive investigator in sleep research. Initially serving as a Liaison Psychiatrist, Fisher began to pursue research in psychoanalysis. Given a small room adjacent to Ward A and meager funds, he undertook work that over the years contributed greatly to the understanding of dreams. Much later (1963), Fisher would discover that REM sleep was associated with nocturnal penile tumescence, an observation that would become an important laboratory test in the evaluation of male erectile dysfunction.[17] Fisher would come to be considered "one of, if not the most, preeminent psychoanalytical experimental researchers of our time."[18]

William Dement was attracted to Fisher's work and came to Mount Sinai for his training. As a medical student, Dement had studied the elicitation of dream recall from rapid (REM) and nonrapid eye movement (NREM) awakenings and had demonstrated that dreams were associated with REM sleep. Dement believed that sleep associated with REM was qualitatively different from the remainder of sleep. He began a series of studies with Fisher concerned with the effect of REM deprivation and the subsequent occurrence of REM periods; the results attracted much attention.[19] Fisher and Dement believed at the time that, if REM deprivation continued long enough, it would initiate a psychosis. Howard Roffwarg joined them for a short time, and they pursued their exciting sleep studies. As the work expanded, the lack of adequate research and animal facilities caused increasing frustration for Dement, who left for Stanford University, where he would become a world-renowned sleep authority.

The Trustees had recognized the lack of laboratory space and adequate clinical facilities and the impact of these deficiencies on patient care, research, and Resident training at the time of the creation of the Department. They had recommended that, when possible, a separate psychiatric facility be built. Kaufman and his staff vigorously pursued this issue almost from the time of his appointment. In 1956, the Trustees finally gave approval, and planning for a new building was begun. In addition to psychiatry, the building would house additional medical and surgical beds. Kaufman planned well for the Department's expansion. On Ward A, he had earlier demonstrated that it was possible to treat private and clinic patients in the same setting. A National Institute of Mental Health training grant was obtained to fund additional Resident positions in both adult and child psychiatry; the adult program was increased from two to three years, and an adolescent program was developed. After several construction delays, the Esther and Joseph Klingenstein Clinical Center (KCC) opened late in 1962 with 103 psychiatry beds, a significant increase from the twenty-three beds on Ward A. The Institute of Psychiatry occupied five floors and stands now as the largest psychiatric unit in any voluntary general hospital in the country, with the largest voluntary psychiatric staff of any general hospital in the world. In January 1963, a fifteen-bed child psychiatry inpatient unit opened in KCC. It remains the only inpatient child psychiatry program in a voluntary hospital in New York City. Later in 1963, a Day and Night Center for partial hospitalization was opened. It was, at the time, one of only two such facilities in the country. There were now 118, mostly voluntary, psychiatrists on staff.

The years prior to the opening of KCC saw the emergence of psychopharmacology, with the development of chlorpromazine for the management of schizophrenia, lithium for mania, and imipramine for depression. Benzodiazepines were also in development for use in anxiety. Psychoanalysis, still the cornerstone of therapy at Mount Sinai, was beginning to lose some of its luster. On the other hand, drug therapy allowed admission of more disturbed patients to the inpatient service. Drug therapy also impacted psychiatric research, increasing the emphasis on studies of the role of the brain and of genetic and biological factors in major psychiatric disorders. The role of neurotransmitters and receptors in psychiatric disorders came under study. This not so subtle shift in research interests toward basic science was occurring throughout Mount Sinai and was a major impetus to the development of the Mount Sinai School of Medicine, which received its charter in 1963. As the school planned to admit its first students in 1968, Kaufman was appointed Chairman and the first Esther and Joseph Klingenstein Professor of Psychiatry and was also appointed Dean of the Page and William Black Post Graduate School of Medicine.

The dramatic increase in bed complement in KCC stimulated expansion of outpatient services, especially the Aftercare Clinic, which had been in existence for many years. The Individual Therapy Clinic became an important site for Resident training, which was headed by David Kairys. Aaron Stein was appointed Director of the Division of Group Therapy. The inception of Medicare and Medicaid led to a substantial increase in visits to the psychiatric emergency room, which underwent a major reorganization in 1969 to provide twenty-four-hour coverage by Residents and Attending staff.

With the Department becoming ever more visible, the Liaison Service expanded once again, and Lawrence Roose was appointed the coordinator of the program in 1965. It had great appeal to the practicing psychiatrists, and many were recruited; Residents were now assigned to the program. The liaison concept was adopted into the Medical School curriculum with the Department's involvement in the Introduction to Medicine course and into the multidisciplinary and system-oriented teaching of the preclinical years. Emily Mumford, a sociologist, joined the Department in 1966 as an educational consultant and played an important role in the formulation of the first Medical School curriculum. A Division of Behavioral Science was established and became a resource for the entire institution.

Planning was now under way for the Medical School building; unfortunately, Kaufman did not push for space for the Department in the emerging structure. Kaufman retired in 1970, and Joseph was appointed the Acting Chair. Active in many aspects of psychiatry and psychoanalysis throughout his career, Kaufman received many awards and honors. He was President of the American Psychoanalytic Association (1949–1951) and Vice President of the American Psychiatric Association (1963–1964). Following his death in 1977, he received many posthumous tributes. In its day, Kaufman's psychiatry program served as a model for the evolution of general hospital psychiatry at its best.

In July 1971, Marvin Stein was appointed Psychiatrist to the Hospital and Professor and Chairman of Psychiatry in the School of Medicine. Stein had been an early Mental Health Career Investigator in the Research Development Program of the National Institute of Mental Health (NIMH). He had also held academic appointments at the University of Pennsylvania, Cornell University, and the State University of New York Downstate Medical Centers where he served as Chairman. Service on major national committees dedicated to developing a stronger scientific basis for psychiatry and the psychoanalytic process had placed Stein in an important policy and administrative role in the emerging field of biological psychiatry.

As noted earlier, hospital-based psychiatry at this time was undergoing major changes. Inpatient care was now being provided for large numbers of chronically ill patients with major psychiatric disorders, such as schizophrenia and manic-depressive illness. However, because of changes in reimbursement, psychiatric hospital lengths of stay were decreasing quickly. At Mount Sinai, the average stay went from sixty to thirty days within a very few years. As a result, Stein had to first undertake a major reorganization of the clinical service before he could embark on his ultimate goal, the development of an academic department. The inpatient service was reconfigured to provide rapid evaluation and treatment of patients during a relatively brief hospital stay. A team approach was utilized, offering a variety of treatment modalities. Full-time Attendings were placed in charge of the inpatient units to provide for the clinical and teaching needs, leading inevitably to friction with the voluntary staff, some of whom resigned.

To reach out to the surrounding community and to furnish a care site for both clinic and private patients, the outpatient service was also strengthened. Full-time positions were created, and Arthur Schwartz was named Director of Psychiatric Ambulatory Care. In 1972, the Psychiatric Emergency Room was incorporated into the organizational structure of the ambulatory care program. One year later, Arthur Meyerson was appointed full-time Director of the Acute Care Service. Both Schwartz and Meyerson were analytically trained and research oriented. A comprehensive program was initiated that offered crisis intervention, admission to hospital when needed, and outpatient treatment. The program was moving from its former primary emphasis on psychosomatic illness to the management of the major psychiatric disorders.

Concurrent with these changes in the clinical components of the program, the Department introduced a research orientation. Fundamental to the conduct of research are personnel, space, and funding. As is usually the case, finding the right people was the easiest. Raul Schiavi, who had worked with Stein in the latter's three posts, moved with him to Mount Sinai. Trained in medicine and psychiatry, Schiavi had already achieved considerable status as a scientist, publishing on the psychosomatic aspects of asthma and the effect of hypothalamic lesions on anaphylaxis. While a Fellow in Paris working with Roger Guillemin, he had published one of the earliest papers on the physiological effects of LH-releasing factor. He had also worked with Stein on the role of central nervous system (CNS) mechanisms in immune processes. Schiavi then began investigations relating to CNS control of gonadal function and sexual behavior; these studies would form the basis of a lifetime of clinical and laboratory research in sexual behavior.

For Stein, finding research space was a nightmare, and funding was made difficult because he had to use a significant amount of his available new dollars to strengthen the clinical program. Planning for the Annenberg Building had begun in the mid-1960s, and, at the time, with KCC still new, Kaufman had not requested any additional space in Annenberg, especially since he was not oriented toward laboratory research. Consequently, there was essentially no research space for Stein and Schiavi on their arrival. The sudden and tragic death in 1972 of Solomon Berson, Chairman of Medicine, suddenly made available the space that had been promised to him. After a series of negotiations involving other departments, Psychiatry was assigned a substantial amount of space for laboratories and offices on Annenberg 22.

In 1972, Schiavi began to devote his total effort at Mount Sinai to his interest in sexual behavior and obtained clinical training at the Payne Whitney Clinic in the treatment of sexual dysfunctions under Helen Singer Kaplan, a leader in the field of human sexuality. With his research and clinical background, Schiavi began to develop a human sexuality program at Mount Sinai that would provide therapy, education, and research in sexual function and dysfunction. The research produced a number of landmark papers. Collaborating with Fisher, Schiavi published a pioneering study on the value of nocturnal penile tumescence in the differential diagnosis of erectile disorders.[20] Looking at genetic abnormalities, Schiavi published the first, and possibly the only, double-blind control study that utilized sexual and hormonal data from men with sex chromosome anomalies.[21] His research looked at diabetic males and the effects of the aging process. In 1999, Schiavi published the authoritative text on sexuality in the aging male, drawing on his clinical and research experience at Mount Sinai.[22] Acknowledged as one of the leading figures in the study of human sexuality, Schiavi received national and international recognition for his work.

With specific drug therapy now available for many mental illnesses, psychiatry was moving quickly toward biological psychiatry and behavior therapy and away from analysis. Because a correct psychiatric diagnosis was now paramount, Arthur Rifkin, a well-known investigator in psychopharmacology and a member of the staff since 1979, would play an important role. Rifkin was given the responsibility for training the staff in the new diagnostic criteria.

Liaison Psychiatry, a bedrock of the Department for decades, had been incorporated into a newly established Consultation Service in 1975. One year later, it received a vital stimulus when Howard Zucker, a long-time member of the Department, planned a model liaison service on a medical unit. Richard Gorlin, Chairman of Medicine, was totally supportive, and the two made rounds together with students and House Staff. The program was an unqualified success; it led to a course in Humanistic Medicine, culminating in the production of a highly acclaimed movie describing the program. In 1979, James Strain was recruited as the full-time Director of the Division of Liaison and Consultative Psychiatry. Committed to an academic program, Strain established relationships with several departments and began studies on the co-morbidity of medical and psychiatric illness.

With the building efforts in patient care and teaching coming to fruition, it was once again time to turn to expanding the research effort. In 1979, Kenneth Davis and a group of young investigators from the Department of Psychiatry at Stanford University were recruited to expand the research endeavor of the Department to include the investigation of underlying neurobiological mechanisms in psychiatric disorders. A graduate of the Mount Sinai School of Medicine, where he had won the Elster award for the highest academic achievement in his medical school class, Davis trained at Stanford University and then received a Career Development Award from the Veterans Administration to investigate cholinergic mechanisms in neuropsychiatric disorders. Studies involving the clinical implications of acetylcholine-dopamine interactions demonstrated that, when central cholinergic activity is increased, manic symptoms are suppressed. This work was awarded the prestigious A. E. Bennett Award of the Society of Biological Psychiatry.

Joined by Richard Mohs, a cognitive psychologist, the Stanford team conducted the first well-controlled study in which a drug was able to improve the storage and retrieval functions of long-term memory in humans.[23] These findings had great significance and implications for some of the memory disorders of the elderly, including Alzheimer's disease, an area that Davis and his colleagues pursued at Mount Sinai. Indeed, the very first trials in the world in which the acetylcholinesterase inhibitors were given to patients with Alzheimer's disease were conducted by Davis, Mohs, and their colleagues. The work was initiated at Stanford and completed at Mount Sinai. The work constituted the critical proof of concept studies that led to the development of an entire class of drugs, the first drugs approved for the treatment of Alzheimer's disease and to date the only such compounds.

Davis was appointed Chief of the Psychiatry Service at the Bronx Veterans Administration Medical Center, and Thomas Horvath, an outstanding clinician and teacher, was appointed Associate Chief responsible for clinical services and teaching. Horvath, an exceptionally gifted administrator, would eventually go on to become the Chief of Psychiatry for the entire VA system. Within five years of coming to Mount Sinai, Davis had developed a program that was recognized as a major undertaking in biologic psychiatry research. Davis and his colleagues made considerable progress in studies concerned with the pharmacology, biology, and phenomenology of both Alzheimer's disease and schizophenia. Indeed, this group received the first national award designating it a Schizophrenia Biological Research Center. The group's research on schizophrenia provided the first direct evidence for the involvement of dopamine in schizophrenic patients.[24] Measuring the relationship between dopamine metabolism and psychiatric symptoms led Davis to reconceptualize the role of dopamine in schizophrenia. The ensuing paper became one of the most cited works on schizophrenia of the past decade.[25]

The research group devised and established the rating scale that has become the international standard for the assessment of drugs in the study of Alzheimer's disease[26] and the very methodology for studying drugs in Alzheimer's disease. The group also demonstrated that cholinesterase inhibitors can be a symptomatic treatment for Alzheimer's disease.[27] In 1983, the Mount Sinai School of Medicine was designated by the National Institute on Aging as one of the first of five Alzheimer's Disease Research Centers, with the goals of conducting research into the causes, mechanisms, and treatment of Alzheimer's disease and related illnesses and of providing clinical care to patients and families; the enterprise was another major advance in the development of the Department. The Alzheimer's Center has received continuous funding since its inception.

Throughout Stein's tenure as Chairman, he was able to pursue his own research interests and was among the first to demonstrate the interaction among brain, behavior, and the immune system.[28] Steven Schleifer, a Mount Sinai Medical School graduate, joined the full-time faculty and with Stein and other colleagues conducted a pioneering prospective study that documented suppression of lymphocyte stimulation following bereavement in a group of men whose wives had died of cancer.[29] This suggested a possible mechanism for the increased morbidity and mortality among the bereaved.

The pioneering studies of Stein and Davis and their colleagues were instrumental in moving the Department away from an emphasis on psychoanalysis and psychosomatic illness to work on the major psychiatric disorders. By the mid-1980s, having met his mandate to develop a major academic Department of Psychiatry with a well-organized clinical service, quality educational programs, and a broad-based, well-funded research enterprise, Stein stepped down from the Chair to devote himself to his own research. During this period, he was President of the American Psychosomatic Society and the Academy of Behavioral Medicine Research. Stein's outstanding achievements in psychiatry as a leading clinician, scientist, and administrator have brought worldwide distinction to him and to the Medical Center.

Kenneth Davis was appointed Chairman in 1987 and, like his predecessor, has taken the Department to a new plateau. The recipient of many awards, including the American Psychiatric Association Award for Research in Psychiatry, Davis was recently elected to membership in the Institute of Medicine, National Academy of Science. He and his associates have been at the forefront in the delineation of the role of amyloid in Alzheimer's disease[30] and were among the first to report the cloning and chromosomal location of the amyloid precursor protein,[31] one of the most important discoveries in Alzheimer's research in the past fifteen years.

The Department's research endeavors have moved into the areas of molecular genetics, neurochemical-based neuropathology, and the use of sophisticated imaging techniques. A Positron Emission Tomography laboratory has been established under the direction of Monte Buchsbaum. Studies have been carried out on more than one thousand psychiatric and neurological patients. A Brain Bank, directed by Daniel Perl, Professor of Pathology, and Vahram Haroutunian, of the Department of Psychiatry, provides the capability to perform neurochemical determinations almost at will. Neuritic plaque formation and amyloid deposition have been identified as among the earliest lesions in Alzheimer's disease.[32] Microarray studies have identified more than eighty different genes that are abnormally expressed and regulated in the brains of schizophrenic patients,[33] opening up significant avenues for new research.

Although significant accomplishments have emanated from the Department's concentrated research efforts, these have not come at the expense of patient care. The Clinical Service has flourished and expanded. Under the direction of Jeremy Silverman, family studies of Alzheimer's disease and schizophrenia have found that the role of genetic risk factors for late-onset Alzheimer's is reduced, while another study has found that surviving dementia-free to age ninety and beyond may be a phenotype for genetic protective factors. The psychobiologic aspects of personality disorders have been extensively studied by Larry Siever, who has been instrumental in finding the important link between serotonin and impulsive and aggressive behavior. Rachel Yehuda has led an internationally recognized group in the examination of posttraumatic stress disorders, and, following the September 11, 2001, disaster, was asked by the *New England Journal of Medicine* to summarize the status of the biology and treatment of stress disorders. A program investigating obsessive-compulsive disorders has led to the development of new treatment modalities, under the direction of Eric Hollander.

With the turn of the millennium, the Department added an important new component in health services research by recruiting a new professor, Susan Essock. Essock has conducted the most extensive and influential work on the question of which modes of treatment are most effective in schizophrenia. She now directs trials that address this and related questions and that bring together multiple sites and collaborators from all over the country.

Over the 150-year history of Mount Sinai, Psychiatry has moved from a small Division in the Department of Neurology to one of the major clinical and academic Departments of Psychiatry in the world. Whereas for almost a century it was dominated by psychoanalysis, the Department today recognizes that psychiatry is a pluralistic field. It includes a wide variety of theoretical viewpoints and practices, and interests range from exciting and innovative clinical approaches to a consideration of neurobiology at the molecular genetic level in psychiatric disorders. Having begun with one full-time member in 1945, the Department now has more than 150 full-time staff, a large voluntary clinical faculty, and three endowed professorships, currently filled by Davis, Deborah Marin, and Nik Robakis. Psychiatry at Mount Sinai is a far cry from what Bernard Sachs knew, but he would have been proud of the growth and development of neuropsychiatry as it exists today. It is the goal of the Department that the continued acquisition of knowledge will make it possible to achieve an integrated theory of mental and emotional processes and to apply that theory to the treatment and prevention of mental illness.

Adapted from a manuscript by Marvin Stein, M.D., Esther and Joseph Klingenstein Professor of Psychiatry Emeritus. Dr. Stein was Chairman of the Department from 1971 to 1987.

30

Department of Radiation Oncology

WITHIN THE FIRST two decades after the discovery of x-rays by Roentgen in 1895 and of radioactivity and radium by Antoine Henri Becquerel (1896) and Marie Curie (1898), major centers for radiation therapy appeared in Stockholm, Paris, London, Manchester, and New York. Mount Sinai purchased its first x-ray machine in 1900. The earliest roentgenograms were taken by members of the House Staff, but in 1901 a separate department was established; the x-ray machine was used for both diagnostic and therapeutic purposes. Initially, therapy proceeded with caution as "results with x-ray therapy have been encouraging, but not such as to warrant great enthusiasm."[1] Nonetheless, a wide range of conditions were treated, including lupus, sarcoma of the ovary, carcinoma of the breast, and carcinoma of the tongue.

At that time [1900–1910] it was the current practice to treat appropriate cases of fibroids of the uterus with X-ray. The equipment and technique were extremely undeveloped. Ten to fifteen women would stand at varying distances from a centrally located tube and exposed to the raying. These were repeated daily over months of time until amenorrhea developed. In spite of the lack of filter and the impossibility of gauging the dosage accurately, only three serious burns occurred.[2]

In 1912, seven years after he first began using radiant energy as treatment in the dermatology clinic, Samuel Stern was appointed Mount Sinai's first official Radiotherapist. Stern published extensively on the use of radiation therapy to treat a number of conditions, including epithelioma, cancer of the larynx, carcinoma of the cervix, Hodgkin's disease, splenic leukemia, rheumatism, eczema, and psoriasis. He was especially interested in the success of x-rays in treating hypertrichosis (superfluous hairs), which although not a serious disease was emotionally debilitating in those so afflicted.[3–6]

An ongoing problem for the Division, as well as for the nation, in the early years was the limited availability of radium. Prior to 1913, all radium was processed in Europe; supply in the United States was scarce, cost was enormous, and therefore the number of patients that could be treated was limited. Even after radium began to be processed in the United States, it was still expensive,[7] a fact frequently noted in the Hospital's *Annual Reports*. In 1920, for instance, the Chief of Radiology, Leopold Jaches, lamented the fact that a substantial number of patients had to be referred to other New York hospitals because Mount Sinai did not have its own radium. He maintained, "We need our own radium and our own emanations in order that we may do justice to our patients and to the community dependent upon us."[8] Later that year, a fund was established with the goal of raising $250,000 to purchase radium. By 1925, the Department had obtained a sufficient supply of "emanations" through a contract with the Radium Corporation of America. Consequently, there was a 60 percent increase in the number of patients treated with radium that year.

Like many of the early pioneers in radiation therapy, Stern was exposed to a large amount of radiation. Once, in order to determine that radium was indeed physiologically active, he recounts that he exposed his arm to it for four hours, with a resulting ulceration that took six months to heal and left some permanent destruction of the tissue.[9] Stern died in 1927 at the age of fifty-two; the cause of his early demise is unknown.

In 1927, under the direction of Max Mayer, Mount Sinai opened the first hospital-affiliated birth control clinic in the United States for therapeutic purposes only. X-ray was used with excellent results to induce abortion in women with life-threatening comorbidities such as tuberculosis and severe cardiac disease.

After Stern's death, William Harris was appointed Radiotherapist to the Hospital. Since there were no organized radiation teaching centers in the United States at the time, Harris had traveled to Europe in the 1920s to study radiation therapy after completing his internship at Mount Sinai. In Paris, he developed a close relationship with Henri Coutard, the originator of many new methods of radiation therapy, who was especially interested in the treatment of cancer of the larynx, which later became Harris's special interest, as well.[10] With the active cooperation of Rudolf Kramer, Chief of the Department of Otolaryngology, Harris undertook the study of radiation therapy as the primary treatment for carcinoma of the larynx and obtained almost as high a cure rate as was accomplished by surgery. Mount Sinai was a pioneer radiation center in this country in establishing radiation therapy as the treatment of choice for laryngeal cancer, in that it preserved the voice as well as being curative.[11]

Despite the fact that, in the 1930s, radiation therapy was still a largely untested field in medicine, radiation therapy was employed in practically every medical specialty both at Mount Sinai and across the nation. Although it was most frequently applied in the treatment of malignant disease, often in conjunction with surgery, its application in treating benign conditions was also extensive, much more so than it is today. It played a major role in dermatology; many dermatologists acquired their own x-ray equipment. Prior to the advent of antibiotics, small doses of radiation were often used to favorably affect such inflammatory conditions as cellulitis, abscesses, carbuncles, parotitis, erysipelas, lymphadenitis, and actinomycosis. At Mount Sinai in the early 1930s, studies were conducted and published on the radiation therapy of bronchiectasis.[12] In orthopaedics, radiation therapy was almost routine for bursitis and painful joints and especially for ankylosing spondylitis (Marie-Strumpell disease). In gynecology, it was used to induce therapeutic abortion, to treat meno-metrorrhagia and carcinoma of the ovary, and also for sterilization. Additionally, irradiation of the pituitary was performed to alleviate menopausal symptoms.[13] In otolaryngology, radiation of lymphoid tissue at the eustachian tube orifices in the nasopharynx was a common practice, not only in children but also in young adults.

While the therapeutic use of radiation grew rapidly, concerns about the effects of exposure to employees working with the radioactive materials also began to increase, though admittedly at a much slower rate. In 1936, x-ray machines were made safer with the addition of shockproof and rayproof devices, and in 1938 the Hospital began to convert radium to a more workable element that eliminated the prolonged handling of radium applicators by employees. However, it was not until the 1940s that routine measurement of the stray radiation received by hospital employees was instituted.

In 1939, following the death of Leopold Jaches, Chief of the Department of Radiology, the Division of Radiation Therapy became a separate Department, with Harris as Chief. The need for physicists to assist in the management of radiation of all forms had been recognized by

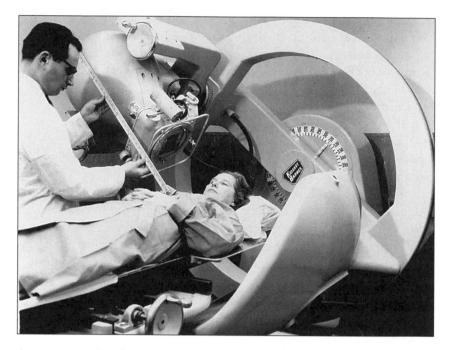

A treatment using the new rotating cobalt unit in the Radiotherapy Center, c. 1967. The machine emitted two million volts and cost $27,500.

Jaches as early as 1920. It was not until nine years later, however, that Carl Braestrup was appointed on a part-time basis.[14]

Over the years, the physicists became principal players in practically all phases of activity in radiation therapy, especially in the development of treatment plans. Credit must also be given to the x-ray equipment manufacturers who engineered outstanding technical improvements. In the 1940s and 1950s, fundamental technical advances were made in supervoltage machines like the betatron and in the development of new radioactive isotopes. Cobalt-60 teletherapy became a major source of radiant energy following World War II and dominated the field of radiation for several decades. By the mid-1960s, the linear accelerator in voltages varying from 2 to 50 megavolts eventually surpassed all other sources of radiation and became the workhorse of the Radiation Therapy Department.

Mount Sinai had to wait for new construction to create a more spacious area for these new machines. This move occurred in 1959, when the Department transferred to a much larger area in the basement of the then Guggenheim building at 1184 Fifth Avenue. A Picker Cobalt-60 teletherapy unit, capable of rotation, thereby lessening skin reactions, was installed. Also, a 24- megavolt betatron was installed in an adjacent room.

Harris died in April 1953, and direction of the Department was taken over by Sidney Silverstone, who had joined the Department in 1938. In the decades that followed, much of Silverstone's research focused on cancer of the cervix. He undertook special studies to determine radiation doses and dose distribution at the periphery of x-ray fields.[15] He also designed a colpostat and tandem for the safer handling of radium in the therapy of cervical cancer and devised a technique for measuring radium doses at six specific points in the pelvis.[16] Silverstone established the first postgraduate course in radium therapy in the United States; it was presented annually for many years.

In 1958, Silverstone began collaboration with Joseph Goldman, the otolaryngologist, to introduce the concept of high-dose preoperative radiation followed by surgery in patients with advanced cancer of the larynx. This combined procedure resulted in a striking improvement over the results previously obtained with either radiotherapy or surgery alone.[17] Silverstone was the last voluntary physician to head the Department, but after his retirement, he remained active in practice, teaching, and research for another four decades. He died December 4, 2001, at ninety-three years of age.

In 1958, John Boland was appointed the first full-time Director of the Department. Recruited from the Christie Hospital, in Manchester, England, he brought many of that institution's concepts with him, including the use of plaster casts for stabilizing treatment fields and definitive treatment protocols for specific sites and stages of disease. He started the Mount Sinai School of Radiotherapy Technology in 1962 with a grant from the United States Public Health Service. The first of its kind in the United States, the school ran an intensive two-year program to train radiotherapy technologists. The school became a catalyst for medical and technical professional bodies to approve a basic curriculum for national use. However, in 1970, it was forced to close due to lack of funding.

In 1967, Boland established the Radiotherapy Research Unit under the direction of Arvin S. Glicksman. This group began investigations into the effects of ionizing radiation on collagen metabolism and

participated in national multicenter studies on Hodgkin's disease, carcinoma of the lung, and head and neck cancer. While at Mount Sinai,
Glicksman joined forces with other radiotherapy departments across
the country to publish some of the earliest reports on computerized radiotherapy treatment planning, which has now become standard in radiotherapy departments around the world.[18] The groundwork for what
would become three-dimensional treatment planning also started at
Mount Sinai, on the basis of the work of this collaborative network.[19]
Three-dimensional planning was the forerunner of most of the sophisticated treatment techniques that have emerged in the last part of the
twentieth century.

In the 1960s, there was a general outcry from the public for radiation safety. In radiation therapy, this impetus was reflected in the development of afterloading techniques. Radium techniques were re-
designed to utilize inactive dummy sources in the actual placement of
applicators, followed by substitution of the dummies by the radioactive
sources under strictly controlled conditions of safety, usually in the patient's room. Afterloading thus reduced radiation exposure to personnel during the implantation of radioactive materials and increased the
accuracy of placement of radioactive sources.

As Chairman, Boland fostered the continued development of
brachytherapy (internal radiation therapy using a radioactive source
placed within the body or a body cavity for the treatment of malignancies.) One of the unique contributions of the Mount Sinai Radiotherapy Department was to convert the cumbersome Heyman multiple capsule technique for cancer of the corpus uteri into a simple and
safe afterloading procedure. Silverstone developed a brass capsule
similar in size and shape to the capsules used in the Heyman Packing
Technique for cancer of the corpus uteri but with a simple needle wire
attached to one end of the capsule instead of the heavy, twisted, chain-
like wire used in the original Heyman capsule. Norman Simon, who
had joined Silverstone and the Department in 1949, used plastic instead of brass for the capsules and developed long needle wires made
with a miniaturized cesium source at one end for afterloading. The in-
sertion of the capsules with inactive dummy wires could be done at a
leisurely pace in the operating room, in contrast to the original cumbersome technique that required the procedure to be performed in
haste behind a heavy lead screen. Then, transfer of the radioactive cesium wires was done in the patient's room. Simon patented the tech-

nique and assigned the patent to Mount Sinai.[20–22] Simon and the Department were also involved in the early use of iridium-192 as a radium substitute.[23]

Silverstone and Simon worked tirelessly as a team in all phases of research. Silverstone was the Director of the Hoffman Fund, which provided the Department with a substantial financial reserve. In 1971, Simon chaired an international meeting on the subject of afterloading with speakers from across the globe, generating intense enthusiasm and interest. It was at this meeting that most of the participants voted to phase out radium and radon in favor of the newer and safer radioactive isotopes. Simon became interested in the foreign associations of radiation therapy and became active in their yearly meetings. Through his influence, Mount Sinai was represented at all of these meetings which were held throughout the world, including Europe, India, and South America. Simon was also active in the protection of the environment from radiation.

In the 1970s, a new 4-megavolt linear accelerator was installed in the Department. Its high penetration and speed greatly reduced exposure time. During this period, the Department established an independent three-year residency training program, separating from the earlier combined program with Radiology. By this time, the majority of the work done by the Department was in oncology; two-thirds of new cancer cases at the Hospital were referred to the Department. In the late 1970s, the Department began to have financial and administrative difficulties, resulting in a loss of productivity and personnel.

In 1983, one year after Boland stepped down, William Bloomer was appointed Chairman. During the next few years, Bloomer and Mount Sinai embarked on a major renovation and expansion of the radiation oncology program and facilities. New state-of-the-art linear accelerators and treatment planning simulators were installed, medical physics services expanded, and new faculty recruited. A successful community outreach program was accomplished with the purchase of an ambulatory radiation oncology facility in Queens. In 1984, Bloomer established a laboratory to study the effects of radiation on the cell and the relationship between sunlight and the development of skin cancer. Additional research during his tenure focused on the use of carriers to escort radioactive substances into the nucleus of cancer cells and the methods by which cells undergo mutation and malignant change and repair DNA damage.[24]

In 1988, the Department began using computer modeling of radioactive implants to simulate the location and action of the implant before the patient actually received the exposure. This technique predicted, analyzed, and improved the dose distribution of radiation with fewer complications. That same year, in collaboration with the Department of Obstetrics and Gynecology, an aberrant structure in the estrogen receptor gene in tumor tissue was isolated in women with breast cancer.[25]

In an effort to formally acknowledge the fact that the main focus of the Department was oncology, its name was officially changed in 1989 to the Department of Radiation Oncology, concomitant with the arrival of Brenda Shank as Chairperson. The first female department chair at Mount Sinai, Shank had extensive experience and expertise in total body irradiation techniques. She succeeded in bringing all equipment up-to-date and also enlarged the Department, introduced total body irradiation techniques,[26] and rejuvenated the residency program.

Shank's nine-year tenure was marked by many interdepartmental and collaborative initiatives, involving the management of prostate and breast cancer, brain tumors, and gynecologic malignancies. A statistical model was designed to determine the risk of axillary node involvement in breast cancer patients.[27] Shank was also the principal investigator of a "patterns of care process survey" to evaluate the characteristics of radiation oncology practice after breast conservation surgery in the United States.[28]

In recent years, the Radiobiology Laboratory established a technique that enables the rapid and accurate screening of large patient populations for genetic mutations and polymorphisms in a variety of cancer-related genes. This work focuses on alternations in the ataxia telangiectasia-mutated (ATM) gene, which plays a key role in the response of cells to mutation. Evidence has been obtained that breast cancer patients who are carriers of a mutated copy of the ATM gene are more susceptible to the development of subcutaneous tissue effects following radiation therapy. These results suggest that possession of an ATM mutation may be a relative contraindication to breast conservation management using conventional doses and that lower treatment doses should be used with these patients. Work is currently in progress to extend these studies to prostate cancer patients.

Following Shank's departure in 1998, Richard Stock was appointed Chairman of the Department. The second graduate of the Mount Sinai

School of Medicine to chair a department in the school, Stock has been a pioneer in the field of prostate brachytherapy. In collaboration with the Department of Urology, he helped develop an ultrasound-guided technique to insert radioactive seeds into the prostate to treat prostate cancer.[29] Utilizing transrectal ultrasound, Stock and his collaborators devised a new technique for performing interstitial implants in the treatment of gynecologic malignancies.[30] Departmental studies also include a long-term analysis of treatment efficacy and morbidity.

It is now one hundred years since the first patients at Mount Sinai were treated with radiation. If here today, Samuel Stern, the Hospital's first radiotherapist, would be amazed at the panoply of sophisticated techniques and equipment at the ready to manage the complexities of current radiation oncologic care.

Adapted from an unpublished article by Sidney M. Silverstone, M.D.

31

Department of Radiology

THE ORIGINS OF the Department of Radiology provide us with a prime example of Mount Sinai's perpetual need for more space. When the Hospital purchased its first x-ray machine in 1900, it was set up in the synagogue, a portion of which had already been converted to an operating room. There, the staff could use the machine as long as there were no religious services in progress. Eugene H. Eising, who was House Surgeon at the time, took the first x-ray plate. The resulting picture revealed a fracture of the upper thigh in a male patient. Eising and Walter Brickner were the first radiographers appointed to the Hospital. The initial success of the two radiographers was reflected in the *Annual Report* for 1901, which concluded that "All cases that have been studied on the operating or post-mortem table have verified our x-ray findings . . . and of the very large number of cases submitted to x-ray exam, not one has to our knowledge suffered the slightest burn."[1] Unfortunately, like many of the early experimenters with x-rays, Eising and Brickner were not so lucky. Both men acquired severe burns from repeatedly testing the machine by placing their left hand in front of the tube.

In fact, as early as 1905, Brickner brought the matter of the safety of x-rays for the medical staff before the Medical Board:

> The frightful, even fatal skin injuries that have been suffered by several x-ray workers are quite familiar through the medical and lay press. That frequent exposure to the x-rays is also capable of effecting deeper injuries is just being discovered. Several members of the board are already familiar with the damages that the x-ray work have inflicted upon my person. . . . The employment of shields and screens, therefore even if altogether practical in active diagnostic work, does not give sufficient promise of protection.[2]

Following Brickner's recommendations, the Board adopted proposals to distribute the x-ray work between the x-ray staff and the rest of the physician staff so that the x-ray workers would be exposed to less radiation. However, it was another thirty-five years before routine measurements of the stray radiation received by hospital employees were conducted by the Physics Department.[3]

Brickner served as Chief of the Department of Roentgenology until 1908, when he was appointed Assistant Attending Surgeon, and Leopold Jaches replaced him. Jaches emigrated to the United States from Latvia in 1892. He studied law and was admitted to the New York Bar in 1898, having become an American citizen the previous year. Later, he studied medicine, graduating from medical school in 1903, and became one of the pioneers of x-ray in America. During World War I, he was in charge of the X-ray Division of the United States Army in France. As Chief at Mount Sinai, Jaches would develop the Department "from small beginnings . . . into a large diagnostic and therapeutic institute."[4] By 1909, the rest of the Hospital was beginning to realize the importance and utility of radiology. According to the *Annual Report* for 1909, "The services of this department have been utilized to a much larger degree by the surgeons and physicians of the hospital, and by the profession, and this department is gaining in importance, as the value of this service and its practical application in the practice of surgery and medicine are more largely recognized."[5] As a reflection of this growing importance, the Department moved into larger quarters in the basement of the medical building the following year. By 1920, the total operating costs of the Department were $20,119, up from $3,370 in 1910, and the number of examinations increased from 1,724 to 10,777 in the same period. As the number of patients examined continued to climb, the Department decided in 1930 to begin using full-time lay technicians for diagnostic work, which up until then had been performed by interns.

The 1920s were marked by a series of scientific achievements by members of the Department. Since radiography was fast becoming an important tool for many of the medical specialties, members of the Department were integrally involved in advances occurring throughout the Hospital. In 1923, Jaches and Harry Wessler published *Clinical Roentgenology of Diseases of the Chest*,[6] which was long considered the standard American work on the subject. In 1926, an x-ray unit was installed in the operating room to permit visualization of the kidneys during the removal of kidney stones. Three years later, Mount Sinai's own Moses Swick formulated Uroselectan, which permitted the visualization and examination of the urinary tract without cystoscopy.[7] This compound led the way for later advances in the visualization of the heart, vascular system, and brain. Jaches frequently collaborated with Swick in the roentgen diagnosis of urinary diseases.[8] Also in the 1920s, the radiologist Arthur Bendick assisted Isidor C. Rubin, of the Department of Gynecology, with his pioneer work in the visualization of the uterus and the fallopian tubes.[9] In 1937, the internship in radiology at Mount Sinai was recognized as part of the course required for the degree of Doctor in Medical Sciences in Radiology at Columbia University.

Jaches died in 1939, after more than thirty years as Chief of Radiology; Marcy L. Sussman succeeded him. That same year, Sussman performed the first angiocardiogram at Mount Sinai.[10] This led to his becoming the head of the Cardiovascular Research Group, a collaborative effort that included cardiologists, radiologists, pediatricians, and thoracic surgeons. Achievements of the group include the first angiographic demonstration of a coarctation of the aorta[11] and the development of one of the first rapid film changers for use in angiography.[12] By 1950, two thousand angiograms had been performed.[13] Sussman served as Chief for ten years and was responsible for training several of the outstanding radiologists of the future, including Bernard S. Wolf, who would succeed Sussman when Sussman resigned his position in 1949.

Under the leadership of Wolf, the Department attained international recognition. Trained in physics and radiation therapy, Wolf entered the United States Army during World War II as a captain and was assigned to the Manhattan Project, working on the development of the atomic bomb. He was one of the first physicians to enter Hiroshima at the end of the war to measure residual radioactivity. Returning to Mount Sinai, Wolf was appointed Associate Radiotherapist and simultaneously served as Director of the Atomic Energy Commission in its New York City office from 1947 until he took up his position as Director of the Department of Radiology in 1949. At the time the Department was relatively small, consisting at most of three to five Attending Radiologists. Wolf was able to attract a group of individuals whose productivity as both full-time and voluntary staff radiologists became the envy of many far larger radiology departments. In addition, Wolf fostered a passion for teaching that has been inherited by every member of the Department for the past half century.

Wolf was a prolific writer, publishing more than two hundred articles on a wide range of radiologic subjects.[14] One of the great leaders in the world of radiology, Wolf was a prodigious worker and a perennial

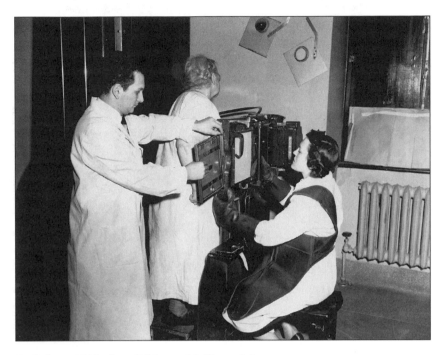

Radiology, 1940s. Joan J. Lipsay, M. D., at right.

student. An inspiration to all who came in contact with him, he was a constant source of support for his staff. Through his work, he helped define the radiographic anatomy of the esophagus, including hiatus hernia, and the esophagogastric junction. He introduced the use of the barium pill (sometimes referred to as "Wolf pills") to detect minimal esophageal strictures. Wolf's collaborations, over a period of many years, with Richard Marshak and Mansho Khilnani on the physiologic and anatomic details of the esophagus and gastrointestinal tract and on the various aspects of inflammatory bowel disease were unique. Much of what we take for granted today was first articulated during this era by these three men.

A dominant figure in radiology for more than thirty years, Richard H. Marshak belongs to a group of Mount Sinai physicians who are remembered equally for their scientific achievements and for their colorful personalities. After completing residencies in pathology and radiology, Marshak was invited by Burrill Crohn to join his private practice as

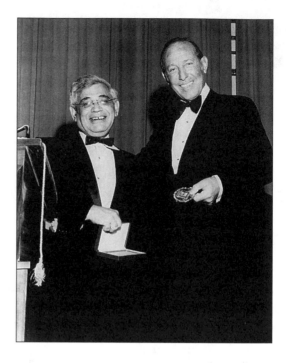

Bernard Wolf, M.D., Chairman of the Dept. of Radiology (1949–1977) presenting the Jacobi Medallion of the Alumni Association to Richard Marshak, M.D., 1972.

a consulting radiologist. Consequently, Marshak saw hundreds of patients with gastrointestinal disorders. This experience, coupled with his amazing abilities as a teacher and a writer, would lead him and his colleagues to their groundbreaking work on the radiologic descriptions of regional enteritis and would inspire further studies on small bowel and colonic radiology. They would go on to describe the radiologic manifestations of sprue, malabsorption, protein-losing enteropathy, parasitic small bowel infection, vascular disease of the small bowel, lymphoma and other small bowel tumors, segmental colitis, toxic megacolon, and numerous other disorders. Marshak's seminal work in this field during the 1950s and 1960s would help to "elevate the small bowel from an untouchable area in diagnostic radiology to a status equal in importance to the remainder of the G.I. tract."[15]

Marshak's remarkable scientific accomplishments and innate intellectual gifts produced a man with a powerful ego. Almost everyone, however, would agree that he was entitled to it. He was known as a radiological evangelist and an indefatigable lecturer, "who could literally caress the film and feel the diagnosis."[16] Unfortunately, this would turn out to be a necessary skill when the ravages of diabetes resulted in Marshak's almost complete loss of vision. However, with the assistance of his long-time associate Daniel Maklansky, himself a gifted radiologist and teacher, Marshak continued to give lectures, describing in detail slides he could barely see.

One of the unsung heroes of the Department was Mansho Khilnani, a superb diagnostic radiologist with a keen analytic mind. He attended medical school at Calcutta University and worked in refugee camps on the India-Pakistan border before coming to the United States in 1951. To review films with Khilnani was to get a lesson in anatomy, pathology, and x-ray diagnosis. An unassuming individual, Khilnani never received the national and international recognition due him. Yet, those who worked with him recognized him as a giant in the field of radiology.

Maklansky has characterized Wolf, Marshak, and Khilnani as follows: "Although they had different personalities, they all shared a passion for excellence, a remarkable dedication to their work, and intellectual and mental energy to allow them to pursue their goals relentlessly until achieved."[17]

John E. Moseley served Mount Sinai for four decades (1943–1983) as its first pediatric radiologist. Internationally recognized for his expertise in bone radiology, he was often requested by anthropologists to study x-rays of ancient bones. Invited to Peru for the opening of the Museum of Paleopathology, he had the opportunity to review x-rays of Peruvian mummies; his report became part of a conference on Human Paleopathology, sponsored by the National Academy of Sciences in 1965. Moseley's conferences with radiologists and pediatricians were amalgamated into the textbook *Bone Changes in Hematologic Disorders*.[18] He also provided the original description of the "spinnaker sail" sign, indicating a pneumomediastinum in the newborn,[19] and was a co-author of the first publication to depict the changes of the lateral spine in Trisomy-21.[20] A warm individual with a fine sense of humor, Moseley became involved in many of his community's projects, including the Harlem Cancer Committee and the local Sickle Cell Anemia Association.

For decades, Charles Newman and Claude Bloch, associates in practice, were invaluable members of the Department. Bloch edited "Radiologic Notes" in the Mount Sinai journals for a number of years; Newman, who would endow a Professorial Chair in the Department, was another superb teacher of students and residents.

Yun Peng Huang joined the Department after completing neuro-surgery training at Mount Sinai in 1961. His contributions to neuroradiology over the next thirty-five years were remarkable. In collaboration with Wolf, he provided the first anatomic delineation of the venous drainage system of the posterior fossa, a noteworthy achievement.[21] His insightful observations guaranteed his reputation as a world-class neuroanatomist.

A most productive member of the Department from 1970 to 1986 was Murray Baron, the first interventional radiologist to perform intra-arterial angiographic studies at Mount Sinai. His angiographic-anatomic correlation of the changes that occur with endocardial cushion abnormalities was a major accomplishment.[22] Harold Mitty, the current Chief of Interventional Radiology and Urologic Radiology, has spent his entire career at Mount Sinai. A founding member of the Society of Cardiovascular Radiology, he also served as President of the New York Roentgen Society and serves on numerous radiologic journal editorial boards. The author or co-author of more than 150 publications, Mitty runs a fellowship program that is highly sought after by budding interventional radiologists. From the earliest days of ultrasound imaging, Hsu-Chong Yeh has provided outstanding diagnostic services, and in his writings he has made significant contributions to the field.

Recruited to Mount Sinai by Wolf in 1961, Jack Rabinowitz left after five years on the staff to become Chief of Radiology at Brooklyn-Cumberland Medical Center, Kings County Hospital, and then Chairman of the Department at the University of Tennessee. He returned "home" in 1978 to become Chairman at Mount Sinai, succeeding his mentor. During Rabinowitz's tenure, the Department assumed responsibility for radiologic care at City Hospital Center at Elmhurst, Queens Hospital Center, and the Bronx Veterans Administration Medical Center. The residency training program, which included rotations to all of the institutions as well as Mount Sinai, increased to more than forty Residents. There was also a concomitant increase in faculty. Many of the graduating Residents have remained on the faculty: Kathleen Halton is now in charge of the Resident training program; David Mendelson, in addition to his expertise in chest and body imaging, has played a major role in the Medical Center's efforts to upgrade computer technology. Karen Norton, the pediatric radiologist, and Robert Shapiro, in ultrasound, among others, have joined Peter Som, an acknowledged expert in head and neck radiology, and George Hermann, whose clinical activities include mammography and bone imaging. Rhona Keller has provided stellar gastrointestinal radiologic services for many years.

Rabinowitz occupied many prestigious positions during his sixteen years as Chairman. He served as President of the New York Roentgen Society and was Editor-in-Chief of *Radiology Today* during its entire existence, as well as a reviewer for the *American Journal of Radiology*. For twenty-five years he was an examiner for the oral examinations for the American Board of Radiology and was Chief Proctor for the written boards. Rabinowitz is the author of two books and fourteen chapters, as well as more than 125 papers. His initial description of the roentgen significance of the pulmonary ligament was an important contribution to the radiologic literature.[23]

During Rabinowitz's tenure, efforts commenced to enlarge and modernize the Department of Radiology. With the opening of the state-of-the-art Radiology Imaging Center in the summer of 1994, Mount Sinai became New York City's preeminent source for ambulatory, comprehensive radiologic services. Offering a full range of technologically advanced diagnostic capabilities in a single location, the Center has enhanced the delivery of patient care, as well as providing the requisite tools to train tomorrow's radiologists and facilitating imaging research.

In 1995, Burton P. Drayer was appointed the Dr. Charles M. and Marilyn Newman Professor and Chairman of the Department. A nationally recognized authority on the use of Computed Tomography (CT) and Magnetic Resonance Imaging (MRI) for the diagnosis of neurological disorders, Drayer came to Mount Sinai from the Barrow Neurological Institute in Phoenix, where he was Chairman of the Division of Neuroimaging and Director of MRI. His clinical research interests focus on the normal aging brain and on the use of innovative imaging techniques for the early detection of Alzheimer's disease, Parkinson's disease, and brain infarction. The author of nearly two hundred publications, he has written extensively on improving diagnostic specificity in multiple sclerosis and primary brain tumors. Drayer played a leading role or was the initiator of a variety of techniques that are routinely utilized in animal models and patients for applying functional concepts to anatomic CT and MR imaging: intrathecally enhanced CT Cisternography, xenon-enhanced CT scanning for regional cerebral blood flow, brain iron detection using standard MRI, and carotid and intracranial MR Angiography.

Drayer holds leadership positions in several radiologic associations; he is Chairman of the Task Force on Appropriateness Criteria for Neuroradiology of the American College of Radiology, Editor of *Neuroimaging Clinics of North America*, and Chairman of the Public Relations Committee of the Radiological Society of North America. In 2000, he served as President of the American Society of Neuroradiology (ASNR). He was the founder of the Research Foundation of the ASNR and served as Chairman of the Foundation's Board from 1995 to 2001. Drayer is currently (2002) President-Elect of the New York Roentgen Ray Society.

Drayer is developing programs to build a service-oriented, user-friendly Radiology Department of the future. The goals of this "Radiology 2000" initiative include radically altering the Radiology inpatient physical plant and equipment to match the quality of the Radiology Imaging Center; transforming Radiology into a digital filmless image and information management department that pursues clinical excellence; providing a resource of data management and clinical expertise for the entire Health System; expanding basic science and research activities; and reevaluating the education of physicians-in-training to prepare them for the changing world of healthcare.

32

Department of Rehabilitation Medicine

THE GREAT MEDICAL AUTHORS of ancient times, including Hippocrates and Galen, mention in their writings the use of physical agents to treat disease and to improve health and human function. Physical agents such as heat, cold, water, sun rays, exercise and massage have been widely used on an empirical basis throughout the ages, with electricity being added more recently. Niels Finsen, an Icelandic physician who practiced in Denmark, received the Nobel Prize for Medicine in 1903 for his work on the effects of ultraviolet rays on animal organisms. Unfortunately, few scientific studies were done on other physical agents, so the use of many agents gradually fell out of favor by the medical profession; their use was often regarded as a form of quackery.

It was in this atmosphere that the Department of Physical Therapy of the Mount Sinai Hospital Dispensary was established on December 5, 1910. Prior to this time, the Physical Therapy Services had been under the supervision of the Orthopaedic Division. In 1911, an inpatient section was created as an independent unit with an allocation of only one bed. A second would be added a few years later. Despite the small size of the Department, its Chief, Heinrich Wolf, gained a seat on the Medical Board. Wolf noted: "As far as I know, no other institution in the United States had at that time acknowledged in like manner the importance of this branch of medicine. It was, I believe, the work of Dr. S. S. Goldwater, then Director of the Hospital, which placed the Department on a par with the others."[1] Treatment provided by the medical staff of the Department consisted mostly of applying hot air and performing massage for such medical conditions as bone fractures, joint diseases, and constipation, reportedly with good results. Wolf believed that The Mount Sinai Hospital was the first hospital to acquire a modern diathermy apparatus and one of the first to use artificial fever in the treatment of disease.[2]

There is little information available about the Department's activities prior to 1935, when William Bierman, one of the pioneers of physical medicine as a specialty,[3] was appointed Attending Physical Therapist and Director of the Department. Bierman, together with two other founders of the specialty, Frank Krusen and John Coulter, established the Board of Registry of Physical Therapy Technicians in 1934 in order to evaluate and register therapists who were considered qualified.[4] From 1932 to 1938, Bierman served on the editorial board of *Archives of Physical Therapy, X-Ray, and Radium,* the publication that became *Archives of Physical Medicine* in 1945 and *Archives of Physical Medicine and Rehabilitation* in 1953. In 1936, Bierman was elected President of the American Congress of Physical Therapy, now the American Congress of Rehabilitation Medicine. One of the first to advocate the establishment of physical medicine as a specialty, Bierman made that recommendation to the American Medical Association Advisory Council for Medical Specialties.[5] In 1937, Bierman organized the first international conference on fever therapy in New York City. A dynamic leader, Bierman obtained new quarters for the Department in 1938. The facility included a well-equipped gymnasium for therapeutic exercises, hydrotherapy facilities, a wide range of devices for electromagnetic therapies, and three rooms with equipment for fever therapy. At the opening of this new facility, an all-day scientific session was held, with the major presentations made by members of the Department of Physical Therapy. Many of these papers were subsequently published in *The Journal of the Mount Sinai Hospital.*[6] The articles describe the use of different physical agents in the management of diseases, such as ultraviolet light for skin infections, conversive heat and iontophoresis for osteoarthritis, and artificial pyrexia (fever therapy) for achalasia and gonococcal infections. Bierman spent considerable time in research and encouraged his staff to do so, as well. His interests were many, and he was fortunate in having his own research fund to support his work on combining fever therapy with various chemicals in the treatment of subacute bacterial endocarditis in the days prior to antibiotics.

In 1938, Bierman was a founding member of the Society of Physical Therapy Physicians, now known as the American Academy of Physical Medicine and Rehabilitation, and served as its third president in 1940–1941. In 1941, Bierman received the Gold Key Award, the highest honor given by the American Congress of Physical Therapy. His research in heat therapy, electrotherapy and the use of high frequency currents was cited in his award. Bierman was in good company. The

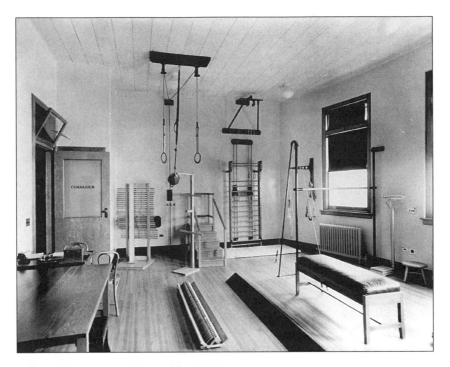

A Rehabilitation Medicine gym, c. 1938.

other recipients of the Gold Key Award that year were President Franklin Delano Roosevelt and Bernard Baruch, the financier and philanthropist. For his contributions to the field of physical medicine, the French government awarded Bierman the rank of Chevalier (Knight) of the Legion of Honor.

During World War II, the focus of physical medicine widened to include the rehabilitation of persons with physical impairments. Howard A. Rusk had introduced into Army Air Corps hospitals the concept of active rehabilitation of injured soldiers, emphasizing physical training as well as psychosocial counseling. This changing philosophy was spurred on in 1943 with the passage of new federal legislation to aid persons with physical disability. The Barden-LaFollette Amendment, commonly known as Public Law 113, appropriated funds for physical restoration and vocational training for persons with physical disabilities. Fever therapy for infectious disease, previously one of physical therapy's most important commodities, all but disappeared as penicillin and then other antibiotics became available.

After the war, Rusk and his colleagues initiated rehabilitation programs for civilians with physical disabilities and began efforts to establish rehabilitation medicine as a new medical specialty with approved residencies. In June 1947, the American Board of Physical Medicine was established and approved by the Advisory Board of Medical Specialties (ABMS). That same year, ninety-three physicians were certified by the Board after passing oral and written examinations, and approximately thirty were certified without examination.[7] Perhaps related to this development, the Department changed its name from Physical Therapy to Physical Medicine in May 1948. In the United States, in 1949, there were a total of only eighty-five house officers in training in physical medicine. There were forty programs: four in military hospitals, ten in Veteran's Administration Hospitals, and only twenty-six in nonfederal hospitals, among them Mount Sinai.[8] In 1950, the name of the certifying Board was changed to Physical Medicine and Rehabilitation, as these two medical specialties merged into one.

During Bierman's tenure, and probably representative of his major interest, most of the treatments provided by the Department continued to involve the use of physical agents. However, even before World War II, there were numerous indications in the Mount Sinai *Annual Reports* that physical exercise and skills training for patients with physical infirmities were gradually becoming more important. During the 1930s and 1940s, Physical Medicine added a corrective exercise class (originally created to help scoliosis patients), an occupational therapy program, and the Rehabilitation Workshop. All of these were started initially by the Department of Social Service. The Social Service Workroom was founded in 1933 to help patients deal with the mental stresses of the Depression. The Social Service Auxiliary sold many of the items produced, even opening a store called The Green Box on Lexington Avenue, and the Workroom became self-supporting. Over time, the Workroom grew to serve different types of patients who produced hand items; it also contracted for services to the Hospital and later to outside groups, as well. These included folding linens, coordinating mailings, and packing surgical kits. By 1955, the character of the Workroom had changed enough for it to be transferred to the Department of Physical Medicine, where it continued to offer paid employment in a sheltered environment for outpatients with disabilities, individuals who were unable to work in a competitive commercial environment but who hoped to gain employment in the future.

An Occupational Therapy program had also been created by the Social Service Department in 1922 to work with patients in the Mental Hygiene Clinic. Two years later, a paid worker was hired for the program, and by 1936 all ward patients were eligible to participate in basic craftwork, with the hope of providing diversion as they recuperated from their illnesses. In 1945, the program began to place greater emphasis on physical rehabilitation; a muscle reeducation program was added for hemiplegic patients two years later. By 1953, the Occupational Therapy program had been taken over by the Department of Physical Medicine.[9]

During his career, Bierman authored three books, many book chapters, and more than one hundred scientific articles.[10] He reached the age of retirement in 1958 but spent the next ten years at the University of California, San Francisco, where he continued to do research, now in biomechanics. He died in 1973.

In January 1959, Lawrence A. Wisham was appointed Chairman of the Department of Physical Medicine. Within a few months, the name of the Department was changed to Physical Medicine and Rehabilitation (PM&R). At the time, Wisham was known for his investigations on the clearance of sodium from human muscle; some of the studies were done at the Bronx Veterans Administration Medical Center in collaboration with Rosalyn Yalow, Mount Sinai's Nobel Laureate.[11] During Wisham's tenure, the Department primarily provided consultation services to inpatients on the acute wards of the Hospital and in various outpatient clinics but did not have its own inpatient service.

On the national scene, during the 1950s and 1960s, a small number of academic medical centers established their own departments of PM&R, which included inpatient hospital beds for the rehabilitation of persons with severe physical disabilities. Teams of rehabilitation professionals were created, consisting of psychiatrists and physical, occupational, and speech therapists, as well as rehabilitation nurses, psychologists, social workers, vocational counselors, and recreational therapists, all working together under the direction of the physician to attain the goals of rehabilitation medicine. The goals were defined as maximizing the function of the disabled person physically, psychologically, socially, and vocationally. In 1965, Congress passed legislation creating Medicare and Medicaid. Through the diligent advocacy of leaders in PM&R, rehabilitation services for both inpatients and outpatients were included in the Medicare/Medicaid healthcare package. Although the level of funding dipped in the 1970s, rehabilitation services have since that time become a standard component of healthcare services in the United States for all persons with a new onset of physical disability.

The Department expanded in the mid-1960s. In the spring of 1964, the Rehabilitation Workshop was moved to improved quarters on the third floor of the Administration Building. In July 1966, the Department, with a training grant from the Vocational Rehabilitation Administration, instituted a three-year residency program in PM&R with eight Residents and Fellows. The reinvigorated training program was a sign of progress, along with the 1966 designation of the Mount Sinai Department as an approved Rehabilitation Center by New York State. Responding to the changing face of the specialty, the Department once again changed its name in May 1968 to the Department of Rehabilitation Medicine.

Demand for inpatient and outpatient rehabilitation services increased steadily in the 1970s creating a continuing need for more space, a problem that was not resolved until 1975, when the Annenberg Building opened. Occupational therapy, physical therapy, and respiratory therapy programs burgeoned. Teaching activities also increased and included Resident training, lectures for the third- and fourth-year medical students, postgraduate courses in arthritis care and electrodiagnosis, and an active undergraduate internship program in occupational and physical therapy in association with schools in the Northeast. Clinical research during Wisham's tenure included studies on the treatment of hip arthritis, a review of the value of rehabilitation for hemophiliac patients, the functional levels of stroke patients, pain measurement and relief, and studies on amputee rehabilitation. Thermography studies were instituted, and additional projects were undertaken, utilizing radioactive sodium uptake and clearance to study changes in dermal blood flow after sympathectomy[12] and the effects of position change on sodium clearance from bone.[13] Looking to place function before form, Frances Dworecka and her colleagues created a new prosthesis that allowed patients with partially amputated hands to retain sensation and to improve function.[14] Patients fitted with the new devices preferred them to conventional cosmetic gloves and mechanical grasping devices. Andrew Fischer designed a tissue compliance meter to measure patient muscle tone and soft tissue consistency. The instrument was seen as a valuable diagnostic aid and proved useful in the management of spastic muscle disorders by enabling the physician or therapist to document objectively the results of differing types of therapy.[15] The various projects were directed by the expanded faculty, including Beatrice Kaplan, Danuta Janiszewski, and Somchat Chiamprasert. The residency, now based at Elmhurst Hospital Center, was directed by Jerry Weissman. The Resident rotations included four hospitals: Elmhurst, Beth Israel Medical Center, the Bronx Veterans Affairs Medical Center (VAMC), and The Mount Sinai Hospital.

Until the mid-1970s, inpatient length of stay (LOS) in rehabilitation units remained relatively long. In a time of rapidly escalating hospital costs and with the significant increase in the number of patients admitted for rehabilitation, insurance companies demanded that rehabilitation centers establish criteria, not only for the admission of patients but also for continued stay; there was also an increased demand for accountability. While the need for rehabilitation services for patients with physical disability was not an issue, the question was raised as to how the value of rehabilitation services could be measured to justify its cost. It was generally agreed that the primary product of rehabilitation therapies was improved function. A variety of functional assessment scales were proposed, but many were found to be too complex to be practical, and others were found not to be scientifically valid, reliable, or reproducible. Finally, one assessment scale, the Functional Independence Measure (FIM), emerged in the early 1980s[16] and has been adopted by virtually all of the major rehabilitation centers. These centers now collect functional data on admission, discharge, and follow-up for each patient.

In 1983, faced with sharply escalating Medicare costs, the U.S. government established the prospective diagnosis-related groups (DRG) payment system, which proved to be a boon for rehabilitation units. By prospectively assigning a specific number of inpatient days at a fixed price for each specific diagnosis, as opposed to the previous per diem payment system, DRGs provided the incentive for hospitals to reduce LOS and thereby reduce cost of care. Rehabilitation medicine and psychiatry services were exempt from the DRG payment system and continued with per diem reimbursement, thereby providing a financial incentive to open up more rehabilitation beds. Needing to shorten acute-care LOS, hospitals discharged patients earlier from the acute-care services and often transferred them to the inpatient rehabilitation medicine services, once again increasing the demand for more rehabilitation beds. Since 1980, the total number of inpatient rehabilitation beds in the United States has more than doubled and is now well in excess of twenty-two thousand. Most of the new rehabilitation beds have been opened within hospitals; relatively few freestanding rehabilitation centers have been built. This, too, has been advantageous for the field, since patients who arrive earlier for rehabilitation after illness or injury tend to be sicker and need continued access to hospital resources for proper management during rehabilitation therapy. At the same time, more young physicians have been attracted to the field of PM&R, which now counts more than five thousand specialists.

By the mid-1980s, it was clear that both the Mount Sinai Medical Center and its Department of Rehabilitation Medicine were about to undergo profound changes. A new hospital building was being planned, and a search committee was established to find a new Chairman for the Department. When Mount Sinai applied to New York State for the requisite certificate of need for the new hospital building, it received the necessary approval from David Axelrod, the Commissioner of Health, with the provision that there would be a reduction in the total number of beds in the Hospital but that fifty beds would be set aside for inpatient rehabilitation.

With Mount Sinai committed to provide comprehensive rehabilitation services for people with physical disabilities and to facilitate rehabilitation research and education, the choice of Kristjan T. Ragnarsson as the next Chairman proved to be an ideal one. Recruited from New York University's Rusk Institute, where he had trained and been a faculty member, Ragnarsson created a world-class Department, renowned for its expertise in the management of spinal cord and brain-injured patients. Remarkable growth occurred in all the various activities of the Department, including expansion of inpatient and outpatient care services, educational programs, and externally funded research.

In December 1986, eight inpatient rehabilitation beds were opened on the seventh floor of the old Semi-Private Surgical (Housman) Pavilion; within a year the number had grown to seventeen beds. Joining Ragnarsson as an Attending Physician for this service was Joseph Carfi, a graduate of the Mount Sinai School of Medicine, who had completed his training in PM&R at the Rusk Institute. When the east tower of the new Guggenheim Pavilion opened in 1990, the Service occupied thirty-six beds; it expanded to fifty in 1992. Two floors of the Klingenstein

Clinical Center (KCC) that had been vacated with the opening of Guggenheim underwent a complete renovation, and in 1996 the Service moved its inpatient units to new state-of-the-art facilities on the second and third floors of KCC. Each unit of twenty-five beds was self-contained, with all rehabilitation services provided on the same floor as the nursing unit. One unit is primarily for patients with spinal cord disorders, while the other offers services for patients with problems caused by stroke and traumatic brain injury. In December 1997, a third self-contained unit, this one on the fifth floor of KCC, was added, primarily to render services to patients with physical dysfunction of nonneurological etiology.

Outpatient rehabilitation services have expanded both on and off the Mount Sinai campus. In 1986, outpatient rehabilitation services were provided only in the subbasement level of 5 East 98th Street; in 1996, the entire outpatient service moved to the current facilities in the new Guggenheim Pavilion. An off-campus facility, the Mount Sinai Sports Therapy Center, opened at 625 Madison Avenue in 1996; this is an elegantly designed outpatient physical and occupational therapy facility, fully equipped with the latest therapeutic devices and staffed by therapists experienced in the treatment of musculoskeletal disorders.

In addition to traditional academic affiliations, the Department has had meaningful interactions with hospitals within the Mount Sinai Health System, providing guidance and assistance in relation to the establishment of new rehabilitation medicine services and recruitment of professional staff, including medical directors. The Department collaborated closely with Jersey City Medical Center and the Liberty Health System in New Jersey, opening, staffing, and operating the thirty-bed Liberty Rehabilitation Institute at Meadowlands Hospital in 1996. In July 1998, twenty-six representatives from twelve system hospitals with rehabilitation medicine services convened for the first time at Mount Sinai to discuss future collaboration and networking. In 2000, Steven Flanagan was appointed Vice Chairman of the Department.

Concurrent with the growth of clinical programs, federally funded rehabilitation research projects have increased significantly. In 1986, the Department was funded by the National Institutes of Health (NIH) for a project on diagnosis and treatment of poststroke depression. In 1987, the Department was designated and funded for five years by the National Institute of Disability and Rehabilitation Research (NIDRR) as a model system of care for traumatic brain injured (TBI) patients. In 1989, the Spinal Cord Damage Research Center at the Bronx VAMC opened under the direction of William A. Bauman, who holds joint appointments in the Departments of Rehabilitation Medicine and Medicine. In 1990, the Department received a designation and federal funding as a spinal cord injury model system of care, the only such system currently operating in New York State. Also in 1990, the Department received additional funding as a comprehensive regional TBI rehabilitation and prevention center. And, in 1993, the Department was designated and funded as a research and training center to assimilate individuals with TBI into the community. More recently, Ragnarsson chaired a National Institutes of Health Consensus Development Panel on Rehabilitation of Persons with Traumatic Brain Injury.[17]

The Spinal Cord Damage Research Center, originally established with funding from Mount Sinai and the Eastern Paralyzed Veterans Association, has been highly productive, as have the other Centers. Total research funding (exclusive of Bauman's funded projects at the VA) varies between $1 million and $2.4 million annually. Instrumental in this success has been the neuropsychologist Wayne A. Gordon, who began his career at the New York University Medical Center but joined Mount Sinai as Director of Research and Associate Director of the Department in 1986.

The Department has had an approved residency training program since 1966. Directed by Adam Stein, who has been at Mount Sinai since 1998, the number of Residents in the program during the past twenty-five years has varied from twenty-four to thirty, depending on the number of affiliated hospitals involved. The residency training program strives to provide exposure to all aspects of the specialty of PM&R. In the past, the major focus was on the management of inpatients with physical disability. Given the changing nature of medical practice, the program has been restructured to include an emphasis on patient care in the outpatient setting.

Like most branches of medicine, Physical Medicine and Rehabilitation is currently facing numerous uncertainties. What is clear, however, is that the fundamental needs of persons with disability will not change and that, with the passage of the Americans with Disabilities Act in 1990, rights of the disabled are legally protected. The elderly population will continue to grow, and more lives will be saved after injury and disease. As a result, there will be more people with diminished functional skill and therefore an increased need for rehabilitation services. In delivering these services, hospitals will increasingly be held accountable and will have to produce optimal results at the lowest possible cost. New and diverse levels of inpatient and outpatient rehabilitation services will have to be created, each unique in scope, focus, intensity, and, importantly, in cost. The services will operate within a continuum of care, convenient and accessible to all patients in need. Partnerships within the health system will increase, building new rehabilitation programs and coordinating these programs into a network of services where high quality of care goes hand-in-hand with effective delivery. Research must continue to find new ways to reduce physical disability and, in collaboration with basic science colleagues, to find a cure for paralysis. Education of students, residents, other health professionals, and the public is essential in order to increase understanding of the needs of and effective treatments for individuals with disabilities. Mount Sinai's formidable Department of Rehabilitation Medicine is ideally positioned to achieve these ambitious goals.

Adapted from an article by Kristjan T. Ragnarsson, M.D., in *The Mount Sinai Journal of Medicine* 66 (1999): 139–144.

33

Department of Urology

PATIENTS WITH GENITOURINARY DISORDERS have been admitted to the Jews' Hospital from its earliest days. Two patients with prostatic hypertrophy and urinary retention were among those admitted in the first nine months of the Hospital's operation in 1855–1856, forty years before specialization began within the Surgical Service. One of them (Patient #68), admitted with urinary infection, succumbed after intermittent catheterization; the other was discharged improved. The earliest surgeries for urological conditions were performed by the Attending Surgeon, Alexander Mott: an orchiectomy under chloroform anesthesia for a "scirrhous" testis, and the drainage of a hydrocele.[1]

Patients with both primary syphilis with penile chancre and secondary syphilis were also among the earliest admissions. The association of genitourinary and venereal disease had been long recognized; the publication of *Genitourinary and Venereal Disease* in 1874 by Van Buren and Keyes[2] is said to have initiated the specialty of urology in the United States. Van Buren, on the staff of Bellevue Hospital, was the son-in-law of Alexander Mott. Two events of 1886 were of great significance to the emerging specialty of urology: in that year, Nitze, in Europe, perfected the cystoscope,[3] and the American Association of Genito-Urinary Surgeons was founded in New York.[4] The Department of Urology at the Mount Sinai Hospital can be said to have had its origin with the establishment of the Skin and Venereal Disease Clinic in 1890 under the leadership of Sigmund Lustgarten and Hermann Goldenberg. Although both were primarily dermatologists who became Chiefs of the Dermatology Service, Goldenberg would also be named Chief of Urology.

In 1895, a Genitourinary Service within the Department of Surgery was created under William Fluhrer. Appointed to the Surgical Staff in 1880, Fluhrer, like all surgeons of the time, was a true "general surgeon," probably as well known for his work on fractures as he was for his urological prowess. In that era, speed was of the essence, and it is alleged that, at one time, Fluhrer performed a leg amputation for gangrene in some twenty seconds. Howard Lilienthal has related a tale of Fluhrer's impatience; upset with the performance of a younger surgeon, Fluhrer took the knife, sharpened it on the sole of his shoe, and took over the procedure.[5] He developed a one-piece bone drill and suture and devised a probe for use in neurosurgery, as well as one for use in performing urethrotomy.[6] One of Fluhrer's major contributions to urology was a urethrotome that he characterized as "an instrument of precision, simple in action and construction, by means of which a stricture anywhere in the urethra can be detected, measured, and cut with accuracy."[7] Elevated to Consultant status in 1902, Fluhrer continued to practice, and in 1916 he published a book on fracture management.[8]

Appointed to the staff in 1899, George Brewer was to make a significant contribution to urology, as well as to Mount Sinai. Best remembered for his description in 1906 of "Brewer's kidney," a fulminating infectious process characterized by multiple septic infarcts,[9] Brewer introduced rubber gloves to the Mount Sinai operating room staff in 1899, his first year on the staff.

Fluhrer was succeeded as Chief of Service by Hermann Goldenberg in 1902. Goldenberg, in addition to his studies on venereal disease, was one of the first to report on the use of the cystoscope to manage urethral polyps.[10] In 1910, Goldenberg relinquished his position as Chief of the Genitourinary Service to become the Chief of the Dermatology Service.

In the early years of the twentieth century, four Mount Sinai surgeons—F. Tilden Brown, Leo Buerger, Edwin Beer, and Maximilian Stern—produced fundamental advances in the rapidly expanding field of cystoscopy. In 1905, F. Tilden Brown, an early Intern at Mount Sinai, developed the Brown cystoscope,[11] the first scope to allow simultaneous bilateral urethral catheterization with collection of urine from each ureter. This allowed for the diagnosis and localization of unilateral renal disease. In 1909, Buerger modified the Brown cystoscope by designing a new and improved optical system. This instrument became known as the Brown-Buerger cystoscope.[12] This was one year after Buerger had described "thrombo-angiitis obliterans,"[13] later known as Buerger's disease. Edwin Beer devised the first pediatric cystoscope in 1911 and was soon able to report its use in children as young as fourteen months of age.[14] Maximilian Stern, appointed to the Urology clinic staff in 1910, developed the prototype for the Stern-McCarthy Resectoscope in 1926.[15]

Little is known about Stern, but he must have been a most inventive individual, since his many publications include "a new type of tube for postoperative suprapubic drainage"; a new apparatus for the use of "heat hyperemia" in urology; a "new method for the localization and measurement" of urethral strictures; the development of an operating urethroscope for the management of urethral strictures; a new plastic procedure for the management of urethral strictures; a "new method for treating remote manifestations of gonorrheal infections"; the description of "an improved technique" of performing epididymectomy (usually for tuberculosis) with preservation of the testicular blood supply; and "new electrodes for the application of diathermy to the prostate."[16]

Edwin Beer was appointed Chief of the Genitourinary Service in 1911 and would later become a giant in the specialty. A disciple of Arpad Gerster, Beer completed his surgical training at Mount Sinai and then spent several years studying in Europe before returning to the staff. Beer's 1910 paper, "Removal of Neoplasms of the Urinary Bladder: A New Method, Employing High-Frequency (Oudin) Current through a Catheterizing Cystoscope,"[17] documented the first description of the successful treatment of tumors of the bladder by transurethral electrocoagulation. Years later, Reed Nesbit, of Ann Arbor, a leader in the field, would comment, "The development of this technique by its brilliant discoverer marked one of the greatest advances in the history of urology: it led not only to radical changes in the therapeutic management of bladder tumors, but also paved the way for subsequent electroresection methods by proving that high frequency current could be employed effectively under water."[18]

In 1914, the Surgical Department was reorganized, and Beer was appointed Attending Surgeon in charge of one of four services. As Chief of the Genitourinary Division, ten of the forty beds on the "Beer" service were reserved for diseases of the kidney, ureters, and bladder. Beer, at that time and subsequently, refused to limit either his activities or those of his associates to urology alone. Although the vast majority of his papers were on urological topics, Beer published extensively on general surgical subjects, as well.[19] His papers on surgery of the spleen[20,21] led Roberto Alessandri[22] to give Beer credit for being a pioneer in the surgery of that organ. A highly skilled surgeon, Beer was also a brilliant writer. His papers are models of clarity, and many read like a short story. He recognized children with "non-neurogenic neurogenic bladder" as having a functional disorder almost fifty years before

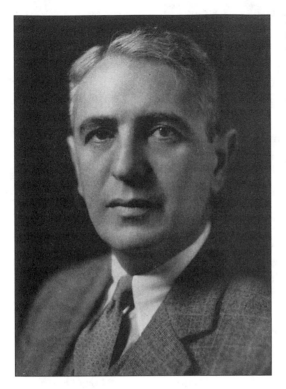

Edwin Beer, M.D., Chief of
the Urological Service,
1911–1937.

the condition was accepted as such (Hinman-Allen syndrome.)[23] In collaboration with Abraham Hyman, Beer published, as the culmination of his lifelong interest in pediatric urology, *Diseases of the Urinary Tract in Children* (1930),[24] the first American text on the subject. His endeavors in the surgical management of prostate and bladder cancer greatly advanced the therapy of these diseases.[25]

Enlisting in the Army Medical Corps in 1917, Beer served overseas with great distinction as a member of Mount Sinai's Base Hospital No. 3; he was also an observer immediately behind the front lines of battle and served with other members of his hospital team at the American Hospital in Paris.[26] Beer returned to the United States and to Mount Sinai in December 1918 and continued with his remarkable career for another twenty years. A member of every prestigious surgical and urological organization, Beer had a substantial impact on all of them.

During Beer's tenure as Chief of Service, the work of Moses Swick revolutionized the specialties of urology and radiology. Joining the

House Staff in 1924, Swick received fellowship funds from Emanuel Libman for study in Berlin upon completion of his training. In collaboration with Arthur H. Binz, an organic chemist who was formulating iodine compounds, Swick developed "Uroselectan," later known in the United States as "Iopax." When injected intravenously, the compound, excreted by the kidneys, allowed for the immediate, safe, and clear visualization of the collecting system of the kidneys, ureters, and bladder.[27,28] Of monumental importance, the development of Uroselectan and intravenous urography was a crucial step in the use of radioopaque materials to diagnose disease. The compound and the technique provided the foundation for the growth of the entire field of diagnostic radiologic arteriography and venography. Swick was honored throughout the world for his contributions, receiving the Billings Medal of the American Medical Association, the Ferdinand Valentine Award of The New York Academy of Medicine, and an honorary degree from the Free University of Berlin, where his work had originally been carried out.

Just as Beer and other urologists generated advances in other branches of surgery, members of the Surgical Services contributed to the expanding field of urology. Harold Neuhof, who made his mark in thoracic surgery, carried out extensive experimental and clinical studies on various aspects of transplantation, including replacing large segments of the bladder with fascia.[29] In this study, he noted that the inner side of the fascia was quickly covered with transitional bladder epithelium. A visionary who was way ahead of his time, Neuhof transplanted a sheep kidney into a human in 1923; the patient survived nine days.[30]

Beer's twenty-six-year tenure as Chief was marked not only by international recognition but also by the astounding growth in his Service. Mount Sinai became a major urological referral center because of the staff's expertise in cystoscopy and intravenous pyelography. The 1930 prediction regarding Swick's innovation that "This new method of visualizing the urinary tract is destined to have wide application and to be of considerable help to the clinician"[31] was certainly borne out by a huge increase in Urology case volume. Expansion of the cystoscopic suite became necessary and was completed in 1933. In that year, more than 1,800 cystoscopic and radiographic examinations were performed. Six years later, that number had increased to almost 2,900 procedures. Transurethral resection of the prostate came into vogue and gradually supplanted open prostatectomy for many patients. By 1935, one thousand cases of bladder tumors had been referred and treated in the Hospital. In 1939, Abraham Hyman was able to report that more than three hundred publications by the members of the staff had appeared over the years covering almost every important phase of urology.[32]

Edwin Beer was, above all, devoted to excellence in all his endeavors. His work achieved worldwide acclaim. In 1927, he was awarded the first gold medal given by the International Society of Urology for his work with electro-fulguration, and ten years later he was awarded the Gold Key by the American Congress of Physical Therapy for his pioneering contributions to the treatment of vesical tumors. Beer retired as Chief in 1937, just one year before his death. He was succeeded by Abraham Hyman. In eulogizing Beer, Ralph Colp, of the Surgical Service, stated,

> Edwin Beer was a born scholar, endowed with a magnificent intellectual background which gave him an unusual clarity of thought whether in surgery or in the field of economics or sociology. He was a great teacher and his surgical approach to any problem was marked with meticulous attention to the slightest detail. . . . He was a mental stimulus and an inspiration to the younger generation of surgeons, who came to rely upon his judgment and advice.[33]

Beer's legacy lives on today in the Edwin Beer Program of The New York Academy of Medicine in support of research in urology.

In 1942, midway through Hyman's tenure as Chief and as a result of his efforts, the Urology Service separated from the Department of Surgery to become an independent Department. With a major interest in urinary infections and genitourinary tumors, Hyman published extensively. The results of his 1934 analysis of 179 patients with tumors of the kidney, 135 of whom had been subjected to nephrectomy with an operative mortality of 9 percent,[34] were unique for their time. In collaboration with William Mencher, in a major publication, in 1935, Hyman reported on the causes of death after urological surgery.[35] He reviewed 165 deaths with 119 autopsies, for an autopsy percentage rate of 72 percent, a rate unheard of today. Not unexpectedly, in the preantibiotic era, infection in one form or another was responsible for the demise of 102 of the 165 patients.

Gordon D. Oppenheimer became Chief of the Urology Department in 1947 upon Hyman's retirement. Internationally known for his work in the description of regional ileitis in 1932 in conjunction with Leon Ginzburg and Burrill Crohn,[36] Oppenheimer had published on a number of general surgical topics. Always interested in research, he conducted multiple studies on the formation, dissolution, and management of renal calculi. In collaboration with Stephan S. Rosenak, of the Surgical Service, Oppenheimer performed early studies on newer aspects of renal dialysis and developed an improved peritoneal dialysis drain.[37] Rosenak, a Hungarian refugee surgeon with appointments in Surgery, Urology, and Chemistry, would play an important role in dialysis research at Mount Sinai. Working with Alfred Saltzman, a house officer, the pair designed a pump suitable for propelling blood without causing hemolysis[38] and developed a new dialysis apparatus for use as an artificial kidney.[39] The apparatus was extensively tested and in use for many years. Oppenheimer also expanded the number and scope of clinical research projects, including studies on the effectiveness of newer antibiotics.

In 1948, Stanley Glickman was appointed to the urology Attending staff. After completing a surgical residency, Glickman opted to go into urology. Accepted for training at the University of Michigan in Ann Arbor, Glickman had the opportunity to work with Reed Nesbit, a highly respected academic urologist. It was to be a most productive relationship. Nesbit and Glickman helped standardize the procedure of transurethral prostatic resection. Intravascular hemolysis accompanied by shock was a well- recognized and not infrequently fatal complication of transurethral resection (TUR). Called the TUR syndrome, it was recognized to result from the use of water as the irrigating solution during cystoscopic resectional procedures. Following laboratory investigations, Nesbit and Glickman identified glycine solution as the solution of choice for bladder irrigation during TUR.[40] A superb technician, Glickman would become one of Mount Sinai's most active urologists for more than three decades.

The Department also collaborated with other departments on numerous research projects. Clinician/researchers devised improved x-ray mats with the Radiology Department and studied the urological aspects of poliomyelitis with the Pediatrics Department. Howard Goldman and Glickman published one of the earliest papers on the urological complications of Crohn's disease.[41]

Oppenheimer recognized the need for a formal training structure and established a two-year residency program in Urology. The program received its initial approval in May 1947.[42] House Staff education was stressed throughout Oppenheimer's tenure; monthly conferences and seminars were instituted for the Residents and staff. The number of beds for the Service was increased in 1954, necessitating an increase in staff. In 1954, the residency program was expanded to include a third year.

Oppenheimer retired in 1963 and was followed by Herbert Brendler, the first full-time Chairman of the Department and a leader in the field of prostatic cancer. Brendler came to Mount Sinai from the New York University School of Medicine, where he had been Chief of the Urology Service at Bellevue Hospital. Brendler reorganized the Department and, in 1966, incorporated the Urology Service at the newly affiliated City Hospital Center at Elmhurst into the Resident training program. Under Brendler's leadership, the ward service was expanded, necessitating another increase in Resident complement so that, by early 1964, the program had grown from three to nine house officers. Brendler put an academic stamp on the educational activities of the Department. The number of conferences, seminars, and rounds were increased and regularized; Residents were encouraged to pursue and publish the results of research projects. A program of visiting professorships was initiated. Chemistry and tissue culture laboratories were established in 1963. By 1965, new research facilities were ready for the Department. These included two chemistry laboratories, a pathology laboratory, a small animal operating room for experimental surgery, tissue and organ culture facilities, a dark room, and a library. In that same year, the Department created a film on selective renal angiography that was well received and was shown at major national medical meetings. Other films were subsequently produced and widely used in many teaching programs. The work on renal angiography[43] led to one of the earliest papers on the perfusion of renal tumors with antineoplastic agents.[44]

The research interests of the Department during the decade of the 1970s centered on urinary infections, genitourinary tract tumors, prostate cancer, and hypertension. Shortly after Brendler's arrival at Mount Sinai, Elliot Leiter was recruited to the staff. Leiter was the first to report on the loss of ejaculation following radical retroperitoneal lymphadenectomy for testis tumors as a result of damage to the sympathetic plexuses.[45] In collaboration with Walter Futterweit, of the Division of Endocrinology, Leiter would later publish a definitive chapter on gender reassignment surgery.[46] For many years, the Department was active in Mount Sinai's kidney transplant program, mounted by the Department of Surgery. Urology participated in the first successful transplant in 1967 and remained an integral part of the program for a number of years, contributing to both the clinical and the research endeavors of the team. Because the Department's research program remained primarily clinical, Urology did not suffer as badly as some departments during the 1970s when there was a cutback in federal research dollars.

With the advent of the Mount Sinai School of Medicine, Brendler was named Chairman of the Department of Urology in the medical school, and faculty positions were created for the staff. Leiter developed the curriculum for the teaching of the genitourinary system. In collaboration with Obstetrics and Gynecology and Psychiatry, he planned and implemented the first course on human sexuality in any medical school. The Department of Urology participated in numerous courses for the medical students and in the Post-Graduate School, including a course to train potential *Mohelim* in ritual circumcision.

The focus of the educational efforts, however, remained on the residency program. In 1969, the residency was expanded to include the Bronx Veteran's Administration Hospital. To meet the needs of the additional site, the number of Residents was increased to fourteen. In 1979, the Urology residency program changed from a three-year to a four-year program, following a preliminary year in general surgery.

Since the days of Beer, pediatric urology has consistently been an area of strength at Mount Sinai. Early in his tenure, Brendler created a formal Division of Pediatric Urology and named Leiter as its first Chief. The Division worked closely with the Department of Pediatrics; joint faculty appointments were tendered, and collaborative clinics, conferences, and lectures were organized. When Leiter left Mount Sinai in 1978 to become Director of Urology at the Beth Israel Medical Center, Michael Gribetz was placed in charge of the Division, a position he held until 1988. Both Leiter and Gribetz were primarily adult urologists. Richard Schlussel, the current Chief of Pediatric Urology, who joined the faculty in 1994, is the first urologist to hold the position whose activities are limited to the care of the pediatric population.

In 1982, Brendler stepped down as Chairman of the Department of Urology. He continued his activities in professional organizations, serving as Editor of the *Journal of Urology* from 1982 to 1984 and as President of the American Urological Association in 1983–1984. Brendler's Presidential Address, discussing the affairs and activities of the organization contained a prophetic remark: "of one thing we may be sure, that is, physicians will be called on more and more to submit to poorly conceived and untested Federal programs designed to curb rising health care costs."[47] Among his many honors, Brendler served six years as Chairman of the Cooperative Study in Prostate Cancer of the NIH.

During the period when a search committee was seeking a new Chairman, the leadership of the Department was split between Elliot Leiter, who became Acting Chairman in the Medical School Department, and Hans Schapira, a longtime stalwart of the voluntary staff, who became Acting Director of the Hospital program.

The search for Brendler's successor was catalyzed with the appointment of James F. Glenn as Chief Executive Officer of the Mount Sinai Medical Center in 1983. A world-renowned urologist, whose textbook was an established work in the field, Glenn had served for many years as Chief of the Division of Urology at Duke University Medical School and as Dean of the Emory University School of Medicine. The next year, Michael J. Droller was appointed Chairman of the Department and Urologist-in-Chief to the Hospital. Following residency and fellowship, Droller joined the faculty of the Johns Hopkins University School of Medicine with appointments in both Urology and Medical Oncology. There he rose through the ranks until his appointment at Mount Sinai. Droller's special interests have been bladder cancer and urologic oncology. He has delineated the different pathways of bladder cancer development and progression, leading to an understanding based upon the tumor's intrinsic biology, of how different treatments might be applied.

Droller instituted a major reorganization of the Department, expanded the clinical services, and recruited faculty with focused interests in the subspecialty areas of urologic oncology, pediatric urology, neuro-urology, endocrinologic urology, endo-urology for stone disease, laparoscopic surgery, female urology, and andrology. He also introduced formal laboratory research into the resident curriculum. As a result, an additional year was added to the residency program to include both research and subspecialty training. Through the efforts of some members of the faculty (Brian Liu, Nelson Stone, Alexander Kirschenbaum and Droller), the Department has become known for its research efforts in elucidating mechanisms of tumor cell invasion in bladder cancer; understanding hormonal and molecular control mechanisms in benign prostatic hyperplasia and prostate cancer; and using radioactive seeds in treating prostate cancer. Droller's text, *The Surgical Management of Urologic Disease: An Anatomic Approach,*[48] published in 1991, has become an accepted standard in the field and has further enhanced Mount Sinai's tradition and reputation in clinical urology.

The Department has taken an active role in the educational and leadership activities of local, regional, and national urologic societies. Members of the faculty have also taken editorial positions in the major urologic journals, adding to the Department's academic luster. In 1985, in recognition of a major gift, the Department was renamed the Milton and Carroll Petrie Department of Urology, and, in 1998, following another endowment, Droller was installed as the Katherine and Clifford Goldsmith Professor of Urology.

Noteworthy initiatives have been undertaken in recent years. Under the direction of Simon Hall, a multidisciplinary Prostate Health Center has been established. The objectives are to combine clinical and laboratory research in translational approaches to prostate health, encompassing a wide range of conditions. Hall's work on gene therapy in prostate cancer combines laboratory and clinical research in the treatment of both regional and metastatic disease. Interdepartmental efforts provide a research directed approach in addressing other specific disease entities. Minority outreach programs and outcomes research complement the other programs in the Prostate Health Center, providing an institutional resource extending beyond traditional departmental lines.

A second initiative is the establishment of a minimally invasive urologic surgery program. Endoscopic and laparoscopic approaches are rapidly replacing traditional open procedures in urology. In concert with the Department of Surgery, Urology, under the aegis of Steven Savage, has brought laparoscopic urologic surgery at Mount Sinai to a leadership position in the Greater New York area. The decreased morbidity, more rapid recovery, and greater patient satisfaction that occur with this surgical modality will increase its application within the Department's therapeutic armamentarium.

The Department continues to build upon its proud history, extending its sights for new opportunities for its physicians and its patients now and in the future.

34

Laboratory Departments

A PATIENT IN The Mount Sinai Hospital of 1890 might have a rudimentary analysis done of his blood or urine, but these tests were handled in an ad hoc setting by a young physician in training. In 1893, the first real laboratory, called the Pathological Laboratory, was established at the Hospital by the physician Henry N. Heineman, who paid for most of the equipment with his own funds. Establishing a pattern that would continue over the years, a young physician, Frederick Mandlebaum, was sent abroad for training in the latest medical science. Upon his return, Heineman resigned in favor of his young Assistant, and Mandlebaum was given control over the Laboratory. Occupying a space not much larger than a closet, this laboratory served as a base for those interested in the further study of the growing sciences of medicine, including bacteriology and chemistry. Activity in this laboratory grew at such a pace that, with Mount Sinai's move to a larger site in 1904, the laboratories were given a separate building, filled with the most modern equipment of the day and underwritten by the Trustee Adolph Lewisohn. Here the staff not only performed the clinical tests needed by the Hospital but also served as a source of expertise and training, providing laboratory space for the medical staff who were interested in conducting research. The facility was used so intensively that, nine years after the new building opened, a plan was put forth for a larger building to house the laboratories.

Over the years, all the laboratory work had been directed by Mandlebaum, and he himself did pioneering work in pathology. At his death in 1926, Louis Gross was hired as the full-time Director to oversee the laboratories; full-time Directors were also employed for each of the three main laboratories: Chemistry, Microbiology, and Pathology. In 1937, when the Director of Laboratories position was eliminated, the three laboratories became independent Departments. This remains the case today with Pathology, but, with the founding of the Mount Sinai School of Medicine in the 1960s, the Chemistry and Microbiology

Departments were subsumed under the Departments of Biochemistry and Microbiology; the clinical laboratory work was separated from the academic and research efforts.

In the mid-1980s, another major change occurred with the creation of the Center for Clinical Laboratories. With this move, the disparate laboratories that performed patient testing, irrespective of their physical location, were gradually amalgamated into one administrative unit, reporting to the Chairman of the Department of Pathology and to Hospital Administration. The Center is now responsible for all patient testing with the exception of anatomic and autopsy pathology. The first Director of the Center was Neville Coleman; Elkin Simson has been the Director since January 1996.

The story of the Department of Pathology is told in another chapter. This section is a brief look at the history and contributions of the Chemistry and Microbiology Departments.

THE CHEMISTRY DEPARTMENT

The Chemistry Laboratory can trace its beginnings to the small corner in the Hospital laboratory at the Lexington Avenue site where Julius Rudisch, M.D., performed basic urinalyses and devised tests to identify sugar while pursuing his interest in diabetes. Formal recognition of the need for a professional lab came in 1902 with the appointment of Samuel Bookman, Ph.D., as an Associate in Physiological Chemistry. He worked with Mandlebaum to design the laboratory space in the buildings on the Fifth Avenue site. The opening of these buildings in 1904 marked the launch of the full spectrum of chemical testing at Mount Sinai. This has been noted as the first department of chemistry in any New York City voluntary hospital.

Bookman received his Ph.D. from the Columbia University School of Mines, with postgraduate work in Berlin. During his tenure at Mount Sinai (1902–1927), the laboratory had only one full-time employee and relied on the unpaid, volunteer efforts of practicing physicians. Bookman routinely served half time, giving more time as needed. Bookman also "arranged for the distribution of private fees amongst his collaborators who, thus, gained greater freedom to pursue their research work."[1] By the time of Bookman's retirement, there were nine Associates and Assistants who devoted a few hours each week, or as much as six hours each day. This staff handled all of the chemical examinations for the Hospital, which by 1927 amounted to more than thirteen thousand analyses. As Bookman noted, "In addition, each assistant was engaged in some research work connected with his branch of medicine [including] general medicine, gastro-intestinal diseases, otology, allergy, surgery and other branches."[2] Bookman himself did research on protein metabolism, the formation of glycocoll in the liver, and the chemical composition of renal and vesical calculi.

In 1926, Mandlebaum died, and Bookman announced his retirement. As noted earlier, the laboratories were then reorganized into departments with full-time Directors, as well as a full-time Director of Laboratories. It is a tribute to the quality of Mount Sinai's laboratory work that the Hospital was able to recruit Michael Heidelberger from Rockefeller University to become the new Director of the Chemistry Laboratory. Heidelberger was already known for his work on the synthesis of tryparsamide, a strong arsenic-based drug. Unfortunately for the Hospital, Heidelberger was recruited by Columbia University and left Mount Sinai after a year and a half. He then went on to found and define the field of immunochemistry.

Harry Sobotka, Ph.D., was appointed Chemist to the Hospital in 1928. Born in Vienna and trained in Munich, Sobotka studied with Richard Willstaetter, a Nobel Laureate in enzyme chemistry, and in 1922 received his Ph.D. with highest honor. By 1924, Sobotka was at the Rockefeller Institute in New York City. He spent two years there and an additional two years at New York University before coming to Mount Sinai as Director of the Chemistry Laboratory in 1928. He served until 1965, when the mandatory retirement policy required his move to Consultant status.

The thirty-seven years Sobotka led the Chemistry Department were times of great advances in the field, both on a theoretical and on a practical level. The goals of the Department continued to be to perform the ever-expanding clinical work of the Hospital in a fast and efficient manner; to train young physicians, technicians, and chemists in chemical investigation; to study chemical compounds and their role in medicine; and to uncover new knowledge of the chemical universe of the human body in health and disease. These goals were ably met during Sobotka's tenure. New techniques and equipment were devised to increase the accuracy of and eventually to automate the chemical tests used. Many educational efforts were begun, including monthly seminars on physiological chemistry, postgraduate courses in clinical chemistry, and training programs in laboratory techniques.

Sobotka, an expert on bile and steroid metabolism, authored two texts in the late 1930s that became the standard on these topics.[3] He also did research on monomolecular layers, vitamins, and liver disease. He was a founding Editor, with Corbet Page Stewart, of Edinburgh, of the first eight volumes of *Advances in Clinical Chemistry* and authored more than three hundred publications on numerous topics.

Sobotka was dedicated to furthering the field of clinical chemistry, and, in doing so, he brought luster to Mount Sinai, as well. He was a founder and the first President of the American Association of Clinical Chemistry and helped establish its journal, *Clinical Chemistry*, in 1954. He was a linguist and a member of many foreign professional associations. He traveled widely, giving lectures, and hosted many visitors from other laboratories. In 1956, he chaired the Program Committee for the International Congress of Clinical Chemists when the meeting was in New York. In 1964, he received an honorary doctorate from the University of Perugia, Italy, and also received the medal of the Société de Chimie Biologique from the French Biological Society. He received many other honors, including the Van Slyke Award of the American Association of Clinical Chemists.

Over the course of Sobotka's years at Mount Sinai, the Department was vibrant; the full-time and volunteer staff expanded dramatically. In 1928, there were two technicians; by 1950, there were ten, and the number continued to grow. In 1937, the Clinical Microscopy Laboratory was placed under Chemistry. Specialized laboratories for various studies were created over the years, including nutrition, enzymes, endocrinology, and gastroenterology. Jacob Chanley, Ph.D., was in charge of the bio-organic chemistry research for many years, working primarily on the nervous system, investigating in particular steroid glycosides.

Another contribution in biochemical research, but one actually accomplished in the Cell Research Laboratory, is the work of Baruch Davis and Leonard Ornstein that formulated the process of polyacrylamide gel electrophoresis to separate proteins.[4] Electrophoresis is the migration of charged molecules, such as proteins, in solution in response to an electric field. As an analytical tool, electrophoresis is simple, rapid, and highly sensitive. It is used analytically to study the properties of a single charged species and as a separation technique. Originally presented at a meeting at The New York Academy of Medicine in

1959, this work, through subsequent papers, became *"Citation Classics,"*[5] and the technique is considered one of the earliest landmarks in the technological development of molecular biology.

The one thorn in Sobotka's side was the ever-present need (common to all Mount Sinai program directors) for more and better space. Though it was allocated more space over the years, the Department grew in a decentralized manner, with departmental laboratories spread over many buildings, some of them quite old. This situation was alleviated in the early 1950s with the opening of the new Atran and Berg research buildings, which provided more than twenty-thousand feet of space to Chemistry. Sobotka retired in 1965 and died unexpectedly at the end of the year.

Ferenc Hutterer, M.D., was appointed Acting Director of the Chemistry Department following Sobotka's death and later became the Director, a position he held until 1975. Hutterer quickly began a reorganization and modernization of the laboratory and its equipment, including acquisition of a new ultraviolet spectrophotometer and an atomic absorption spectrophotometer. He also reorganized to provide twenty-four hour service every day. In 1975, Hutterer was followed as Director by Laszlo Sarkozi, Ph.D., who had already been at Mount Sinai for ten years and who has held the position ever since.

Over the past thirty-five years, the laboratory has experienced exponential growth in the number of tests performed; from 266,000 tests on 64,000 specimens in 1965 to 4,339,148 tests on more than 400,000 specimens in 2000. Thanks to automation, this growth has been accompanied by vastly improved productivity. A sea change occurred in 1997 when the laboratory moved into greatly expanded space in the new East Building, and sample handling became totally automated. This "robotic" laboratory is one of the largest of its kind in the world. Measured in 1965 dollars, the cost per test (salary plus reagents) has been reduced from $0.79 per test to $0.15 per test, despite a greatly increased test menu and greatly reduced turnaround time.[6]

THE MICROBIOLOGY DEPARTMENT

The early history of clinical microbiology at The Mount Sinai Hospital was driven by the intellectual curiosity and interest of internists and surgeons, most of whom lacked advanced microbiology training but who sought to investigate infectious processes in their own patients. Amazingly, these avant-garde investigators studied difficult microbiological problems in the absence of modern-day technologic innovations with enough clarity of vision to achieve results still valid today.

Among these internist pioneers was Emanuel Libman, who, at the end of the nineteenth century, studied bacteriology and pathology in renowned clinics in Berlin, Vienna, and Munich and who, in 1897, published, in German, his description of *Streptococcus enteritis* (later named *Streptococcus Libman*), which causes focal infection of the intestine.[7] Libman isolated this bacterium from the blood of an infant with severe diarrhea. In 1904, Libman, using a gift from Trustee Adolf Lewisohn (a philanthropic mining tycoon) to build a laboratory building at Mount Sinai, established a separate department of bacteriology and serology. Libman went on to study meningococci, streptococci, and *Bacillus pyocyaneus*, known today as *Pseudomonas aeruginosa*, and became an outstanding bacteriologist. Libman's use of blood cultures to diagnose disease was another major contribution in its day.[8] His seminal work, published in 1910, dealt with the pathogenesis of subacute bacterial endocarditis, which he elucidated through bacteriologic (blood cultures), pathologic, and clinical studies.[9]

Leo Loewe, an internist working in the bacteriology laboratory of the Hospital, in 1921 reported the first cultivation of Rickettsia-like bodies from the blood of patients with typhus fever and from the blood and multiple organs of guinea pigs infected with the blood of typhus fever patients.[10] Because of these and other innovative investigations at Mount Sinai, the laboratory services were expanded. Scientists and the other laboratory staff pursued their own studies and also worked with clinicians on topics of interest to them, often facilitating interdepartmental research. In 1932, John Cohen, a surgeon, studied the bacteriology of putrid lung abscesses in great detail and devised and improvised methods for the recovery of anaerobic bacterial species that he suspected played a major role in their causation.[11]

In the 1926 reorganization, Gregory Shwartzman, M.D., was appointed Bacteriologist to the Hospital, a position he held until his retirement in 1957. Shwartzman was born in 1896 in Odessa, Russia, studied at the University of St. Petersburg, and obtained his medical degree from the University of Odessa in 1919 and a Doctor of Surgery degree from the University of Brussels in 1920. In 1927, he undertook graduate studies at the University of London and the University of Edinburgh. Shwartzman held the title of Professor of Microbiology at Columbia University's College of Physicians and Surgeons and served as President of the Mount Sinai Medical Board in 1955–1956. He died July 21, 1965.

Shwartzman is best known for his groundbreaking research on the effect of extracts of *Bacillus (Salmonella) typhosus* culture filtrates on rabbit skin reactivity. In his celebrated 1928 publication in the *American Journal of Experimental Medicine*, he described the development of local skin reactivity induced by the cutaneous injection of a bacterial filtrate, followed twenty-four hours later by an intravenous injection of the same filtrate.[12] The local skin reactivity consisted of severe hemorrhagic necrosis and was fully developed four to five hours after the second injection. The reaction became known as the "Shwartzman phenomenon," a term that is still in use today. In subsequent studies, Shwartzman showed that the toxic activity could be neutralized by antisera prepared against the components of the filtrate. Shwartzman then went on to develop antisera that proved effective against typhoid and meningococcus infections. A 1937 monograph that summarizes his work is a milestone in experimental pathology. In it, Shwartzman also documents his production of degenerative diseases in animals similar to those in human aging that involve the breakdown of bodily processes.[13] In 1934, at the annual meeting of the American Medical Association, Shwartzman presented a summary of his research activities and was awarded the Association's Gold Medal, Class 1. In 1937, he was nominated for the Nobel Prize in Medicine and Physiology but lost out to Albert Szent-Gyorgi, who won for his discovery of Vitamin C. Later, Soffer, Shwartzman, and their colleagues were able to show that the "Shwartzman phenomenon" could be inhibited by adrenocorticotrophic hormone (ACTH).[14]

In 1934, Shwartzman was joined by S. Stanley Schneierson, M.D., who would ultimately succeed him as Director of the Department. Four years later, through Shwartzman's connections, Schneierson spent a year with Maurice Weinberg at the Pasteur Institute in Paris, studying anaerobic bacteria and their infectious processes, two months with Jules Bordet at the Pasteur Institute in Brussels, and three months at the London School of Tropical Medicine. Upon his return to the United States, Schneierson continued his association with Shwartzman until he was inducted into the Navy in 1941. He served with the Marines as the Venereal Diseases Control Officer in the Caribbean and later supervised a hospital and laboratory in Saipan, where he expanded his interest in parasitic diseases and their diagnosis. Upon his discharge from the Navy in 1946, he rejoined Shwartzman as his Assistant, a position he held until the end of 1955, when, upon Shwartzman's illness-related retirement, he was appointed Attending Microbiologist and Acting Director of the Microbiology Department. In 1960, Schneierson was appointed full Director, and, with the establishment of the Mount Sinai School of Medicine a few years later, he became the first Professor of Microbiology.

Under Schneierson's stewardship, the Microbiology Laboratories underwent enormous growth in all of the microbiologic subspecialties: bacteriology, serology, parasitology, mycology, and virology. In this expansion, Schneierson attracted many brilliant clinicians and scientists, including Maxwell Littman, M.D., and Michael A. Pisano, Ph.D. (Mycology); Morton Edelman, M.D., and Clifford Spingarn, M.D. (Parasitology); Jacques Singer, M.D., and Irwin Oreskes, Ph.D. (Serology). The productivity of this group enabled the Microbiology Laboratories of The Mount Sinai Hospital to achieve worldwide recognition. In fact, in 1955, Schneierson was among the first hospital microbiology laboratory directors to establish a full diagnostic virology laboratory offering both serologic and tissue culture testing for virologic diagnosis. Furthermore, in the serology laboratory, the latex agglutination test for rheumatoid arthritis was developed.[15] Along with Littman, Schneierson described the hazard of pigeon droppings in the transmission of the fungus *Cryptococcus neoformans* in New York City (and elsewhere).[16]

Schneierson's intellectual curiosity as a clinician/microbiologist led him to publish eighty-two papers across the specialties of microbiology, as well as the *Atlas of Diagnostic Microbiology*,[17] which became a standard text in medical schools and laboratories. Although his tenure preceded the emergence of infectious diseases as a distinct subspecialty of medicine, Schneierson was often called upon as a consultant and effectively bridged the gap between the microbiology laboratories and the bedside. During the era of the rise of antibiotics, many advances were made at Mount Sinai, and in the Microbiology Laboratory in particular, in the development and applications of these new drugs. Schneierson was a pioneer in initiating bacterial antibiotic susceptibility testing, devising new methods for determining minimal inhibitory concentrations, and monitoring therapy by providing antibiotic serum levels and serum bacteriostatic and bactericidal levels. Paramount among Schneierson's innovative methods were a rapid disc-broth dilution method for the determination of bacterial susceptibility to antibiotics, a two-tube broth dilution method that introduced the concept of antibiotic "break-points," and use of high and low antibiotic concentrations representing normal and bolus antibiotic administration.[18] With the advent of electronic data processing, he developed a punch-card system for identifying bacteria and their antibiotic susceptibility, as well as a system for analyzing antibiotic sensitivity patterns at the Hospital.[19] Both of these systems were the forerunners of today's commercially available computer-generated identification and susceptibility testing methods. Schneierson retired as Director of the Microbiology Department in January 1973 and held the position of Chief of Infectious Diseases at the Bronx Veterans Administration Hospital until his death in 1976.

In 1959, Edward J. Bottone was interviewed and hired as a Bacteriology Technician by Schneierson and the latter's Associate, Cecele Herschberger. It is unlikely that any of the three could ever have imagined that Bottone, brought up in the neighborhood immediately surrounding Mount Sinai, a high school graduate just discharged from the United State Army, would become the Director of the Department of Microbiology fourteen years later, succeeding Schneierson.

Bottone remained at Mount Sinai for a year as a Technician before assuming a similar position elsewhere. In 1962, when Mount Sinai affiliated with Greenpoint Hospital in Brooklyn, New York, a member hospital of the Health and Hospital Corporation of New York's municipal hospital system, Bottone was offered the position of Supervisor of Bacteriology at the new affiliate. He and Schneierson, who had now become Bottone's "professional father," set up a formidable diagnostic microbiology laboratory. In 1964, Mount Sinai shifted its affiliation to the City Hospital Center in Elmhurst, Queens, and Bottone and Schneierson continued their collaboration at that institution for five years, after which Schneierson brought Bottone back to Mount Sinai as his Assistant upon Herschberger's retirement.

Encouraged by Schneierson, Bottone completed his baccalaureate studies in 1965 and obtained his doctorate in 1973. Upon Schneierson's retirement in 1973, Bottone was appointed Acting Director of the Microbiology Department and then Director, in 1975. The establishment, in 1976, of a postdoctoral training program in Medical and Public Health Laboratory Microbiology, under the auspices of the American Academy of Microbiology, was a highlight of Bottone's tenure. Through the program, Bottone trained twenty clinicians and scientists, many of whom went on to distinguished careers of their own. Because of the talented students in this program, the Microbiology Laboratory not only excelled in the provision of superb laboratory support services but also established itself as a center for research excellence across the subspecialties of microbiology.

Bottone's particular research interests have centered about characterizing infrequently encountered human pathogens and their disease potential. His early studies on *"Yersinia enterocolitica-like"* bacteria gained him international recognition and led to the development of a separate species designation *Yersinia intermedia* for the rhamnose-positive strains which he isolated and described.[20] He further established the symbiotic relationship between free-living amoebae of the genus *Acanthamoeba* and environmental gram-negative bacterial species that co-exist in contact lens care systems as a prelude to *Acanthamoeba* corneal ulcer formation in contact lens wearers.[21] Bottone received a patent for a *Bacillus pumilis* strain that he isolated that produces an antifungal compound active against the opportunistic fungal pathogens *Aspergillus* and *Mucoraceae*.[22]

Bottone, who has held faculty appointments as Professor of Microbiology, Pathology, and Medicine, directed the Microbiology Laboratories of the Hospital through 1993, at which time he joined the Division of Infectious Diseases of the Department of Medicine as Director for Consultative Microbiology. Widely respected for his contributions to microbiology, Bottone was honored by the New York City Branch of the American Society for Microbiology for Distinguished Achievements in Clinical Microbiology. In 1995, Bottone was honored by the American Society for Microbiology with the bioMerieux Vitek Sonnenwirth Memorial Award for his contributions and leadership in clinical microbiology. In 1991, Bottone was elected to Alpha Omega Alpha, the honorary medical fraternity, by the Mount Sinai students, and he was also the first recipient of the Faculty Council Award for Excellence in Academics of the Mount Sinai School of Medicine.

Since 1994, the laboratories have been directed by John Boyle, Ph.D. (1995–1998), Stephen Jenkens, Ph.D. (1999–2001), and currently by Philip Tierno, Ph.D. Henry D. Isenberg, Ph.D. has served as a consultant.

The continued growth and development of the Laboratory Departments will play a significant role in Mount Sinai's future.

Afterword

The Years of the Giants

MOUNT SINAI HAS always been full of stories about "the Giants" who roamed the halls long ago. It is interesting that these stories always relate to a time in the past, regardless of when they are told. Interns in the 1890s heard tales of the Giants, as did Interns of every succeeding generation. This changeable aspect of the Giants does not diminish the fact that there truly were leaders of medicine here. But it does point to the importance of this story in providing a common history for the people of Mount Sinai: the feeling that this is a special place with a tradition of excellence and high standards. The impact of this story has been greatest on the medical staff, in particular the young doctors who have come to Mount Sinai for training, some of whom became Giants to the next group. This is their story.

From very early on in the institution's history, obtaining a House Staff position at Mount Sinai was extremely desirable. It was also extremely difficult. From the beginning in 1872, prospective candidates would take the annual entrance examination to compete for a handful of House Staff positions. By the early 1900s, the number of applicants exceeded one hundred per year. Many of these young doctors came from City College and then Columbia University's College of Physicians and Surgeons or, less often, the New York University School of Medicine. Because many hospitals at the time did not welcome Jewish interns, Mount Sinai had a large pool of Jewish candidates from which to choose and was able to select only the most qualified.

From 1872 to around World War II, Mount Sinai had "mixed" internships lasting two and a half years. During this time, the general medicine Interns spent six months on the surgery wards, and the surgical Interns spent six months on the medical wards. The last six months of internship were spent as "House Physician" or "House Surgeon," respectively, or as Senior Physician or Surgeon; the term varied over time.

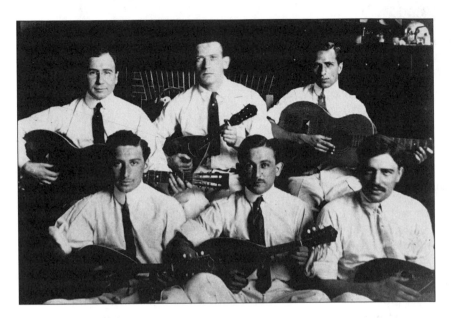

House Staff, 1891.

Departments established their own residency training programs over the years that were in addition to the general preparation of the internship. Throughout these two and a half years, the House Staff expected work to be their life. Internship was all- consuming, and such constant, close, and intense contact with colleagues from around the Hospital enabled the staff to coalesce into a tightly knit and intellectually stimulating group. Inevitably, there were some personality clashes and disagreements, but, for the most part, relationships remained amicable.

After the internship, many young doctors began climbing the career ladder at Mount Sinai, jockeying to obtain Out-patient Department assignments. Many accepted volunteer positions in the laboratories as they built their private practice on the side. Mount Sinai staff were expected to be highly involved in scientific research. To this end, some physicians were chosen for fellowships following their internships so that they could pursue postgraduate study or spend time in the laboratories, concentrating entirely on research before starting a practice. Until the mid 1920s, it was typical for many fellowship recipients to go abroad to study. As Reuben Ottenberg put it, "Postgraduate teaching in

America was in the horse and buggy stage. If a man wished technical training in any specialty, he generally went abroad."[1] The Emanuel Libman Fellowship Fund was one such fellowship. It was established in 1924 to "Encourage, aid, assist, foster, conduct, and endow medical and allied scientific research and investigation and to increase medical and allied scientific knowledge and education."[2] Moses Swick, who while in Berlin developed Uroselectan to visualize the urinary tract and kidneys, was just one of the physicians to make an important scientific contribution while on a Libman fellowship. Numerous other fellowships had already been established by the Trustees to encourage research, beginning with the George Blumenthal, Jr., Fellowship in Pathology, instituted in 1907.

One reason that the Mount Sinai community stayed so close was because of the Mount Sinai Hospital Alumni Association, a group of physicians who had trained at the Hospital. Created in 1896, The Associated Alumni of The Mount Sinai Hospital sponsored medical talks, provided funds for the care of sick alumni and support for the library, and, on the lighter side, held an annual banquet.[3] The banquets were known for their raucous skits where House Staff poked fun at senior members of the Attending staff. These performances were often accompanied by the publication of ribald programs in a newsletter format, written by alumni, including *The Gewalter* and *The Pornographic*. The humor present in these publications and theatrics reflected the "boys' club" nature of the Association. In fact, invitations to the annual banquet were not extended to female members of the Alumni or to spouses until 1931. (Although Mount Sinai had graduated perhaps the first woman from an internship program in the United States, in 1885, the Board of Trustees later banned women from serving on the House Staff until 1921.)

Another enduring tradition created by the Alumni Association was the establishment of the Jacobi Medallion. Conceived and designed by William Hitzig, it was first awarded in 1952 to commemorate the one hundredth anniversary of The Mount Sinai Hospital. The Jacobi Medallion is given in recognition of distinguished achievement in the field of medicine or for extraordinary service to the Alumni or the Hospital. Originally awarded solely to physicians, medallions have occasionally been given to nonphysicians who have rendered outstanding service to the institution. Recipients of the medallion personify the Alumni Association's commitment to Mount Sinai.[4]

Another award given at Mount Sinai is the Gold-Headed Cane. This is the highest honor given to a Mount Sinai physician. Bernard S. Oppenheimer, the renowned cardiologist and Chief of the First Medical Service, created this award in 1941 and selected the first recipient the next year. He modeled the actual cane and its meaning from a centuries-old tradition of the Royal College of Physicians in London. At Mount Sinai, the cane is given to the physician or surgeon who best represents the values of Mount Sinai on a professional and personal level. The cane has been passed only a handful of times in the intervening years. The current holder of the cane, in association with any other living prior holders, chooses the next recipient at the point when the holder reaches retirement or emeritus status. The physicians so honored include Eli Moschcowitz (1942), George Baehr (1945), Ralph Colp (1952), Solomon Silver (1955), Morris B. Bender (1972), Arthur H. Aufses, Jr. (1982), David Sachar (1996), and Donald Gribetz (2000).

In the end, the best way to acquire a sense for the life of a young doctor and the life of The Mount Sinai Hospital during the first half of the twentieth century, the "years of the Giants," is through the words of those who were there. Following are brief excerpts from interviews and writings of Mount Sinai physicians over the years. After each entry is a date in parentheses noting when the physician graduated from the House Staff.

It was, according to all standards, the outstanding Jewish institution and in those days, it was most difficult for anyone of the Jewish persuasion to get into one of the outstanding gentile hospitals such as Presbyterian, New York, Roosevelt and the like, or even St. Luke's. *Percy Klingenstein, M.D. (H.1919)*[5]

In my time there was one place, really, where a Jewish boy could get a decent surgical training. In those days, you either got an internship at Mount Sinai, or you didn't get a decent training, because Mount Sinai Hospital was the only first rate Jewish hospital around at that time, and it towered over the other ones like a Matterhorn. Getting an appointment on the staff at Mount Sinai—I don't think that anyone today can realize just what that meant. It was an entrance; it was an admission card to the Promised Land. It carried in the Jewish community at that time, a weight of reputation that I don't think one could get today if one went both to the Mayo, the Lahey Clinic, and Houston and a few other places put together. It really was Sinai, almost as holy as the original Mount Sinai. *Leon Ginzburg, M.D. (H.1925)*[6]

Accordingly, the competition for positions was intense:

The competition at that time was extremely keen and an internship at Mount Sinai Hospital was considered a very real prize. *Percy Klingenstein, M.D. (H.1919)*[7]

The examinations for internship were extremely severe . . . and anybody who could get a place at Mount Sinai was regarded as . . . extremely capable. *Burrill B. Crohn, M.D. (H.1910)*[8]

In those days there was a very difficult examination, I would say, consisting of two parts, really. There was a six-hour written examination, three hours in the morning, three hours in the afternoon. We were locked in the big Blumenthal Auditorium with a little time for lunch. Then, after those papers were marked, [the 39 men with the highest marks] were called back. [The men] were again locked into the auditorium. We drew lots, who would be called in to the committees for an oral examination. That oral examination consisted of appearing before three committees of a Senior attending, each with his acolytes, so to speak. *Samuel Klein, M.D. (H.1931)*[9]

The rigorous examination process foreshadowed the intensity of life as an intern:

You were assigned to a ward, and as a Wardsman you were under the direction of a Junior, a Senior and a House Physician. We had a night off from 5:30 to midnight three times a week. You had to be back by midnight no matter what was going on. And on Sunday you had half a day. You had rounds every day and Sunday morning. We made rounds until 12:30 and then lunch off, on alternate Sundays. . . . The intern, the wardsman had to do everything when the patient arrived. . . . We had no technicians, which meant that when you arrived, they gave you, as a present, a stethoscope, a hammer for reflexes, a tuning fork, a little cell counting device for blood counts. We had to do the tests in the lab on the 5th floor, blood counts, urines, sed rates, stool exams, and hemoglobin. . . . Those were our chores, besides the fact that we also had to examine every new patient that came in. . . . Unfortunately, on Mondays there were 6 to 10 admissions. You had to examine the patients, write them up and check with the senior at midnight and go over the physical examination at 2:00 in the morning. The hours were terrible. In the morning, you did all the stat work, finished up the blood counts, and the work that wasn't done. We drew all the bloods. We also did the transfusions. . . . We would have 3 rounds. We would make rounds in the morning with the charge nurse. The interns were busy doing all the laboratory work, but the senior was making rounds so they would be ready for the afternoon rounds. The rounds were made in the afternoon then, everybody joined the attending staff. We got through with that, we then got together, just our House staff, for 5 o'clock rounds. And we sat down to discuss what had been decided to do for patient so and so for the next day. And then, upon that point, somebody would say, 'Let's get off for the evening.' Then at midnight we would make rounds again! Even after dinner, whoever was on call then made rounds, just to catch up. So we had another batch of rounds made by either the Senior or the House Physician on both floors. *Henry Dolger, M.D. (H.1938)*[10]

The chiefs [chief resident] came alive after the 9:00 P.M. meal, made an assessment of your newly admitted patients, and pronounced: "I will meet you and your patients in the fluoroscopy room at 11:00 P.M." This set off a frantic search for the elevator, which had been shut down at 8:00 P.M. Fluoroscopy was on the 3rd floor, ward K on the 5th. If we could not break into the elevator, up and down the stairs we would go with dyspneic Mrs. Schwartz and Mrs. Brown. With our patients finally tucked or tied into bed, the chief resident assumed a professional air. If Mrs. Schwartz had arthritis, he would ask, "Tell me about the arthritides." If Mrs. Brown was anemic we would talk about the anemias, until 3 or 4:00 A.M. . . . Some of us managed a few hours sleep before the 7:00 A.M. bugle for the next day, but most joined the endless, on-going poker game, which had started in antiquity. *Alvin S. Teirstein, M.D. (H.1956)*[11]

Poor performance was not tolerated:

It was unthinkable to miss or be late for medical x-ray conference, grand rounds, clinical pathology conference, or mortality conference. *Alvin S. Teirstein, M.D. (H.1956)*[12]

There was no such nonsense as a casual atmosphere. You stood up when they [the attendings] arrived. *Henry Dolger, M.D. (H.1938)*[13]

Then [A. V. Moschcowitz] said to me, "You know, on my service you can do anything you want to do, as long as you do it my way." That was my initiation at Mount Sinai Hospital. *Ralph Colp, M.D. (H.1923)*[14]

My knuckles [were] raw from the daily raps he [Dr. Garlock] administered because of my poor retraction. *Alvin S. Teirstein, M.D. (H.1956)*[15]

Dr. Berg had a rather high-pitched voice, and he would let go with certain pet phrases of his. He'd say to the assistant, "Doctor, you're about as much good as a fifth wheel on a wagon." *Leon Ginzburg, M.D. (H.1925)*[16]

Initially, all Interns lived at the hospital and were not allowed to marry:

When a resident got married, his residency terminated that weekend—no argument, no explanation. *Harry C. Saltzstein, M.D. (H. approx. 1915)*[17]

It will be of interest to compare briefly the career of the house staff man 15 years ago, and during the past few years. Of diversion in the old days there was no lack. Your Chairman entered the Hospital just after a brilliant poker era. Then came the progressive whist era . . . the chess and checker crowd . . . the mandolin players (good and bad) and then even "crap shooters." At one time there was much revolver shooting, or rather attempted shooting. *Emanuel Libman, M.D., (H.1896) in a 1912 speech to Alumni.*[18]

House staff quarters were all together in a building, which was over the outpatient department. On the top floor we had a pool table and a piano. We had a roof with chairs, where during the summer time we went to cool off, because there was no air conditioning. We also had rest period on Tuesdays and Thursdays from 2 to 3, when we could take a nap in the afternoon. And we would all go upstairs. You had a phone in your room. You were given six uniforms and a laundry service. . . . Uniforms were made in a Federation of Jewish Charities workshop called Altro workshops. They were made by patients who were recovering from tuberculosis. They were all white with a dentist's collar . . . the white collar, the jacket, pants, and black shoes. No one had heard of sneakers, no beard, no jewelry, and the uniform had to be starched and creased. You couldn't have dirt or stains. *Henry Dolger, M.D. (H.1938)*[19]

An ominous sign of my forthcoming life at Mount Sinai greeted me on the day of my arrival. I was, and almost remain, the average-sized everything. . . . I learned the basic level of Mount Sinai efficiency when Mel Kahn, my somewhat outsized co-intern, emerged smiling from the uniform room with a year's supply of what appeared to be Gucci fitted whites. Mount Sinai did not have my size. *Alvin S. Teirstein, M.D. (H.1956)*[20]

We had a dining room where the intern staff would come for breakfast, lunch, and dinner, served by 2 waitresses. In the next adjoining room was the attending dining room where they came and had lunch. Then at night, no one really stayed for dinner. Everybody came back at midnight. This was laid out for us. First a big platter of cold cuts, quart jars of chocolate milk, lots of Danish pastry, rye bread and sliced deli, tea and coffee, all that sort of stuff. You could also order fried eggs. Ruby served us as the housemother. I always ate 12 fried eggs and a quart of chocolate milk. *Henry Dolger, M.D. (H.1938)*[21]

By the late 1930s, Interns were allowed to marry, but they did not spend much time at home:

I remember my future mother-in-law asking Dr. Friesner if it would hurt her son's medical career if he got married. Dr. Friesner said to go ahead, so we were married in 1937, but while he was on the house staff I was only allowed to be in his room if the door was kept open. *Wife of Gerson Jonas Lesnick, M.D. (H.1941)*[22]

During the next six years Mount Sinai was my home. Although we were married, Alice and I viewed that time as an extended courtship. Kissing her goodnight at our door after she had joined me for the "free" 9:00 P.M. meal, I returned to night call—every other night, after every other night. To this day we subtract three years from the duration of our marriage, in memory of those every-other-night and weekend duties. . . . I cannot recall a single vacation during those years. Vacations were a time to sleep and eat, to get acquainted with your family and what few remaining friends you had. I never saw a house staff officer returning from vacation with a tan. At $25 a month and all you could eat at the 9:00 P.M. meal, the Central Park boat pond was the Caribbean. If the ever-present sallow house staff complexion turned to tan, you suspected Addison's disease. *Alvin S. Teirstein, M.D. (H.1956)*[23]

Following internship and possibly a fellowship, it was time for the physicians to start their own practice and begin the climb up the hospital ladder. This was not easy however:

Practice in those days was very slow. The first year, I made $914. The second year, I earned $1,040 and married. *Burrill B. Crohn, M.D. (H.1910)*[24]

Well, nobody sent cases to young people. . . . There were two kinds of patient: the wealthy patient who went to the professor, and the very poor people who went to the ward . . . so that it was very difficult for a young man to develop a reputation. . . . Some people fell by the wayside, for one reason or another, and they left the hospital to look for greener pastures. Others didn't want to stay in New York and starve, literally almost, waiting for practice, because your practice depended terribly upon your position in the hospital. *Samuel Klein, M.D. (H.1931)*[25]

You didn't automatically become a member of the attending staff. You could apply for privileges only after you had served six months to a year in the clinic. *Henry Dolger, M.D. (H.1938)*[26]

Promotions in this hospital were very slow, except under extraordinary circumstances, namely, the sudden death of a chief or some other misadventure whereby the chief's tenure was terminated or something like that. But in those days, it was a long time waiting for an appointment. No one ever was appointed following a residency or internship. There was always a hiatus, a wait of four, five, six, seven years. That was routine. It was very disheartening. And then when one got the adjunctship, it was a long, long wait again for the associate, and that depended, of course, on the time the higher-ups retired, or as I say per misadventure, they left the hospital. Of course we had misgivings. We all worried and we struggled and we competed, and we just hoped we'd go up the ladder. *Samuel Klein, M.D. (H.1931)*[27]

In those days, if you were an Adjunct Physician and you didn't make the promotion to Associate, you were dropped. You had six years to prove yourself worthy by doing work that was original, of clinical or some scientific value, and if you didn't do it you were finished. *Henry Dolger, M.D. (H.1938)*[28]

Consequently, the scientific fervor established during internship continued to grow:

They'd be in their office part time, part time in the hospital, and research at night. All these papers were written on their own time. . . . When I made observations about the eye in diabetes, I made them myself. I took the records of 200 patients. I analyzed them and studied them at night. I left my home, my kids, and I'd be in the record room from 8:00 till 11:00. When I got home I'd sit down and would write until 3:00 in the morning. This was the way it was always done. *Henry Dolger, M.D. (H.1938)*[29]

I recall, in my early years of marriage, I apologized almost every night to my wife after dinner, saying, "I'm sorry. I have to pay calls." And every night I'd go out and pay two or three calls because my afternoons were so busy in the laboratory that practice had to be performed in between, before and after the laboratory sessions in the afternoon. *Burrill B. Crohn, M.D. (H.1910)*[30]

You queried me as to payment, and I said it never entered our minds. We were expected to develop our curiosity, our scientific curiosity, and make contributions on our own time. *Henry Dolger, M.D. (H.1938)*[31]

I spent every afternoon in the laboratory of biological chemistry, under Dr. Sam Bookman, as a volunteer. That was the type of personnel—all of us working as volunteers, no salaries ever. In fact, the entire 60 years or so that I spent at Mount Sinai, I've never had any remuneration of any type. *Burrill B. Crohn, M.D. (H.1910)*[32]

In the end, remuneration came from the knowledge that they belonged to an extraordinary community:

The operation of the hospital was still so small, and the staff was so small that we all had a common interest. . . . I sat with the surgical res-

ident or the x-ray resident and exchanged mutual experiences on patients we got to know. If something went wrong on Ward U, we all
shared the experience. *Henry Dolger, M.D. (H.1938)*[33]

And I spent the most exciting and most interesting year of my life in
the laboratory, preparing for medicine, doing all the surgical pathology, doing the autopsies with Dr. Libman, all the bacteriology for the
whole hospital. *Burrill B. Crohn, M.D. (H.1910)*[34]

We made rounds every day of the week. And every day I would have
some brilliant person who developed a technique in doing blood
transfusions or taking care of ulcers, or people like that who developed the first typhoid fever treatment. *Henry Dolger, M.D. (H.1938)*[35]

The ferment of this devil's cauldron of genius, this witches brew of talent, is hard to imagine unless you lived through those years at the hospital. *Bernard E. Simon, M.D. (H.1942)*[36]

I look back in awe at the intense medical dedication and exchange of
knowledge. This highly integrated intellectual atmosphere was, in a
sense, a seminary, because there was a kind of forced, intellectual
heightening of your medical prowess and powers, and it made us into
really exceptional physicians. *Henry Dolger, M.D. (H.1938)*[37]

Dr. John Bookman (H.1940), in a postcard to his parents from a Japanese prisoner-of-war camp, wrote: "Don't forget to keep my place at
Mount Sinai open."

Appendix A

Directors* of The Mount Sinai Hospital, 1855–

Julius Raymond, 1855–1865
M. J. Bergman, 1865
Gabriel Schwarzbaum, 1866–1872
Doctor Treusch, 1872–1875
Leopold B. Simon, 1875–1878+
Theodore Hadel, 1878–1892
Leopold Minzesheimer, 1892–1898+
S. L. Fatman, 1898–1903
S. S. Goldwater, M.D., 1903–1929
Joseph Turner, M.D., 1929–1948
Martin Steinberg, M.D., 1948–1969
S. David Pomrinse, M.D., 1969–1975
Samuel Davis, 1975–1981
Barry Freedman, 1982–1995
Wendy Z. Goldstein, 1995–1998
Jeffrey Menkes, 2000–

Presidents of the Mount Sinai Medical Center, 1965–

George James, M.D., 1965–1972+
Hans Popper, M.D., Ph.D., 1972–1973
Thomas C. Chalmers, M.D., 1973–1983
James F. Glenn, M.D., 1983–1987
John W. Rowe, M.D., 1987–2000
Nathan Kase, M.D., 2001–2002
Kenneth I. Berns, M.D., Ph.D., 2002–

Deans of the Mount Sinai School of Medicine, 1965–

George James, M.D., 1965–1972
Hans Popper, M.D., Ph.D., 1972–1973
Thomas C. Chalmers, M.D., 1973–1983
James F. Glenn, M.D., 1983–1984 [Acting]
Lester B. Salans, M.D., 7/1–9/1/84
James F. Glenn, M.D., 9/84–1/85 [Acting]
Nathan Kase, M.D., 1985–1997
Arthur Rubenstein, M.D., 1997–2001
Nathan Kase, M.D., 2001– [Interim]

Chairmen** of The Mount Sinai Hospital Board of Trustees, 1852–

Sampson Simson, 1852–1855
John I. Hart, 1855–1856
Benjamin Nathan, 1856–1870+
Emanuel B. Hart, 1870–1876
Adolph Hallgarten, 1876–1879
Harris Aronson, 1879+
Hyman Blum, 1879–1896
Isaac Wallach, 1896–1907
Isaac Stern, 1907–1910
George Blumenthal, 1911–1938
Leo Arnstein, 1938–1944
Waldemar Kops, 1944–1945+
George B. Bernheim, 1945–1948
Alfred L. Rose, 1948–1956
Joseph Klingenstein, 1956–1962
Gustave L. Levy, 1962–1976+
Alfred R. Stern, 1977–1985
Frederick A. Klingenstein, 1985–1995
Stephen M. Peck, 1995–2002
Peter May, 2002–

* Until 1917, this position was called the Superintendent.
+ Died in office.
** Until 1969, this title was President of the Board of Trustees.

Appendix B

Jacobi Medallions Awarded by The Mount Sinai Alumni.

1952
Leo Edelman*
Elmer S. Gais
Joseph H. Globus
Abraham Hyman
Arthur M. Master
Sadao Otani
The Mount Sinai Hospital
(in honor of its 100th anniversary)

1953
William M. Hitzig
Harry Rosenwasser
Gregory Shwartzman
Israel Strauss
Ms. Bella Trachtenberg

1954
David Beck
Richard Lewisohn
Bernard S. Oppenheimer
Bela Schick

1955
Ralph Colp
Reuben Ottenberg
Jonas Salk
Harry Weiss
Kaufman Schlivek (posthumous)

1956
George Baehr
Samuel Karelitz
Eli Moschcowitz

1957
Paul Klemperer
Israel S. Wechsler
David Wexler

1958
Bernard H. Eliasberg
Isidor C. Rubin

1959
Solomon Silver
Moses Swick

1960
Murray H. Bass
Harold Neuhof
Mr. Eugene Metzger

1961
Morris B. Bender
Coleman B. Rabin
Mr. Joseph Klingenstein

1962
Burrill B. Crohn
John H. Garlock
Samuel Rosen

1963
Max Ellenberg
Leon Ginzburg

1964
Morris A. Goldberger
M. Ralph Kaufman

1965
Milton Mendlowitz
Robert A. Nabatoff
Mr. Gustave L. Levy

1966
Eugene Braunwald
Albert Cornell
Joseph L. Goldman
Lester R. Tuchman

1967
Dr. and Mrs. Arthur H. Aufses, Sr.
Mr. George Lee
Percy Klingenstein

1968
Irving B. Goldman
Alan F. Guttmacher
Samuel M. Peck

1969
Joseph Harkavy
Gordon D. Oppenheimer
Isidore Snapper
Martin R. Steinberg

1970
Alan H. Barnert
Ms. Claire Hirschfield

Saul Jarcho

1971
Mr. James Felt (posthumous)
Joseph A. Gaines
Max L. Som

1972
Richard H. Marshak
S. David Pomrinse
George L. Engel

1973
J. Lester Gabrilove
Alvin J. Gordon
Hans Popper
Frederick H. Theodore

1974
Henry D. Janowitz
Albert S. Lyons
Mr. Ira A. Schur
Norman Simon

1975
Mr. Sheldon R. Coons
Henry Dolger
Jean Pakter
Robert Turell
Louis R. Wasserman

1976
Irving J. Selikoff
Robert S. Siffert
Louis E. Siltzbach
Mr. Alfred R. Stern

1977
Sidney W. Gross
Mr. Alfred L. Rose
Bernard S. Wolf
Tsai-Fan Yu

1978
David A. Dreiling
Arthur M. Fishberg
Bernard E. Simon
Rosalyn S. Yalow, Ph.D.

1979
Arthur H. Aufses, Jr.
Simon Dack
Alfred P. Fishman
Peter Vogel

1980
Mr. and Mrs. Jack and Jane Aron
Lester R. Cahn
Jacob Churg
Arthur R. Sohval

1981
Lester Blum
Thomas C. Chalmers
Samuel H. Klein
Ralph E. Moloshok

1982
Ellen Fuller Zwiefach, R.N.
Horace L. Hodes
Ezra M. Greenspan
Barry Stimmel

1983
Mortimer and Richard Bader
John DeHoff
Leonard I. Malis
Lotte Strauss

1984
David R. Coddon
Samuel K. Elster
Charlotte Friend, Ph.D.
Sidney M. Silverstone

1985
James F. Holland
Robert S. Litwak
Gabriel P. Seley
Jerome D. Waye

1986
Yun Peng Huang
Paul A. Kirschner
Gene H. Stollerman
Alvin S. Teirstein

1987
Robert M. Berne
Ephraim Donoso
Bernard C. Meyer
Melvin D. Yahr

1988
Eugene W. Friedman
Mr. Milton H. Sisselman
Leonard Steinfeld
Edwin A. Weinstein

1989
Kurt W. Deuschle
Frederick H. King
Burton I. Korelitz
Gail Kuhn Weissman, R.N.

1990
Mr. William T. Golden
Donald Gribetz
Saul B. Gusberg
Jack Klatell

1991
Edward J. Bottone, Ph.D.
Richard Gorlin
Edwin D. Kilbourne
Gerson J. Lesnick
Daniel H. Present

1992
Hugh F. Biller
Janice Gabrilove
Mamoru Kaneko
Mr. Frederick A. Klingenstein
Fenton Schaffner

1993
Kurt Hirschhorn
Sherman Kupfer
Louis S. Lapid
Richard E. Rosenfield

1994
Seymour Gendelman
Nathan G. Kase
Isadore Kreel
David B. Sachar

1995
Valentin Fuster
Irwin Gelernt
Panayotis Katsoyannis, Ph.D.
Harry Spiera
Ms. Helen Wilson

1996
Robert Butler
Carmel J. Cohen
Arthur Figur
Marvin Stein

1997
Ruth Abramson
Gerald Friedman

Sheldon Glabman
Marvin F. Levitt
John W. Rowe

1998
Barry S. Coller
Mr. Barry R. Freedman
Samuel L. Guillory
Kristjan T. Ragnarsson

1999
Janet Cuttner
Mr. Andrew Heineman
Terry Ann Krulwich, Ph.D.
Steven M. Podos

2000
Bernard Cohen
Charles M. Miller
Jack G. Rabinowitz
Nathaniel Wisch

2001
Ms. Patricia S. Levinson
Roger N. Levy
Arthur H. Rubenstein
Mark H. Swartz

2002
Kenneth L. Davis
Jonathan L. Halperin
Philip Landrigan
Lloyd F. Mayer
Gary Rosenberg, Ph.D.

* All recipients are M.D.s unless otherwise noted.

Notes

NOTES TO THE PREFACE AND ACKNOWLEDGMENTS

1. H. Popper, "Foreword: Dr. Sadao Otani: His contributions to American pathology," *Mount Sinai J Med* 39 (1972): 1.

2. J. Hirsh and B. Doherty, *The First Hundred Years of The Mount Sinai Hospital of New York, 1852–1952* (New York: Random House, 1952).

3. *Amer J Med* 13 (Nov. 1952).

4. See Appendix A for a listing of the Senior leadership over the years.

5. See the Introduction for citations.

NOTES TO THE INTRODUCTION

1. J. Hirsh and B. Doherty, *The First Hundred Years of The Mount Sinai Hospital of New York* (New York: Random House, 1952).

2. For a history of the School of Nursing, see J. B. Nowak, *The Forty-Seven Hundred: The Story of the Mount Sinai Hospital School of Nursing* (Canaan, N.H.: Phoenix, 1981).

3. The history of nursing at Mount Sinai has recently been updated. See M. G. Lewis and S. M. Barker, *The Sinai Nurse: A History of Nursing at the Mount Sinai Hospital, New York, New York, 1852–2000* (West Kennebunk, Maine: Phoenix, 2001).

4. For a review of the history of the Social Work Services Department at Mount Sinai, see H. Rehr, G. Rosenberg, and S. Blumenfield, *Creative Social Work in Health Care* (New York: Springer, 1998).

5. *Mount Sinai Unit in the World War; with Scenes at Base Hospital No. 3 A.E.F. at Vauclaire, Dordogne, France* (New York: Mount Sinai Hospital, 1919).

6. Hirsh and Doherty, *First Hundred Years*, 1952.

7. K. M. Ludmerer, "The origins of Mount Sinai School of Medicine," *J Hist Med Allied Sci* 45 (1990): 469–89.

8. B. J. Niss and N. Kase, "An overview of the history of the Mount Sinai School of Medicine (CUNY), 1963–1988," *Mt Sinai J Med* 56 (1989): 356–66.

9. The Mount Sinai Hospital, *Annual Report for 1905*, p. 49.

NOTES TO CHAPTER I

1. *Minutes of the Medical Board*, 1872. Mount Sinai Archives.

2. See the chapter on the Division of Pulmonary Medicine for more on Meyer.

3. See the chapter on the Division of Endocrinology for more on Rudisch.

4. See the chapter on the Department of Pathology for more information.

5. As cited in *The Story of the First Fifty Years of the Mount Sinai Hospital, New York, 1852–1902* (New York: The Mount Sinai Hospital, 1944), p. 78.

6. See the chapter on the Department of Pathology for a more complete description of these works and the citations.

7. See the Division of Gastroenterology for more about Manges's contributions.

8. C. D. Haagensen, "An exhibit of important books, papers, and memorabilia illustrating the evolution of the knowledge of cancer," *Am J Cancer* 18 (1933): 107–8.

9. E. Libman, "Weitere Mittheilungen uber die Streptokokken-Enteritis bei Saulingen," *Centralbl fur Bakt* 22 (1897): 376–82.

10. E. Libman, "On some experience with blood-cultures in the study of bacterial infections," *Johns Hopkins Hosp Bull* 17 (1906): 215–28.

11. See the chapter on the Division of Cardiology for more on Libman's work and the citations.

12. *Time*, June 10, 1935, v.25, no. 23; *The New Yorker*, April 8, 1939, p. 24–29; J. M. Block, "My most unforgettable character," *Reader's Digest*, December 1964: 107–12.

13. See the chapter on the Department of Surgery for more on Berg.

14. See the chapter on the Division of Cardiology for Oppenheimer's clinical contributions.

15. See the Afterword for more details and for the holders of the Gold-Headed Cane.

16. Interview with George Baehr, February 6, 1939. Historian's Office, MSH. Files, 1852–1955: box 1, f.9.

17. L. Loewe, S. A. Ritter, and G. Baehr, "Cultivation of rickettsia-like bodies in typhus fever," *JAMA* 77 (1921): 1967–69.

18. G. Baehr, "Glomular lesions of subacute bacterial endocarditis," *Proc NY Soc Path* 11 (1911): 123–30; *J Exp Med* 15 (1912): 330–47.

19. P. Klemperer, A. D. Pollack, and G. Baehr, "Diffuse collagen disease: acute disseminated lupus erythematosus and diffuse scleroderma," *JAMA* 119 (1942): 331–32.

20. G. Baehr, P. Klemperer, and A. Schifrin, "A diffuse disease of the peripheral circulation (usually associated with Lupus erythematosus and endocarditis," *Trans Assoc Am Physicians* 50 (1935): 139–55.

21. L. Chargin et al. various papers in *Arch Dermatol and Syph* (August 1940). See also the chapter on the Department of Dermatology.

22. E. Moschcowitz, "Eosinophilia and anaphylaxis," *NY Med J* 93 (1911): 15–19.

23. E. Moschcowitz, "Acute febrile pleiochromic anemia with hyaline thrombosis of terminal arterioles and capillaries: An undescribed disease," *Arch Int Med* 36 (1925): 89–93.

24. E. Moschcowitz, "Hypertension of the pulmonary circulation: Its causes, dynamics, and relation to other circulatory states," *Am J Med Sci* 174 (1927): 388–406.

25. E. Moschcowitz, *Biology of Disease* (New York: Grune and Stratton, 1948).

26. "Mount Sinai in 1938," memo by Alvin J. Gordon. Mount Sinai Archives, biographical file.

27. The Mount Sinai Hospital, *Annual Report for 1946*, p. 31.

28. A. A. H. van den Burgh and I. Snapper, "Die Farbstoffe des Blutserums," *Arch f klin Med* 110 (1913): 540–61.

29. The Mount Sinai Hospital, *Annual Report for 1949*, p. 19.

30. A. B. Gutman and T. F. Yu, "Benemid (p-di- –propylsulfamyl-benzoic acid) as uricosuric agent in chronic gouty arthritis," *Trans Assoc Am Physicians* 64 (1951): 279–88. See also the chapters on The Division of Nephrology and the Division of Rheumatology.

31. See the chapter on the Division of Nephrology for more on the work of Sherman Kupfer.

32. B. Stimmel and J. Rabin, "The ability to remain abstinent upon leaving methadone maintenance: A prospective study," *Am J Drug Alcohol Abuse* 1 (1974): 379–92; B. Stimmel and K. Adamsons, "Narcotic dependency in pregnancy. Methadone maintenance compared to use of street drugs," *JAMA* 235 (1976): 1121–24; B. Stimmel, J. Goldberg, E. Rothkopf, and M. Cohen, "Ability to remain abstinent after methadone detoxification. A six-year study," *JAMA* 237 (1977): 1216–20.

33. R. S. Yalow and S. A. Berson, "Assay of plasma insulin in human subjects by immunologic methods," *Nature* 184 (1959): 1648–49; S. A. Berson and R. S. Yalow, "Quantitative aspects of the reaction between insulin and insulin-binding antibody," *J Clin Invest* 38 (1959): 1996–2016.

34. R. S. Yalow, "Radioimmunoassay: A probe for the fine structure of biologic systems," *Science* 200 (1978): 1236–37.

35. See the chapters on the Division of Liver Disease and the Department of Pathology for more on Schaffner.

36. See the chapter on the Division of Cardiology for more on Richard Gorlin.

37. B. Coller, ed., *Progress in Hemostasis and Thrombosis*, vol. 8 (Orlando: Grune and Stratton, 1986), Vols. 9 and 10 (Philadelphia: W. B. Saunders, 1989,

1991). E. Beutler, M. A. Lichtman, B. Coller, and T. J. Kipps, eds., *Williams Hematology*, 5th ed. (New York: McGraw-Hill, 1995), and E. Beutler et al., eds., *Williams Hematology*, 6th ed. (New York: McGraw-Hill, New York, 2000). See also the chapter on the Division of Hematology.

NOTES TO CHAPTER 2

1. W. B. Fye, *American Cardiology: A History of a Specialty and Its College* (Baltimore: Johns Hopkins University Press, 1996), p. 489.

2. H. Lilienthal, "In the beginning," *J Mt Sinai Hosp 8* (1942): 321–22.

3. See the Afterword for more about the Gold-Headed Cane.

4. B. S. Oppenheimer and M. A. Rothschild, "Electrocardiographic changes associated with myocardial involvement," *JAMA* 69 (1917): 429–31.

5. For a more detailed description of Libman's accomplishments outside the field of cardiology and of his contributions to the Hospital, see the chapters on "The Leadership" and the Department of Pathology.

6. E. Libman and H. Celler, "The etiology of subacute infective endocarditis," *Am J Med Sci* 140 (1910): 516–27; E. Libman, "Demonstration of the cardiac lesions of subacute bacterial endocarditis," *Proc NY Path Soc* 11 (1911): 118–23, E. Libman, "A study of the endocardial lesions of subacute bacterial endocarditis, with particular reference to healing or healed lesions: with clinical notes," *Am J Med Sci* 144 (1912): 313–27.

7. E. Libman and B. Sacks, "Atypical verrucous endocarditis," *Proc NY Path Soc* 23 (1923): 69–74, E. Libman and B. Sacks, "A hitherto undescribed form of valvular and mural endocarditis," *Arch Int Med* 33 (1924): 701–37. See also the chapter on the Department of Pathology.

8. E. Libman, "Some observations of thrombosis of the coronary arteries," *Trans Assoc Amer Phys* 34 (1919): 138–40.

9. W. H. Welch, "Introduction," *Contributions to the Medical Sciences in Honor of Dr. Emanuel Libman, by His Pupils, Friends, and Colleagues* (New York: International Press, 1932), p. xix.

10. B. S. Oppenheimer and M. A. Rothschild, "Value of electrocardiogram in the diagnosis and prognosis of myocardial disease," *Trans Assoc Am Phys* 39 (1924): 247–57.

11. H. A. Mann, "A method of analyzing the electrocardiogram," *Arch Int Med* 25 (1920): 283–94.

12. M. A. Rothschild and M. Kissin, "Production of the anginal syndrome by induced general anoxemia," *Am Heart J* 8 (1933): 729–44; M. A. Rothschild and M. Kissin, "Induced general anoxemia causing S-T deviation in the electrocardiograph," *Am Heart J* 8 (1933): 745–54.

13. A. M. Master and H. Jaffe, "Rheumatoid (infectious) arthritis and acute rheumatic fever," *JAMA* 98 (1932): 881–82; A. M. Master and A. Romanoff,

"Treatment of rheumatic fever patients with and without salicylates," *JAMA* 98 (1932): 1978–82.

14. H. Mann, "Interpretation of bundle branch block by means of the mono-cardiogram," *Am Heart J* 6 (1931): 447–57.

15. William Hitzig was also the individual who conceived of and designed the Jacobi Medallion of the Alumni Association, awarded for the first time in 1952 at the time of the Hospital's one hundredth anniversary. See the Afterword for more on the Jacobi Medallion.

16. W. Hitzig, "Measurement of circulation time from antecubital veins to pulmonary capillaries," *Proc Soc Exp Bio Med* 31 (1934): 935–38.

17. A. M. Master and E. T. Oppenheimer, "A simple exercise tolerance test for circulatory efficiency with standard tables for normal individuals," *Amer J Med Sci* 177 (1929): 223–42.

18. A. M. Master, "P-wave changes in acute coronary artery occlusion," *Am Heart J* 8 (1933): 462–70.

19. A. M. Master and E. T. Oppenheimer, "A study of obesity," *JAMA* 92 (1929): 1652–56.

20. A. M. Master, H. L. Jaffe, and S. D. Dack, "The basal metabolic rate in a patient with coronary artery thrombosis when placed on an 800 calorie diet," *J Mt Sinai Hosp* 1 (1935): 263–65.

21. A. M. Master, H. L. Jaffe, and S. Dack, "The treatment and the immediate prognosis of coronary artery thrombosis (267 attacks)," *Am Heart J* 12 (1936): 549–62.

22. See the chapter on the Department of Urology for more on Swick.

23. M. L. Sussman, A. J. Gordon, S. A. Brahms, et al., "The technique of cardiac catheterization and angiography as employed at the Mount Sinai Hospital," *J Mt Sinai Hosp* 17 (1951): 272–94.

24. A. M. Master, R. Gubner, S. Dack, and H. L. Jaffe, "The diagnosis of coronary occlusion and myocardial infarction by fluoroscopic examination," *Am Heart J* 20 (1940): 475–85.

25. A. M. Master, R. Friedman, and S. Dack, "The electrocardiogram after standard exercise as a functional test of the heart, *Am Heart J* 24 (1942): 777–93.

26. S. Jarcho, "Research on cardiovascular disease and congenital heart disease at the Mount Sinai Hospital," *J Mt Sinai Hosp* 17 (1951): 269–71.

27. *Journal of the Mount Sinai Hospital*, 17 (1951): 272–343.

28. S. Blumenthal, S. Brahms, and M. L. Sussman, "Tricuspid atresia with transposition of the great vessels successfully treated by surgery," *J Mt Sinai Hosp* 17 (1950): 328–35. The operation was performed by Arthur S. W. Touroff. See the chapter on the Department of Cardiothoracic Surgery.

29. The Mount Sinai Hospital, *Annual Report for 1950*, p. 19.

30. A. M. Master, H. H. Marks, and S. Dack, "Hypertension in people over forty," *JAMA* 121 (1943): 1251–56.

31. A. M. Master, L. I. Dublin, and H. H. Marks, "The normal blood pressure range and its clinical implications." *JAMA* 143 (1950): 1464–70.

32. A. J. Gordon, E. Braunwald, and M. M. Ravitch, "Simultaneous pressure pulses in the human left atrium, ventricle, and aorta," *Circ Res* 2 (1954): 432–33.

33. L. Gross and C. K. Friedberg, "Nonbacterial thrombotic endocarditis. Classification and general description," *Arch Int Med* 58 (1936): 620–40.

34. L. Gross and C. K. Friedberg, "Lesions of the cardiac valves in rheumatic fever," *Amer J Path* 12 (1936): 855–909.

35. C. K. Friedberg, *Diseases of the Heart* (Philadelphia: W. B. Saunders, 1949).

36. H. L. Moscovitz, E. Donoso, I. J. Gelb, and W. Welkowitz, "Intracardiac phonocardiography: Correlation of mechanical, acoustic, and electric events of the cardiac cycle," *Circulation* 18 (1958): 983–88.

37. The ideal clinician-scientist, Mendlowitz remains active in his laboratory in the twenty-first century. See the Web site www.mountsinaihistory.org for a list of Mendlowitz's most important papers.

38. See also the chapter on the Division of Endocrinology.

39. R. Gorlin and S. G. Gorlin, "Hydraulic formula for calculation of area of stenotic mitral valve, other cardiac valves and central circulatory shunts," *Am Heart J* 41 (1951): 1–29.

40. V. Fuster, D. N. Fass, M. P. Kaye, et al., "Arteriosclerosis in normal and von Willebrand pigs: Long-term prospective study and aortic transplantation study," *Circ Res* 51 (1982): 587–93.

41. J. H. Chesebro, V. Fuster, L. R. Elveback, et al., "Effect of dipyridamole and aspirin on late vein-graft patency after coronary bypass operations," *N Engl J Med* 310 (1984): 209–14.

42. L. Badimon, V. Turitto, J. A. Rosemark, et al., "Characterization of a tubular flow chamber for studying platelet interaction with biologic and prosthetic materials: deposition of indium 111-labeled platelets on collagen, subendothelium, and expanded polytetrafluoroethylene," *J Lab Clin Med* 110 (1987): 706–18.

43. M. E. Goldman and B. P. Mindich, "Intraoperative cardioplegic contrast echocardiography for assessing myocardial perfusion during open heart surgery," *J Am Coll Cardiol* 4 (1984): 1029–34.

44. J. A. Ambrose, S. L. Winters, A. Stern, et al., "Angiographic morphology and the pathogenesis of unstable angina pectoris," *JACC* 5 (1985): 609–16.

45. J. A. Gomes, S. L. Winters, D. Stewart, et al., "A new noninvasive index to predict sustained ventricular tachycardia and sudden death in the first year after myocardial infarction: Based on signal-averaged electrocardiogram radionuclide ejection fraction and Holter monitoring," *JACC* 10 (1987): 349–57.

46. T. A. Sanborn, H. A. Mitty, J. S. Train, and S. J. Dan, "Infrapopliteal and below-knee popliteal lesions: Treatment with sole laser thermal angioplasty. Work in progress," *Radiology* 172 (1989): 89–93.

47. M. Heras, J. H. Chesebro, W. J. Penny, et al., "Effects of thrombin inhibition on the development of acute platelet-thrombus deposition during angioplasty in pigs. Heparin versus recombinant hirudin, a specific thrombin inhibitor," *Circulation* 79 (1989): 657–65.

48. J. J. Badimon, L. Badimon, and V. Fuster, "Regression of atherosclerotic lesions by high density lipoprotein plasma fraction in the cholesterol-fed rabbit," *J Clin Invest* 85 (1990): 234–41.

49. M. B. Taubman, B. J. Rollins, M. Poon, et al., "JE mRNA accumulates rapidly in aortic injury and in platelet-derived growth factor-stimulated vascular smooth muscle cells," *Circ Res* 70 (1992): 314–25.

50. G. C. Flaker, J. L. Blackshear, R. McBride, et al., "Antiarrhythmic drug therapy and cardiac mortality in atrial fibrillation," *J Am Coll Cardiol* 20 (1992): 527–32.

51. J. F. Toussaint, G. M. LaMuraglia, J. F. Southern, V. Fuster, and H. L. Kantor, "Magnetic resonance images lipid, fibrous, calcified, hemorrhagic, and thrombotic components of human atherosclerosis in vivo," *Circulation* 94 (1996): 932–38.

52. S. G. Worthley, G. Helft, V. Fuster, et al., "High resolution ex vivo magnetic resonance imaging of in situ coronary and aortic atherosclerotic plaque in a porcine model," *Atherosclerosis* 150 (2000): 321–29.

53. Z. A. Fayad, V. Fuster, J. T. Fallon, et al., "Noninvasive in vivo human coronary artery lumen and wall imaging using black-blood magnetic resonance imaging," *Circulation* 102 (2000): 506–10.

54. Z. A. Fayad, J. T. Fallon, M. Shinnar, et al., "Noninvasive in vivo high-resolution magnetic resonance imaging of atherosclerotic lesions in genetically engineered mice," *Circulation* 98 (1998): 1541–47.

55. V. Fuster, Message from the Director, 2001.

NOTES TO CHAPTER 3

1. See the chapter on the Department of Pediatrics for more on Schick and citations.

2. See the chapter on the Laboratory Departments for more on Shwartzman's work and citations.

3. J. Harkavy, "Spasm-producing substance in the sputum of patients with bronchial asthma," *Arch Int Med* 45 (1930): 641–46.

4. J. Harkavy, S. Hebald, and S. Silbert, "Tobacco sensitiveness in thromboangiitis obliterans," *Proc Soc Exp Biol & Med* 30 (1932): 104–7.

5. J. Harkavy, "Vascular Allergy: Pathogenesis of Bronchial Asthma with Recurrent Pulmonary Infiltrations and Eosinophilic Polyserositis," *Arch Int Med* 67 (1941): 709–34.

6. J. Harkavy, *Vascular Allergy and Its Systemic Manifestations* (Washington, D.C.: Butterworth, 1963).

7. H. A. Abramson, "A stable hydrogen peroxide aerosol," *Science* 96 (1942): 238.

8. H. A. Abramson, "Combined penicillin and hydrogen peroxide aerosol therapy in lung infections," *Ann Allergy* 4 (1946): 199–206.

9. See the chapter on the Department of Pediatrics for more on Peshkin.

10. S. Siegal, "Benign paroxysmal peritonitis," *Ann Int Med* 23 (1945): 1–21.

11. S. M. Peck, S. Siegal, A. W. Glick, and A. Kurtin, "Clinical problems in penicillin sensitivity," *JAMA* 138 (1948): 631–38.

12. A. B. Gutman, "In memoriam. Kermit E. Osserman, M.D., 1909–1972," *Mt Sinai J Med* 39 (1972): 216–20. This article is the basis for the material about Osserman. See also S. A. Berson, "Contributions of the Mount Sinai Hospital to the study and care of patients with myasthenia gravis," *Mt Sinai J Med* 38 (1971): 602–8, for an annotated bibliography of sixty-eight of the most important papers by the Hospital staff on the subject.

13. K. E. Osserman and G. Genkins, "Studies in myasthenia gravis: Review of a twenty-year experience in over 1200 patients," *Mt Sinai J Med* 38 (1971): 497–537.

14. A. H. Rule and P. Kornfeld, "Studies in myasthenia gravis: Biologic aspects," *Mt Sinai J Med* 38 (1971): 538–72.

15. K. E. Osserman and L. E. Kaplan, "Rapid diagnostic test for myasthenia gravis. Increased muscle strength, without fasciculations, after intravenous administration of edrophonium (tensilon) chloride," *JAMA* 150 (1952): 265–68.

16. See the chapter on the Department of Surgery for more information.

17. A. J. L. Strauss, B. C. Seegal, K. C. Hsu, et al., "Immunoflourescence demonstration of a muscle-binding, complement-fixing serum globulin fraction in myasthenia gravis," *Proc Soc Exp Biol Med* 105 (1960): 184–91.

18. K. E. Osserman, *Myasthenia Gravis* (New York: Grune and Stratton, 1958).

19. See the chapters on the Division of Infectious Diseases and the Division of Nephrology for more on Mount Sinai's contributions to the problem of AIDS and for appropriate citations.

20. L. Mayer, S. P. Kwan, C. Thompson, et al., "Evidence for a defect in 'switch' T cells in patients with immunodeficiency and hyperimmunoglobulinemia M," *N Engl J Med* 314 (1986): 409–13.

21. C. Cunningham-Rundles, K. Kazbay, J. Hassett, et al., "Brief report: Enhanced humoral immunity in common variable immunodeficiency after long-term treatment with polyethylene glycol-conjugated interleukin-2," *N Engl J Med* 331 (1994): 918–21.

NOTES TO CHAPTER 4

1. J. Rudisch, "A new method for detecting and determining glucose in the urine," *International Contributions to Medical Literature* (1900): 1–9.

2. J. Rudisch and E. A. Aronson, "Statistics of cases of diabetes in the Mount Sinai Hospital during the years 1890–1900," *Mount Sinai Hospital Reports* 2 (1899–1900): 26–29.

3. The Mount Sinai Hospital, *Annual Report for 1917*, p. 22.

4. H. Dolger, "Clinical evaluation of vascular damage in diabetes mellitus," *JAMA* 134 (1947): 1289–91.

5. Proceedings of the Seminar on Degenerative Lesions in Metabolism, October 5, 1947. Mount Sinai Archives. Henry Dolger biographical file.

6. E. A. Weinstein and H. Dolger, "External ocular muscle palsies occurring in diabetes mellitus," *Arch Neurol Psych* 60 (1948): 597–603.

7. H. Dolger, "Clinical experience with orinase," *Metabolism* 5 (1956): 947–52.

8. S. A. Mirsky, D. Diengott, and H. Dolger, "Hypoglycemic action of sulfonylureas in patients with diabetes mellitus," *Science* 123 (1956): 583–84.

9. H. Dolger and B. Seeman, *How to Live with Diabetes* (New York: W. W. Norton, 1958).

10. M. Ellenberg and K. E. Osserman, "The role of shock in the production of central liver necrosis," *Am J Med* 11 (1951): 170–78.

11. M. Ellenberg and H. Rifkin, *Diabetes Mellitus: Theory and Practice* (New York: McGraw-Hill, 1970).

12. A. Jacobi, "Exophthalmic goitre occurring in a child, and followed by St. Vitus' dance," *Med Rec NY* 16 (1879): 1–4.

13. L. J. Soffer, *Diseases of the Adrenals* (Philadelphia: Lea and Febiger, 1946).

14. L. J. Soffer, J. L. Gabrilove, H. P. Laqueur, et al., "Effects of anterior pituitary adrenocorticotropic hormone (ACTH) in myasthenia gravis with tumor of thymus," *J Mt Sinai Hosp* 15 (1948): 73–82.

15. L. J. Soffer, *Diseases of the Endocrine Glands* (Philadelphia: Lea and Febiger, 1951).

16. S. Feitelberg, P. E. Kaunitz, L. R. Wasserman, and S. B. Yohalem, "Use of radioactive iodine in diagnosis of thyroid disease," *Am J Med Sci* 216 (1948): 129–35.

17. M. Eller, S. Silver, S. B. Yohalem, and R. L. Segal, "The treatment of toxic nodular goiter with I-131: 10 years experience with 436 cases," *Ann Intern Med* 52 (1960): 976–1013.

18. S. Silver, P. Poroto, and E. B. Crohn, "Hypermetabolic states without hyperthyroidism (nonthyrogenous hypermetabolism)," *Arch Int Med* 85 (1950): 479–82; S. Silver and M. H. Fieber, "Blood levels of I-131 after tracer doses in the diagnosis of hyperthyroidism," *Proc Soc Exp Biol Med* 75 (1950): 570–73; S. Silver, S. B. Yohalem, and M. H. Fieber, "Blood iodine and I-131 excretion in diagnostic

problems of hyperthyroidism," *J Mt Sinai Hosp* 17 (1951): 781–86. See also the chapter on the Department of Physics.

19. E. H. Quimby, S. Feitelberg, and S. Silver, *Radioactive Isotopes in Clinical Practice* (Philadelphia: Lea and Febiger, 1958).

20. See Afterword for more on the Gold-Headed Cane.

21. L. J. Soffer, *Diseases of the Endocrine Glands*.

22. See the chapter on the Division of Cardiology for more on Mendlowitz. See also the Web site www.mountsinaihistory.org for the citations to the most important of these papers.

23. S. E. Gitlow, M. Mendlowitz, S. Khassis, et al., "The diagnosis of pheochromocytoma by determination of 3-methoxy, 4- hydroxymandelic acid," *J Clin Invest* 39 (1960): 221–26.

24. S. E. Gitlow, L. Ornstein, M. Mendlowitz, et al., "A simple colormetric test for pheochromocytoma," *Am J Med* 28 (1960): 921–26.

25. See the chapter on "The Leadership" for more on Berson.

26. D. T. Krieger, M. J. Perlow, M. J. Gibson, et al., "Brain grafts reverse hypogonadism of gonadotropin releasing hormone deficiency," *Nature* 298 (1982): 468–71.

27. W. Futterweit and L. Deligdisch, "Effects of androgens on the ovary," *Fertil Steril* 46 (1986): 343–45.

28. See the Web site www.mountsinaihistory.org for selected citations of Davies's work.

NOTES TO CHAPTER 5

1. J. H. Baron and H. D. Janowitz, "Gastroenterology and Hepatology at The Mount Sinai Hospital, 1852–2000," *Mt Sinai J Med* (Theme Issues) 67, no. 1 (2000): 2–94; 67, no. 3 (2000): 174–244; 68, no. 3 (2001): 79–116.

2. *Case Book No. 1, 1855–1856*, The Jews' Hospital. Mount Sinai Archives.

3. Ibid.

4. J. H. Baron, "Morris Manges and Edmund Aronson," *Mt Sinai J Med* 67 (2000): 9–11. See the chapter on "The Leadership" for more on Manges.

5. M. Manges, *Translation of C. A. Ewald, The Diseases of the Stomach* (New York: Appleton, 1892).

6. Berg was a staunch advocate of separate surgical services and credited the collaborative innovations on the intestinal service for Mount Sinai's preeminence in gastrointestinal surgery. See the chapter on the Department of Surgery.

7. L. B. Meyer and B. B. Crohn, "Acute glanders: Report of a case, with a review of the literature and a complete bacteriologic report," *JAMA* 1 (1908): 1593–95.

8. B. B. Crohn and H. Rosenberg, "The sigmoidoscopic picture of chronic ulcerative colitis (non-specific)," *Am J Med Sci* 170 (1925): 220–28.

9. B. B. Crohn, *Affections of the Stomach* (Philadelphia: W. B. Saunders, 1927).

10. B. B. Crohn, L. Ginzburg, and G. D. Oppenheimer, "Regional ileitis," *JAMA* 99 (1932): 1323–28.

11. L. Ginzburg and G. D. Oppenheimer, "Non-specific granulomata of the intestines (inflammatory tumors and strictures of the bowel)," *Ann Surg* 98 (1933): 1046–62. See the chapters on the Department of Surgery and the Department of Urology for more on Ginzburg and Oppenheimer, respectively.

12. A. Winkelstein, "A new therapy for peptic ulcer: Continuous alkalinized milk drip into the stomach," *Am J Med Sci* 185 (1933): 695–703.

13. A. Winkelstein, "Peptic esophagitis: New clinical entity," *JAMA* 104 (1935): 906 9.

14. F. Hollander, E. E. Jemerin, and V. Weinstein, "An insulin test for differentiating vagal from non-vagal stomach pouches," *Fed Proc* 1 (1942): 116.

15. H. D. Janowitz, H. Colcher, and F. Hollander, "Inhibition of gastric secretion of hydrochloric acid in vivo by carbonic anhydrase inhibition," *Nature* 170 (1952): 449.

16. S. Rosenthal, "To make a difference: The founding of the Crohn's and Colitis Foundation of America," *Mt Sinai J Med* 68 (2001): 113–16.

17. D. Sachar, personal communication, August 3, 1998.

18. J. D. Waye, "The evolution of gastrointestinal endoscopy at the Mount Sinai Hospital," *Mt Sinai J Med* 68 (2001): 106–9.

19. R. H. Hunt and J. D. Waye, *Colonoscopy: Techniques, Clinical Practice, and Color Atlas* (London: Chapman and Hall, 1981).

20. D. Sachar, personal communication, 2001.

21. A. Lindner, R. H. Marshak, B. S. Wolf, and H. D. Janowitz, "Granulomatous colitis: A clinical study," *New Engl J Med* 269 (1963): 379–85; S. Meyers, J. S. Walfish, D. B. Sachar, et al., "Quality of life after surgery for Crohn's disease: A psychosocial survey," *Gastroenterology* 78 (1980): 1–6; S. Meyers and H. D. Janowitz, "The 'natural history' of Crohn's disease. An analytic review of the placebo lesson," *Gastroenterology* 87 (1984): 1189–92.

22. A. J. Greenstein, H. D. Janowitz, and D. B. Sachar, "The extra-intestinal complications of Crohn's disease and ulcerative colitis: A study of 700 patients," *Medicine* 55 (1976): 401–12.

23. D. B. Sachar, H. Smith, S. Chan, et al., "Erythrocytic sedimentation rate as a measure of clinical activity in inflammatory bowel disease," *J Clin Gastroenterol* 8 (1986): 647–50.

24. S. Otani and I. Snapper, "On the incidence of carcinoma in chronic ulcerative colitis," *J Mt Sinai Hosp* 19 (1952): 275–88.

25. A. J. Greenstein and H. D. Janowitz, "Cancer in Crohn's disease. The

danger of a by-passed loop," *Am J Gastroenterol* 64 (1975): 122–24; A. J. Greenstein, D. B. Sachar, A. Pucillo, et al., "Cancer in Crohn's disease after diversionary surgery. A report of seven carcinomas occurring in excluded bowel," *Am J Surg* 135 (1978): 86–90; A. J. Greenstein, D. B. Sachar, H. Smith, et al., "A comparison of cancer risk in Crohn's disease and ulcerative colitis," *Cancer* 48 (1981): 2742–45.

26. L. Ginzburg, K. M. Schneider, D. H. Dreizin, and C. Levinson, "Carcinoma of the jejunum occurring in a case of regional enteritis," *Surgery* 39 (1956): 347–51.

27. See the chapter on the Department of Radiology.

28. See the chapter on the Department of Surgery.

29. J. J. Deren, J. G. Porush, M. F. Levitt, and M. T. Khilnani, "Nephrolithiasis as a complication of ulcerative colitis and regional enteritis," *Ann Int Med* 56 (1962): 843–53; D. H. Present, J. G. Rabinowitz, P. A. Banks, and H. D. Janowitz, "Obstructive hydronephrosis. A frequent but seldom recognized complication of granulomatous disease of the bowel," *N Engl J Med* 280 (1969): 523–28.

30. L. J. Werther, A. Schapira, O. Rubenstein, and H. D. Janowitz, "Amyloidosis in regional enteritis. 5 cases in 17 autopsies," *Am J Med* 29 (1960): 416–23.

31. S. Meyers, H. D. Janowitz, V. V. Gumaste, et al., "Colchicine therapy of the renal amyloidosis of ulcerative colitis," *Gastroenterology* 94 (1988): 1503–7.

32. P. Salomon, A. A. Kornbluth, and H. D. Janowitz, "Treatment of ulcerative colitis with fish oil n-3-omega-fatty acid: An open trial," *J Clin Gastroenterol* 12 (1990): 157–61.

33. D. H. Present, B. I. Korelitz, N. Wisch, et al., "Treatment of Crohn's disease with 6-mercaptopurine. A long-term, randomized, double-blind study," *N Engl J Med* 302 (1980): 981–87.

34. N. Hirschhorn, J. L. Kinzie, D. B. Sachar, et al., "Decrease in net stool output in cholera during intestinal perfusion with glucose-containing solutions," *N Engl J Med* 279 (1968): 176–81.

35. A. J. Greenstein, D. B. Sachar, B. S. Pasternack, and H. D. Janowitz, "Reoperation and recurrence in Crohn's colitis and ileocolitis. Crude and cumulative rates," *N Engl J Med* 293 (1975): 685–90.

36. D. B. Sachar, D. M. Wolfson, A. J. Greenstein, et al., "Risk factors for postoperative recurrence of Crohn's disease," *Gastroenterology* 85 (1983): 917–21.

37. A. J. Greenstein, P. Lachman, D. B. Sachar, et al., "Perforating and nonperforating indications for repeated operations in Crohn's disease: Evidence for two clinical forms," *Gut* 29 (1988): 588–92; D. B. Sachar, K. Subramani, K. Mauer, et al., "Patterns of postoperative recurrence in fistulizing and stenotic Crohn's disease. A retrospective cohort study of 71 patients," *J Clin Gastroenterol* 22 (1996): 114–16.

38. Alexander Richman was a superb practicing gastroenterologist at Mount Sinai for almost his entire career. See the chapter on the Division of Liver Diseases for more about him.

39. S. H. Itzkowitz, E. J. Bloom, W. A. Kokal, et al., "Sialosyl-Tn. A novel mucin antigen associated with prognosis in colorectal cancer patients," *Cancer* 66 (1990): 1960–66; S. H. Itzkowitz, A. Marshall, A. Kornbluth, et al., "Sialosyl-Tn antigen: Initial report of a new marker of malignant progression in long-standing ulcerative colitis," *Gastroenterology* 109 (1995): 490–97.

NOTES TO CHAPTER 6

1. R. Ottenberg, "Transfusion and arterial anastomosis," *Ann Surg* 47 (1908): 486–505.

2. Reuben Ottenberg biographical file. Mount Sinai Archives.

3. R. Ottenberg, "Studies in isoagglutination. Transfusion and the question of intravascular agglutination," *J Exp Med* 13 (1911): 425–38.

4. R. Ottenberg, "The etiology of eclampsia: Historical and critical notes," *JAMA* 81 (1923): 295–97.

5. A. A. Epstein and R. Ottenberg, "A simple method of performing serum reactions," *Proc NY Path Soc* 8 (1908–09): 117–23.

6. R. Ottenberg and N. Rosenthal, "A new and simple method for counting blood platelets," *JAMA* 69 (1917): 999.

7. R. Ottenberg and H. Weiss, "Relation between bacteria and temperature in subacute bacterial endocarditis," *J Inf Dis* 50 (1932): 61–68.

8. R. Ottenberg, "Occlusion of the internal carotid artery: clinical diagnosis and therapy," *J Mt Sinai Hosp* 22 (1955): 99–103.

9. L. J. Unger, "A new method of syringe transfusion," *JAMA* 64 (1915): 582–84.

10. R. Lewisohn, "A new and greatly simplified method of blood transfusion. A preliminary report," *Medical Record (N.Y.)* 87 (1915): 141–42.

11. R. Lewisohn "The development of the technique of blood transfusion since 1907," *J Mt Sinai Hosp* 10 (1944): 605–22.

12. Ibid.

13. R. Lewisohn and N. Rosenthal, "Prevention of chills following transfusion of citrated blood," *JAMA* 100 (1933): 466–69.

14. E. Moschcowitz, "Acute febrile pleiochromic anemia with hyaline thrombosis of terminal arterioles and capillaries; an undescribed disease," *Arch Intern Med* 36 (1925): 89–93.

15. N. Brill, G. Baehr, and N. Rosenthal, "Generalized giant lymph follicle hyperplasia of lymph nodes and spleen; a hitherto undescribed type," *JAMA* 84 (1925): 668–71.

16. M. W. Wintrobe, *Hematology, the Blossoming of a Science: A Story of Inspiration and Effort* (Philadelphia: Lea and Febiger, 1985).

17. R. L. Rosenthal, O. H. Dreskin, and N. Rosenthal, "New hemophilia-like disease caused by a deficiency of a third plasma thromboplastin factor," *Proc Soc Exp Biol Med* 82 (1953): 171–74.

18. S. L. Lee, F. Rosner, N. Rosenthal, and R. L. Rosenthal, "Reticulum cell leukemia. Clinical and hematologic entity," *NY State J Med* 69 (1969): 422–29.

19. "In Memoriam: Nathan Rosenthal, 1890–1955." *J Mt Sinai Hosp* 22 (1955): 261–63.

20. D. Stats and L. R. Wasserman, "Cold hemagglutination—an interpretive review," *Medicine* 22 (1943): 363–424.

21. D. Stats, "The sedimentation differential agglutination test," *Blood* 5 (1950): 950–63.

22. F. A. Bassen and A. L. Kornzweig, "Malformation of the erythrocytes in a case of atypical retinitis pigmentosa," *Blood* 5 (1950): 381–87.

23. The Mount Sinai Hospital, *Annual Report for 1938*, p. 10.

24. N. Rosenthal, L. R. Wasserman, H. Abel, et al., "The organization of the blood bank at the Mount Sinai Hospital," *J Mt Sinai Hosp* 8 (1941): 210–31.

25. The Mount Sinai Hospital, *Annual Report for 1954*, p. 55.

26. P. Levine, L. Burnham, E. M. Katzin, and P. Vogel, "The role of isoimmunization in the pathogenesis of erythroblastosis fetalis," *Am J Obstet Gynecol* 42 (1941): 925–37.

27. R. Rubin, J. Niemetz, and S. Estren, "Use of animal AHG concentrates (factor VIII) in the treatment of life-threatening hemorrhage in patients with factor VIII antibodies," *Ann NY Acad Sci* 240 (1975): 362–69.

28. S. Estren, E. A. Brody, and L. R. Wasserman, "The metabolism of vitamin B12 in pernicious anemia and other megaloblastic anemias," *Advance Int Med* 9 (1958): 11–44.

29. C. Friend, "Cell-free transmission in adult Swiss mice of a disease having the character of a leukemia," *J Exp Med* 105 (1957): 307–18. See also the chapter on the Department and Division of Neoplastic Diseases.

30. R. E. Rosenfield and M. A Gilman, "An improved small centrifuge for rapid blood typing and matching tests," *Amer J Clin Path* 26 (1956): 201–4.

31. R. E. Rosenfield, F. H. Allen, Jr., S. N. Swisher, and S. Kochwa, "A review of Rh serology and presentation of a new terminology," *Transfusion* 2 (1962): 287–312.

32. R. E. Rosenfield, P. Vogel, and R. R. Race, "Un nouveau cas d'anti-Fy^a dans un serum humain," *Rev d'Hem* 5 (1950): 315–17; M. E. Nichols, R. E. Rosenfield, and P. Rubinstein, "Monocloncal Anti-K14 and Anti-K2," *Vox Sang* 52 (1987): 231–35.

33. R. E. Rosenfield, "A-B hemolytic disease of the newborn. Analysis of 1480 cord blood specimens, with special reference to the direct antiglobulin test and to the group O mother," *Blood 10* (1955): 17–18.

34. S. H. Cherry and R. E. Rosenfield, "The clinical management of erythroblastosis fetalis utilizing amniocentesis and intrauterine fetal transfusion," *NY State J Med* 66 (1966): 43.

35. G. V. Haber, A. Bastani, P. D. Arpin, and R. E. Rosenfield, "Rh Null and pregnancy complicated by maternal anti- 'total Rh'. I. Anti-Rh29 (Rh)," *Transfusion* 7 (1967): 389.

36. The Mount Sinai Hospital, *Annual Report for 1964*, p. 19.

37. L. M. Aledort, S. Puszkin, E. Puszkin, et al., "Control of platelet contraction," *Ser hematol* 6 (1973): 410–17.

38. D. Shaw, "Hemophilia agency aware of AIDS risk in '82, files indicate," *Houston Chronicle*, Oct. 24, 1994, Sec. A, p. 2.

39. N. I. Berlin and L. R. Wasserman, "Polycythemia vera: a retrospective and reprise," *J Lab Clin Med* 130 (1997): 365–73. See the Web site www.mountsinaihistory.org for more of Wasserman's publications.

40. W. Stremmel, G. Strohmeyer, F. Borchard, et al., "Isolation and partial characterization of a fatty acid binding protein in rat liver plasma membranes," *Proc Natl Acad Sci USA* 82 (1985): 4–8; P. D. Berk, H. Wada, Y. Horio, et al., "Plasma membrane fatty acid-binding protein and mitochondrial glutamic- oxaloacetic transaminase of rat liver are related," *Proc Natl Acad Sci USA* 87 (1990): 3484–88. See the chapter on the Division of Liver Diseases for more on Berk.

41. See, for example, Y. Nemerson and M. P. Esnouf, "Activation of a proteolytic system by membrane lipoprotein: The mechanism of action of tissue factor," *Proc Nat Acad Sci USA* 70 (1973): 310–14.

42. E. K. Spicer, R. Horton, L. Bloem, et al., "Isolation of cDNA clones coding for human tissue factor: primary structure of the protein and cDNA," *Proc Nat Acad Sci USA* 84 (1987): 5148–52. Other groups also published their work on this in 1987. See E. Bachli, "History of tissue factor," *Brit J Haemotol* 110 (2000): 248–55.

43. M. W. Wintrobe, *Hematology, the Blossoming of a Science*, p. 339.

44. S. M. Fruchtman, E. Scigliano, V. Ross, et al., "Bone marrow transplantation at The Mount Sinai Hospital" *Mt Sinai J Med* 61 (1994): 3–12.

45. S. M. Fruchtman, L. Isola, A. Hurlet, et al., "Autologous cord blood infusion for severe aplastic anemia (SAA)," Abstract # 2872, *Blood* 98 (2001): 687.

46. G. F. Atweh, M. Sutton, I. Nassif, et al., "Sustained induction of fetal hemoglobin by pulse butyrate therapy in sickle cell disease," *Blood* 93 (1999): 1790–97.

47. Department of Medicine: Division of Hematology, Mount Sinai School of Medicine. http://www.mssm.edu/medicine/hematology/introduction .shtml> [Accessed March 21, 2001].

NOTES TO CHAPTER 7

1. See the chapters on the Departments of Neurosurgery, Medicine, and Pathology for more on Elsberg, Brill, and Libman and for the appropriate citations.

2. L. Loewe, S. A. Ritter, and G. Baehr, "Cultivation of rickettsia-like bodies in typhus fever," *JAMA* 77 (1921): 1967–69. See also chapter 1, "The Leadership," for more on Baehr.

3. See the chapter on the Department of Cardiothoracic Surgery.

4. Letter to the Directors of The Mount Sinai Hospital, 1983. Director's Office Files. Mount Sinai Archives.

5. See the chapter on the Department of Cardiothoracic Surgery.

6. See the chapter on the Department of Dermatology.

7. See the chapter on the Laboratory Departments for more on Schneierson and for citations.

8. S. Z. Hirschman, S. J. Vernace, and F. Schaffner, "D.N.A. polymerase in preparations containing Australia antigen," *Lancet* 1 (1971): 1099–103.

9. S. Z. Hirschman, M. Gerber, and E. Garfinkel, "DNA purified from naked intranuclear particles of human liver infected with hepatitis B virus," *Nature* 251 (1974): 540–42; S. Z. Hirschman, P. Price, E. Garfinkel, et al., "Expression of cloned hepatitis B virus DNA in human cell cultures," *Proc Natl Acad Sci USA* 77 (1980): 5507–11.

10. S. Z. Hirschman and C. W. Chen, "Peptide nucleic acids stimulate gamma interferon and inhibit the replication of the human immunodeficiency virus," *J Investig Med* 44 (1996): 347–51.

11. F. P. Siegal, C. Lopez, G. S. Hammer, et al., "Severe acquired immunodeficiency in male homosexuals, manifested by chronic perianal ulcerative herpes simplex lesions," *N Engl J Med* 305 (1981): 1439–44. See also the chapter on the Division of Clinical Immunology.

12. E. Donegan, M. Stuart, J. C. Niland, et al., "Infection with human immunodeficiency virus type 1 (HIV-1) among recipients of antibody-positive blood donations," *Ann Intern Med* 113 (1990): 733–39.

13. B. J. Luft, R. Hafner, A. H. Korzun, et al., "Toxoplasmic encephalitis in patients with the acquired immunodeficiency syndrome. Members of the ACTG 077p/ANRS 009 Study Team," *N Engl J Med* 329 (1993): 995–1000; J. M. Jacobson, J. S. Greenspan, J. Spritzler, et al., "Thalidomide for the treatment of oral aphthous ulcers in patients with human immunodeficiency virus infection. National Institute of Allergy and Infectious Diseases AIDS Clinical Trials Group," *N Engl J Med* 336 (1997): 1487–93.

14. E. M. Connor, R. S. Sperling, R. Gelber, et al., "Reduction of maternal-infant transmission of human immunodeficiency virus type 1 with zidovudine treatment. Pediatric AIDS Clinical Trials Group Protocol 076 Study Group," *N*

Engl J Med 331 (1994): 1173–80. See also the chapter on the Department of Obstetrics, Gynecology, and Reproductive Sciences.

15. J. I. Tokars, D. M. Bell, D. H. Culver, et al., "Percutaneous injuries during surgical procedures," *JAMA* 267 (1992): 2899–904; J. I. Tokars, D. H. Culver, M. H. Mendelson, et al., "Skin and mucous membrane contacts with blood during surgical procedures: Risk and prevention," *Infect Control Hosp Epidemiol* 16 (1995): 703–11.

16. M. H. Mendelson, L. J. Short, C. B. Schecter, et al., "Study of a needleless intermittent intravenous-access system for peripheral infusions: analysis of staff, patient, and institutional outcomes," *Infect Control Hosp Epidemiol* 19 (1998): 401–6.

17. J. J. Rahal, Jr., B. R. Meyers, L. Weinstein, "Treatment of bacterial endocarditis with cephalothin," *N Engl J Med* 279 (1968): 1305–9.

18. B. R. Meyers, G. Wormser, S. Z. Hirschman, A. Blitzer, "Rhinocerebral mucormycosis: Premortem diagnosis and therapy," *Arch Intern Med* 139 (1979): 557–60.

19. B. R. Meyers and P. Wilkinson, "Clinical pharmacokinetics of antibacterial drugs in the elderly. Implications for selection and dosage," *Clin Pharmacokinet* 17 (1989): 385–95.

20. B. R. Meyers, G. Papanicolaou, P. Sheiner, et al., "Tuberculosis in orthotopic liver transplant patients: Increased toxicity of recommended agents; cure of disseminated infection with nonconventional regimens," *Transplantation* 69 (2000): 64–69.

21. J. A. Winston, L. A. Bruggeman, M. D. Ross, et al., "Nephropathy and establishment of a renal reservoir of HIV type 1 during primary infection," *N Engl J Med* 344 (2001): 1979–84. See also the chapter on the Division of Nephrology.

NOTES TO CHAPTER 8

1. *Case Records of the Jews' Hospital, 1855–56.* Mount Sinai Archives.

2. F. Schaffner, "The history of liver disease at the Mount Sinai Hospital," *Mt Sinai J Med* 67 (2000): 76–83. Many of the references cited in this article may be found with annotations on the Web site www.mountsinaihistory.org.

3. P. Klemperer, J. A. Gillian, and G. G. Head, "The pathology of 'icterus catarrhalis,'" *Arch Pathol Lab Med* 2 (1926): 631–52.

4. P. Klemperer, "Chronic intrahepatic obliterating cholangitis," *J Mt Sinai Hosp* 4 (1937): 270–91.

5. See the article by Schaffner, the Web site noted in n. 2, and the chapter on the Department of Pathology.

6. R. Ottenberg and R. Spiegel, "The present status of non-obstructive jaundice due to infectious and chemical agents: causative agents, pathogenesis, inter-relationships, clinical characteristics," *Medicine* 22 (1943): 27–71.

7. H. Sobotka, *Physiological Chemistry of the Bile* (Baltimore: Williams and Wilkins, 1937).

8. I. Snapper and A. Saltzman, "Quantitative aspects of benzoyl glucuronate formation in normal individuals and in patients with liver disorders," *Am J Med* 11 (1947): 327–33.

9. S. S. Lichtman and A. R. Sohval, "Clinical disorders with associated hepatic and renal manifestations, with especial reference to the so-called 'hepatorenal' syndrome," *Am J Dig Dis Nutr* 4 (1937): 26–32.

10. S. S. Lichtman, *Diseases of the Liver, Gallbladder and Bile Ducts*, 3rd ed. (Philadelphia: Lea and Febiger, 1953).

11. H. Popper and F. Schaffner, *Liver: Structure and Function* (New York: Blakiston, 1957).

12. F. Schaffner, "History of liver disease," p. 78.

13. See the Web site cited in n. 2 for selected references.

14. T. L. Fabry and F. M. Klion, *Guide to Liver Transplantation* (New York: Igaku-Shoin Medical Publishers, 1992).

15. P. D. Berk, "Foreword: An institutional perspective on liver transplantation," in Fabry and Klion, *Guide to Liver Transplantation*, pp. v–ix.

16. W. Stremmel, G. Strohmeyer, F. Borchard, et al., "Isolation and partial characterization of a fatty acid binding protein in rat liver plasma membranes," *Proc Natl Acad Sci USA* 82 (1985): 4–8; P. D. Berk, H. Wada, Y. Horio, et al., "Plasma membrane fatty acid-binding protein and mitochondrial glutamic- oxaloacetic transaminase of rat liver are related," *Proc Natl Acad Sci USA* 87 (1990): 3484–88. See also the chapter on the Division of Hematology for more on Berk.

17. B. S. Coller, as quoted in *Inside Mount Sinai*, Issue of April 10–16, 2000, p. 2.

18. F. Schaffner, "History of liver disease," p. 81.

19. H. C. Bodenheimer, Jr., N. F. LaRusso, W. F. Thayer, Jr., et al., "Elevated circulating immune complexes in primary sclerosing cholangitis," *Hepatology* 3 (1983): 150–54.

20. H. C. Bodenheimer, Jr., K. L. Lindsay, G. L. Davis, et al., "Tolerance and efficacy of oral ribavirin treatment of chronic hepatitis C: A multicenter trial," *Hepatology* 26 (1997): 473–77. Bodenheimer was the principal investigator of this multicenter trial. See the Web site cited in n. 2 for additional citations to other clinical trials.

21. S. L. Friedman, F. J. Roll, J. Boyles, and D. M. Bissell, "Hepatic lipocytes: The principal collagen-producing cells of normal rat liver," *Proc Natl Acad Sci USA* 82 (1985): 8681–85.

22. S. L. Friedman, "Seminars in medicine of the Beth Israel Hospital, Boston. The cellular basis of hepatic fibrosis. Mechanisms and treatment strategies," *N Engl J Med* 328 (1993): 1828–35.

NOTES TO CHAPTER 9

1. "60% Cured," *Time*, March 21, 1938. For more on Lewisohn see also the chapters on the Department of Surgery and the Division of Hematology.

2. C. Leuchtenberger, R. Lewisohn, D. Laszlo, and R. Leuchtenberger, "Folic Acid," a tumor growth inhibitor," *Proc Soc Exp Biol* 55 (1944): 204–5; R. Lewisohn, D. Laszlo, R. Leuchtenberger, and C. Leuchtenberger, "The Action of xanthopterin on tumor growth," *Proc Soc Exp Biol* 56 (1944): 144–45. Cecele Leuchtenberger held a B.S. degree and was an Assistant Bacteriologist in the Laboratories; Rudolph Leuchtenberger and Laszlo were physicians with appointments in Pathology.

3. D. Laszlo and C. Leuchtenberger, "Rapid test for tumor growth inhibitors," *Cancer Res* 3 (1943): 401–10.

4. R. Leuchtenberger, C. Leuchtenberger, D. Laszlo, and R. Lewisohn, "Influence of 'folic acid' on spontaneous breast cancers in mice," *Science* 101 (1945): 46.

5. N. B. Bikhazi, A. M. Kramer, J. H. Spiegel, and M. I. Singer, "'Babe' Ruth's illness and its impact on medical history," *Laryngoscope* 109 (1999): 1–2. Subsequent discussion of this case is based on this article.

6. This was not to be. Soon after his retirement, a generous donor bequeathed a sum of money for Lewisohn to establish a new lab. He determined that cell biology would be important in the future, and so a Cell Research Laboratory was opened in 1954, when Lewisohn was eighty years old. He went to the laboratory nearly every day for the next five years.

7. E. M. Greenspan and M. Fieber, "Combination chemotherapy of advanced ovarian carcinoma with the antimetabolite methotrexate and the alkylating agent thio-TEPA," *J Mt Sinai Hosp* 29 (1962): 48–62; E. M. Greenspan, M. Fieber, G. Lesnick, and S. Edelman, "Response of advanced breast carcinoma to the combination of the antimetabolite methotrexate and the alkylating agent thio-TEPA," *J Mt Sinai Hosp* 30 (1963): 246–67; E. M. Greenspan, "Combination of cytotoxic chemotherapy in advanced disseminated breast carcinoma," *J Mt Sinai Hosp* 33 (1966): 1–27.

8. Interview of Ezra Greenspan, M.D., by Arthur Aufses, M.D., March 22, 1999; INT88, Mount Sinai Archives.

9. H. Bruckner, C. J. Cohen, G. Deppe, et al., "Chemotherapy of gynecologic tumors with platinum II," *J Clin Hemat Oncol* 7 (1977): 619–32.

10. See also the chapter on the Division of Hematology.

11. C. Friend, W. Scher, J. G. Holland, and T. Sato, "Hemoglobin synthesis in murine virus-induced leukemic cells in vitro: Stimulation of erythroid differentiation by dimethyl sulfoxide," *Proc Nat Acad Sci USA* 68 (1971): 378–82.

12. M. Weil, O. Glidewell, C. Jacquillat, et al., "Daunorubicin in the therapy

of acute granulocytic leukemia, *Cancer Res* 33 (1973): 921–28; J. W. Yates, H. J. Wallace Jr., R. R. Ellison, and J. F. Holland, "Cytosine arabinoside (NSC 63878) and daunorubicin (NSC 83142) therapy in acute nonlymphocytic leukemia," *Cancer Chemo Reports* 57 (1973): 485–88.

13. D. C. Tormey, J. F. Holland, V. Weinberg, et al., "5-Drug vs 3-drug MER positive chemotherapy for mammary carcinoma," in *Adjuvant Therapy of Cancer III*, ed. S. E. Salmon and S. E. Jones (New York: Grune and Stratton, 1981). pp. 377–84.

14. J. F. Holland and E. Frei III, *Cancer Medicine* (Philadelphia: Lea and Febiger, 1973).

15. J. D. Jiang, J. Roboz, I. Weisz, et al., "Synthesis, cancericidal, and antimicrotubule activities of 3- (haloacetamido)-benzoylureas," *Anticancer Drug Des* 4 (1998): 735–47.

16. B. Lui, Y. Wang, S. M. Melana, et al., "Identification of a proviral structure in human breast cancer," *Cancer Res* 61 (2001): 1754–59.

17. *The Mount Sinai Journal of Medicine* 59 (October 1992).

18. T. Ohnuma, Introduction to the Symposium "Human Cancer: From 'Precurable' to Curable," May 29, 1990, *Mt Sinai J Med* 59 (1992): 373.

19. Ibid.

20. The Mount Sinai Hospital, *Annual Report for 1998*, p. 50.

NOTES TO CHAPTER 10

1. As quoted in G. E. Schreiner, "How end-stage renal disease (ESRD)-Medicare developed," *Am J Kidney Dis* 35, Suppl. 1 (2000): S37–44.

2. A. A. Epstein, "Concerning the causation of edema in chronic parenchymatous nephritis: Method for its alleviation," *Am J Med Sci* 154 (1917): 638–47.

3. Ibid. Reprinted in *Am J Med* 13 (1952): 556–61. Annotation by A. B. Gutman, p. 556.

4. A. P. Fishman, I. G. Kroop, E. Leiter, and C. A. Hyman, "Experiences with the Kolff artificial kidney," *Am J Med* 7 (1949): 15–34.

5. S. Rosenak and P. Siwon, "Experimentelle untersuchungen uber die peritoneale aussscheidung harnpflichtiger substanzen aus dem blute" [Experimental investigation of the peritoneal clearance of urea-bound substances from the blood]. *A Med U Chir* 39 (1926): 391–408.

6. S. S. Rosenak and G. D. Oppenheimer, "An improved drain for peritoneal dialysis," *Surgery* 23 (1949): 832–33. See also the chapter on the Department of Urology.

7. B. S. Oppenheimer, S. S. Rosenak, and G. D. Oppenheimer, "Blood pressure of chronic hypertensive dogs surviving bilateral nephrectomy," *J Mt Sinai Hosp* 19 (1952): 266–74.

8. A. B. Gutman and T. F. Yu, "Benemid (p-(di-n- propylsulfamyl) -benzoic acid) as uricosuric agent in chronic gouty arthritis," *Trans Assoc Am Physicians* 64 (1951): 279–88. See also chapter 1, "The Leadership," and the chapter on the Division of Rheumatology.

9. A. B. Gutman, T. F. Yu, and L. Berger, "Tubular secretion of urate in man," *J Clin Invest* 38 (1959): 1778–81.

10. The Mount Sinai Hospital, *Annual Report for 1957.*

11. S. Kupfer and S. S. Rosenak, "A new parallel tube continuous hemodialyzer," *J Lab Cl Med* 54 (1959): 746–55.

12. S. Kupfer and R. Goyo, "A new easily inserted catheter for intermittent peritoneal dialysis," *JAMA* 200 (1967): 595–97.

13. L. A. Kuhn, F. L. Gruber, A. Frankel, and S. Kupfer, "Hemodynamic effects of extracorporeal circulation," *Circ Res* 8 (1960): 199–206.

14. L. Burrows, P. Stritzke, and S. Kupfer, "The simultaneous measurement of glomerular filtration rate (GFR) and renal plasma flow (RPF) following renal transplantation by use of functional imaging," *Int J Artif Organs* 14 (1991): 667–71.

15. R. M. Stein, D. D. Bercovitch, and M. F. Levitt, "Dual effects of saline loading on renal tubular sodium reabsorption in the dog," *Am J Physiol* 207 (1964): 826–34; R. M. Stein, R. G. Abramson, T. Kahn, and M. F. Levitt, "Effects of hypotonic saline loading in hydrated dog. Evidence for a saline-induced limit on distal tubular sodium transport," *J Clin Invest* 46 (1967): 1205–14; G. Mohammad, V. DiScala, and R. M. Stein, "Effects of salt depletion on sodium and water reabsorption in dogs," *Am J Physiol* 227 (1974): 469–76.

16. A. Lauer, A. Saccaggi, C. Ronco, et al., "Continuous arteriovenous hemofiltration in the critically ill patient. Clinical use and operational characteristics," *Ann Intern Med* 99 (1983): 455–60.

17. J. A. Winston, M. E. Klotman, and P. E. Klotman, "HIV-associated nephropathy is a late, not early, manifestation of HIV-1 infection," *Kidney Int* 55 (1999): 1036–40; J. A. Winston, G. C. Burns, and P. E. Klotman, "Treatment of HIV-associated nephropathy," *Semin Nephrol* 20 (2000): 293–98. See also the chapter on the Division of Infectious Diseases.

18. E. Leal-Pinto, W. Tao, J. Rappaport, et al., "Molecular cloning and functional reconstitution of a urate transporter/channel," *J Biol Chem* 272 (1997): 617–25.

19. M. S. Lipkowitz, E. Leal-Pinto, J. Z. Rappoport, et al., "Functional reconstitution, membrane targeting, genomic structure, and chromosomal localization of a human urate transporter," *J Clin Invest* 107 (2001): 1103–15.

20. B. Hanss, E. Leal-Pinto, L. A. Bruggeman, et al., "Identification and characterization of a cell membrane nucleic acid channel," *Proc Natl Acad Sci USA* 95 (1998): 1921–26.

21. L. A. Bruggeman, M. D. Ross, N. Tanji, et al., "Renal epithelium is a previously unrecognized site of HIV-1 infection," *J Am Soc Nephrol* 11 (2000): 2079–87.

22. M. S. Lipkowitz, B. Hanss, N. Tulchin, et al., "Transduction of renal cells in vitro and in vivo by adeno-associated virus gene therapy vectors," *J Am Soc Nephrol* 10 (1999): 1908–15.

NOTES TO CHAPTER 11

1. A. Meyer, "Recollections of old Mount Sinai days," *J Mt Sinai Hosp* 3 (1937): 295–307.

2. I. Cohen, "Alfred Meyer: An appreciation," *J Mt Sinai Hosp* 10 (1944): 503–7.

3. H. Wessler and C. B. Rabin, "Benign tumors of the bronchus," *Am J Med Sci* 183 (1932): 164–80.

4. H. Wessler and L. Jaches, *Clinical Roentgenology of Diseases of the Chest* (Troy, N.Y.: Southworth, 1923).

5. H. Wessler, "Lung suppuration after tonsillectomy," *Interstate Med J* (Supplement Roentgenology II) 23 (1916): 5–9.

6. R. Kramer and A. Glass, "Bronchoscopic localization of lung abscess.," *Am J Otol Rhin Laryngol* 41 (1932): 1210–20. See also the chapter on the Department of Otolaryngology.

7. H. Neuhof and A. S. W. Touroff, "Acute putrid abscess of the lung: Principles of operative treatment," *Surg Gynecol Obstet* 63 (1936): 353–68. See also the chapter on the Department of Cardiothoracic Surgery.

8. C. B. Rabin, An Interview with Dr. Coleman Rabin held on July 8, 1965 [sound recording]. Interviewed by Albert S. Lyons. INT38, 1965.

9. C. B. Rabin, "Precise localization of pulmonary abscess," *J Thor Surg* 10 (1941): 662–71.

10. C. B. Rabin, "A technique for the more precise localization of pulmonary abscesses," *Am J Roentgenol Radium Ther* 46 (1941): 130–31.

11. P. Klemperer and C. B. Rabin, "Primary neoplasms of the pleura; report of five such cases," *Arch Pathol* 11 (1931): 385–412.

12. H. Wessler and C. B. Rabin: 164–80.

13. C. B. Rabin and H. Neuhof, "A topographical classification of primary cancers of the lung: Its application to operative indication and treatment," *J Thor Surg* 4 (1934): 147–64.

14. C. B. Rabin, *X-Ray Diagnosis of Chest Diseases* (Baltimore: Williams and Wilkins, 1952).

15. C. B. Rabin and M. G. Baron, *Radiology of the Chest* (Baltimore: Williams and Wilkins, 1980).

16. L. E. Siltzbach, "Effects of cortisone in sarcoidosis. A study of thirteen patients," *Am J Med* 12 (1952): 139–60.

17. L. E. Siltzbach and J. C. Ehrlich, "The Nickerson-Kveim reaction in sarcoidosis," *Am J Med* 16 (1954): 790–803.

18. L. E. Siltzbach, "Pulmonary sarcoidosis," *Am J Med* 89 (1955): 556–68.

19. L. E.Siltzbach, "Significance and specificity of Kveim reaction," *Acta Med Scand* (Suppl. 425) 176 (1964): 74–78.

20. L. E. Siltzbach, "An international Kveim test study," *Acta Med Scand* (Suppl. 425) 176 (1964): 178–90.

21. E. H. Robitzek and I. J. Selikoff, "Hydrazine derivatives of isonicotinic acid (Rimifon, Marsalid) in the treatment of active progressive caseous-pneumonic tuberculosis," *Am Rev Tuber* 65 (1952): 402–428.

22. I. J. Selikoff, J. Churg, and E. C. Hammond, "Asbestos exposure and neoplasia," *JAMA* 188 (1964): 22–26.

23. I. J. Selikoff, E. C. Hammond, and J. Churg, "Asbestos exposure, smoking and neoplasia." *JAMA* 204 (1968): 106–12.

24. A. S. Teirstein, M. Chuang, and A. Miller, "Application of the flexible bronchoscope," *Mt Sinai J Med* 42 (1975): 81–94.

25. A. S. Teirstein, M. Chuang, A. Miller, and L. E. Siltzbach, "Flexible-bronchoscope biopsy of lung and bronchial wall in intrathoracic sarcoidosis," *Ann NY Acad Sci* 278 (1976): 522–27.

26. A. S. Teirstein, M. J. Rosen, D. Mildvan, et al., "Management of opportunistic pneumonia in AIDS," *Ann NY Acad Sci* 437 (1984): 461–65.

NOTES TO CHAPTER 12

1. Guillaume Baillou, "Description of the first affection which is given the name of rheumatism," in Baillou, *Liber de Rheumatismo. Opera Medica Omnia* (Geneva: De Tournes, 1762), cited in R. H. Major, *Classic Descriptions of Disease*, 3rd ed. (Springfield, Ill.: Charles C. Thomas, 1945), pp. 212–13.

2. See the chapter on the Department of Orthopaedics for more on Nathan.

3. See the chapter on the Division of Cardiology for citations.

4. G. Baehr, P. Klemperer, and A. Schifrin, "A diffuse disease of the peripheral circulation (usually associated with lupus erythematosus and endocarditis)," *Trans Assoc Am Physicians* 50 (1935): 139–55.

5. See the chapter on the Laboratory Departments for more on Shwartzman and for citations.

6. P. Klemperer, A. D. Pollack, and G. Baehr, "Diffuse collagen disease: Acute disseminated lupus erythematosus and diffuse scleroderma," *JAMA* 119 (1942): 331–32.

7. J. Churg and L. Strauss, "Allergic granulomatosis, allergic angiitis and periarteritis nodosa," *Am J Path* 27 (1951): 277–301.

8. A. B. Gutman and T. F. Yu, "Benemid (p-di-propylsulfamyl-benzoic acid) as uricosuric agent in chronic gouty arthritis," *Trans Assoc Am Physicians* 64 (1951): 279–88. See also chapter 1, "The Leadership," and the chapter on the Division of Nephrology.

9. T. F. Yu and A. B. Gutman, "Efficacy of colchicine prophylaxis in gout. Prevention of recurrent gouty arthritis over a mean period of five years in 208 gouty patients," *Ann Int Med* 55 (1961): 179–92.

10. J. M. Singer and C. M. Plotz, "The latex fixation test. I. Application to the serologic diagnosis of rheumatoid arthritis," *Am J Med* 21 (1956): 888–92; C. M. Plotz and J. M. Singer, "The latex fixation test. II. Results in rheumatoid arthritis," *Am J Med* 21 (1956): 893–96.

11. S. Davison, H. Spiera, and C. M. Plotz, "Polymyalgia rheumatica," *Arthritis Rheum* 9 (1966): 18–23.

12. C. R. Steinman, U. Deesomchok, and H. Spiera, "Proceedings: Detection of antibody to nature DNA (N–DNA): Increased specificity for active SLE by using a synthetic N–DNA antigen free of contaminating single-stranded DNA (ss-DNA)," *Arthritis Rheum* 18 (1975): 284.

13. H. Spiera and R. R. Rothenberg, "Myocardial infarction in four young patients with SLE," *J Rheumatol* 10 (1983): 464–66.

14. H. Spiera, W. Lawson, and H. Weinrauch, "Wegener's granulomatosis treated with sulfamethoxazole-trimethoprim. Report of a case," *Arch Intern Med* 148 (1988): 2065–66.

NOTES TO CHAPTER 13

1. *Case Records of the Jews' Hospital, 1855–1856.* Mount Sinai Archives.

2. J. J. Walsh, *History of Medicine in New York*, 5 vols. (New York: National Americana Society, 1919), 1: 167.

3. *Case Records, 1855–1856.* Mount Sinai Archives.

4. Also spelled "Krakowizer" or "Krakowitzer."

5. The Mount Sinai Hospital, *Annual Report for 1876*, pp. 24–25. Mount Sinai Archives.

6. A. G. Gerster, *Recollections of a New York Surgeon* (New York: Paul B. Hoeber, 1917), p. 209.

7. W. J. Mayo, "Master surgeons of America: Arpad Geza Charles Gerster," *Surg Gynecol Obstet* 40 (1925): 582–84.

8. A. G. Gerster, *The Rules of Aseptic and Antiseptic Surgery: A Practical Treatise for the Use of Students and the General Practitioner* (New York: D. Appleton, 1888).

9. Ibid., p. viii. Italics are Gerster's.

10. A. A. Berg, "An interview with Dr. A. A. Berg on the development of the surgical services at Mount Sinai." Mount Sinai Archives, 1939.

11. W. J. Mayo, "Master surgeons of America."

12. A. G. Gerster, "On the surgical dissemination of cancer," *NY Med J* 41 (1885): 233–36.

13. M. M. Ravitch, *A Century of Surgery: The History of the American Surgical Association*, 2 vols. (Philadelphia: J. B. Lippincott, 1981).

14. A. G. Gerster, *Recollections of a New York Surgeon.*

15. J. A. Wyeth, *With Sabre and Scalpel: The Autobiography of a Soldier and Surgeon* (New York: Harper and Bros., 1914).

16. Lilienthal's early years were spent as a general surgeon. After 1914, when he was placed in charge of the thoracic service, he devoted himself almost entirely to thoracic surgery. The chapter on Cardiothoracic Surgery documents that phase of his career.

17. H. Lilienthal, "Hyperplastic colitis: Extirpation of the entire colon, the upper portion of the sigmoid flexure, and four inches of the ileum," *Amer Med* 1 (1901): 164–65.

18. H. Lilienthal, "Suprapubic prostatectomy in two stages," *NY Med J* 91 (1910): 1279–82.

19. H. Lilienthal, "Transfusion by Lewisohn's citrate method; the first case in a human being in North America," *J Mt Sinai Hosp* 4 (1937–38): 200–2.

20. See the chapter on the Department of Neurosurgery.

21. See the chapter on the Department of Urology.

22. A. A. Berg, Interview, 1939. Mount Sinai Archives.

23. J. C. Gerster, An Interview with Dr. John Gerster, November 16, 1965. Mount Sinai Archives.

24. B. B. Crohn, L. Ginzburg, and G. D. Oppenheimer, "Regional ileitis," *JAMA* 99 (1932): 1323–28.

25. Surgeons of the Mount Sinai Hospital, *The Surgical Technique of Dr. A. A. Berg: A Tribute to Forty Years' Service at the Mount Sinai Hospital* (New York: Mount Sinai Hospital, 1934).

26. A. A. Berg, "The radical operative cure of gastric and duodenal ulcer," *Surg Cl N Am* 8 (1928): 1167–91.

27. A. A. Berg, "The mortality and late results of subtotal gastrectomy for the radical cure of gastric and duodenal ulcer," *Ann Surg* 92 (1930): 340–59.

28. See the chapter on the Division of Hematology.

29. R. Lewisohn, "The frequency of gastrojejunal ulcers," *Surg Gynecol Obstet* 40 (1925): 70–76.

30. See the chapter on Neoplastic Diseases for a more complete discussion and pertinent references.

31. S. R. Kagan, *Jewish Contributions to Medicine in America*, 2d ed. (Boston: Boston Medical Publishing Co., 1939), p. 656.

32. A. V. Moschcowitz, "Femoral hernia: A new operation for the radical cure," *NYS J Med* 7 (1907): 396–400.

33. A. V. Moschcowitz, "The pathogenesis, anatomy, and cure of prolapse of the rectum," *Surg Gynecol Obstet* 15 (1912): 7–21.

34. A. V. Moschcowitz, "Hernia of the large intestine, with special reference to 'sliding hernia,'" *Ann Surg* 59 (1914): 610–20.

35. See the chapter on the Department of Cardiothoracic Surgery for details of the Commission's findings and report.

36. L. Buerger, "Thromboangiitis obliterans: A study of the vascular lesions leading to presenile spontaneous gangrene," *Am J Med Sci* 136 (1908): 567–80.

37. L. Buerger, *The Circulatory Disturbances of the Extremities Including Gangrene, Vasomotor and Trophic Disorders* (Philadelphia: W. B. Saunders, 1924).

38. See the chapter on the Department of Urology.

39. S. Silbert, "Etiology of thromboangiitis obliterans," *JAMA* 129 (1945): 5–9.

40. See the chapter on the Department of Neurosurgery.

41. See the chapter on the Department of Urology.

42. B. B. Crohn, L. Ginzburg, and G. D. Oppenheimer, "Regional iletis." See also the chapter on Gastroenterology for a discussion of the conflict between Crohn and Ginzburg. Although Ginzburg acknowledged that Crohn had "spread the gospel" about regional enteritis throughout the world, he remained bitter to the end in relation to the eponym.

43. R. Colp, "A case of non-specific granuloma of the terminal ileum and cecum," *Surg Clin N Amer* 14 (1934): 443–49.

44. F. Hollander, E. E. Jemerin, and V. Weinstein, "An insulin test for differentiating vagal from non-vagal stomach pouches," *Fed Proc* 1 (1942): 116.

45. See the Afterword for a more complete discussion of the Gold-Headed Cane.

46. J. H. Garlock, "The reestablishment of esophagogastric continuity following resection of esophagus for carcinoma of the middle third," *Surg Gynecol Obstet* 78 (1944): 23–38.

47. J. L. Madden, "Reflections of J. L. Madden, M.D.," *Contemporary Surg* 31 (1987): 28–34.

48. J. H. Garlock, *Garlock's Surgery of the Alimentary Tract* (New York: Appleton-Century Crofts, 1967).

49. Neuhof and Touroff contributed in a very major way to the development of thoracic and cardiac surgery. See the chapter on The Department of Cardiothoracic Surgery for their accomplishments.

50. The introducer was the Chairman, Arthur H. Aufses, Jr., M.D.

51. See the chapter on the Department of Cardiothoracic Surgery for more details.

52. Ibid.

53. J. H. Jacobson and E. L. Suarez, "Microsurgery in anastomoses of small vessels," *Surg Forum* 11 (1960): 243–45.

54. L. Blum and S. J. Megibow, "Exclusion of the dog heart by parabiosis," *J Mt Sinai Hosp* 17 (1950): 38–43.

55. R. A. Nabatoff and D. C. Stark, "Complete stripping of varicose veins with the patient on an ambulatory basis," *Am J Surg* 124 (1972): 634–36.

56. See the chapter on the Department of Cardiothoracic Surgery.

57. L. Burrows and P. Tartter, "Effect of blood transfusions on colonic malignancy recurrence rate," *Lancet* 2, no. 8299 (1982): 662.

58. H. Schanzer, M. Schwartz, E. Harrington, and M. Haimov, "Treatment of ischemia due to 'steal' by arteriovenous fistula with distal artery ligation and revascularization," *J Vasc Surg* 7 (1988): 770–73.

59. A complete description of the accomplishments of the SICU is beyond the scope of this work. It is detailed in A. B. Leibowitz, "The Surgical Intensive Care Unit of The Mount Sinai Hospital: A brief history with focus on its contributions to academic critical care medicine and excellence in patient care," *Mt Sinai J Med* 69 (2002): 25–30. The references are also available at www.mountsinaihistory.org.

60. T. E. Starzl, C. Miller, B. Broznick, and L. Makowka, "An improved technique for multiple organ harvesting," *Surg Gynecol Obstet* 165 (1987): 343–48.

NOTES TO CHAPTER 14

1. *Case Records of the Jews' Hospital, 1855–1856.* Mount Sinai Archives.

2. S. M. Brickner, "Some remarks on anesthesia from ether and chloroform," *Medical News* 67 (1895): 508–11.

3. *Minutes of the Medical Board, 1898.* Mount Sinai Archives.

4. M. L. Maduro and M. P. Denton, "Report of anesthesias," in *Mount Sinai Hospital Reports* (New York: Stettiner Bros., 1903), 563–72.

5. Ibid., p. 569.

6. C. Koller, "Preliminary report on local anesthesia of the eye," *Wiener Medizinische Wochenschaft*, October 25 (1884). Translated and reprinted in *Arch Ophth* 12 (1934): 473–74. See also the chapter on the Department of Ophthalmology.

7. B. M. Duncum, *The Development of Inhalation Anaesthesia—with Special Reference to the Years 1846–1900* (London: Oxford University Press, 1947).

8. Maduro and Denton, "Report of anesthesias," p. 572.

9. Ibid., p. 572.

10. W. Branower, "Artificial respiration by an apparatus which permits measured and controlled volumes and pressures," *J Thor Surg* 5 (1936): 377–83.

11. B. M. Duncum, *The Development of Inhalation Anaesthesia.*

12. C. A. Elsberg, "The value of continuous intratracheal insufflation of air (Meltzer) in thoracic surgery," *Medical Record*, March 19, 1910. Off print available in the Levy Library of The Mount Sinai Medical Center. See also C. A. Elsberg, "Anaesthesia by the intratracheal insufflation of air and ether; a description

of the technic of the method and of a portable apparatus for use in man," *Ann Surg* 53 (1911): 161–68.

13. C. A. Elsberg, "Clinical experiences with intratracheal insufflation (Meltzer) with remarks upon the value of the method for thoracic surgery," *Ann Surg* 52 (1910): 23–29.

14. H. Lilienthal, "The first case of thoracotomy in a human being under anaesthesia by intratracheal insufflation," *Ann Surg* 52 (1910): 30–33.

15. See the chapter on the Department of Neurosurgery.

16. M. Adelman, R. A. Berman, and A. S. W. Touroff, "Automatic controlled respiration: A preliminary report," *Anesthesiology* 10 (1949): 673–76.

17. M. Adelman, S. J. Megibow, and L. Blum, "A method of automatic controlled respiration for anesthesia in the dog," *Surgery* 28 (1950): 1040–42.

18. M. Bien, "General anesthesia in ophthalmic surgery," *Am J Ophthalmal* 29 (1946): 1119–21.

19. M. Bien, "Anesthesia for gastric surgery," *Surg Cl N Am* 27 (1947): 261–64.

20. M. Bien, "General anesthesia in ophthalmic surgery."

21. A. B. Leibowitz, "The surgical intensive care unit of the Mount Sinai Hospital: A brief history focusing on contributions to academic critical care medicine and excellence in patient care," *Mt Sinai J Med 69* (2002): 25–30. See also the chapter on the Department of Surgery.

22. B. Ebido, A. Weinreich, and B. Lipton, "Anesthetic agents and neuropsychiatric complications following extracorporeal circulation," *Bull NY Acad Med* 48 (1972): 545–57.

23. B. Lipton, A. Toth, and J. H. Jacobson, "The hyperbaric chamber and pulmonary oxygen toxicity: A clinical and pathologic study," *Mt Sinai J Med* 40 (1973): 7–19.

24. B. Lipton, A. Weinreich, T. Brondum, and J. H. Jacobson II, "Respiratory failure treated in the hyperbaric chamber with the membrane oxygenator. III. Studies of three membranes at various flow rates and ambient pressures," *Anesthesiology* 34 (1971): 421–26.

25. D. C. C. Stark, "In Memoriam: Barbara Lipton, M.D.," *J. Mt Sinai Hosp* 41 (1974): 719–21.

26. R. B. Roberts and M. A. Shirley, "Reducing the risk of acid aspiration during cesarean section," *Anesth Analg* 53 (1974): 859–68.

27. D. S. Girnar and A. I. Weinreich, "Anesthesia for transcervical thymectomy in myasthenia gravis," *Anesth Analg* 55 (1976): 13–17.

28. D. C. C. Stark and R. B. Roberts, *Practical Points in Anesthesiology*, 1st ed. (New York: Med. Exam. Publ. Co., 1974).

29. J. A. Kaplan, *Cardiac Anesthesia* (New York: Grune and Stratton, 1979).

30. J. A. Kaplan, "Role of ultrashort-acting B-blockers in the perioperative period," *J Cardiothor Anesth* 2 (1988): 683–91.

31. S. N. Konstadt, D. Thys, B. P. Mindich, et al., "Validation of quantitative intraoperative transesophageal echocardiography," *Anesthesiology* 65 (1986): 418–21.

32. E. Cohen, *The Practice of Thoracic Anesthesia* (Philadelphia: J. B. Lippincott, 1995).

33. G. V. Gabrielson, A. V. Guffin, J. A. Kaplan, et al., "Continuous intravenous infusions of phentolamine and esmolol for preoperative and intraoperative adrenergic blockage in patients with pheochromocytoma," *J Cardiothor Anesth* 1 (1987): 554–58.

34. J. M. Kreitzer, L. P. Kirschenbaum, and J. B. Eisenkraft, "Epidural fentanyl by continuous infusion for relief of postoperative pain," *Clin J Pain* 5 (1989): 283–90.

NOTES TO CHAPTER 15

1. Gerster, a true general surgeon, published in all realms of surgery. See the chapter on the Department of Surgery for a more complete account of his life and accomplishments.

2. In addition to being the "Father of Thoracic Surgery," Lilienthal made major contributions to general surgery, especially in his earlier years. See the chapter on the Department of Surgery for details of this facet of his work.

3. A. G. Gerster, *Recollections of a New York Surgeon* (New York: Paul B. Hoeber, 1917).

4. H. Lilienthal, "The Mount Sinai Hospital and its surgeons of the middle eighties; a few recollections," *J Mt. Sinai Hosp* 3 (1937): 229–40.

5. H. Lilienthal, "The first case of thoracotomy in a human being under anaesthesia by intratracheal insufflation," *Ann Surg* 52 (1910): 30–33.

6. See the chapter on the Department of Anesthesiology.

7. H. Lilienthal, "Resection of the lung for suppurative infections with a report based on 31 operative cases in which resection was done or intended," *Ann Surg* 75 (1922): 257–320.

8. H. Lilienthal, "Carcinoma of the thoracic esophagus. Successful resection," *Ann Surg* 74 (1921): 116–17.

9. M. M. Ravitch, *A Century of Surgery: The History of the American Surgical Association*, 2 vols. (Philadelphia: J. B. Lippincott, 1981), p. 575.

10. H. Lilienthal, "Malignant tumor of the lung: Necessity for early operation," *Arch Surg* 8 (1924): 308–16.

11. H. Lilienthal, "Thoracic surgery as a specialty," *Ann Surg* 81 (1925): 1191–97.

12. H. Lilienthal, *Thoracic Surgery: The Surgical Treatment of Thoracic Disease*, 1st ed., 2 vols. (Philadelphia: W. B. Saunders, 1926).

13. See the chapter on the Department of Surgery.

14. Empyema Commission, "Cases of empyema at Camp Lee, Petersburg, Virginia," *JAMA* 71 (1918): 366–73; 443–48.

15. A. V. Moschcowitz, "The treatment of diseases of the costal cartilages," *Trans Am Surg Asso* 36 (1918): 327–49.

16. H. Neuhof and S. Hirshfeld, *The Transplantation of Tissues*, 1st ed. (New York: D. Appleton, 1923).

17. H. Neuhof and H. Wessler, "Putrid lung abscess—its etiology, pathology, clinical manifestations, diagnosis and treatment," *J Thor Surg* 1 (1932): 637–49.

18. H. Neuhof and A. S. W. Touroff, "Acute putrid abscess of the lung: principles of operative treatment," *Surg Gynecol Obstet* 63 (1936): 353–68.

19. E. W. Wilkins, Jr., "Acute putrid abscess of the lung," *Ann Thor Surg* 44 (1987): 560–61.

20. H. Neuhof and A. H. Aufses, Sr., "Cancer of the lung. Interval and late results of operation in relation to topography and gross pathology," *J Thor Surg* 17 (1948): 297–305.

21. A. S. W. Touroff and H. Vesell, "Subacute Streptococcus Viridans endocarditis complicating patent ductus arteriosus," *JAMA* 115 (1940): 1270–72.

22. S. Blumenthal, S. Brahms, and M. L. Sussman, "Tricuspid atresia with transposition of the great vessels successfully treated by surgery," *J Mt Sinai Hosp* 17 (1950): 328–35.

23. See the chapter on the Department of Surgery.

24. See the chapter on the Department of Surgery.

25. I. Kreel, L. I. Zaroff, J. W. Canter, et al., "A syndrome following total body perfusion," *Surg Gynecol Obstet* 111 (1960): 317–21.

26. P. A. Kirschner, "Mediastinoscopy: Experiences with fifty cases," *J Mt Sinai Hosp* 34 (1967): 559–73.

27. P. A. Kirschner, K. E. Osserman, and A. E. Kark, "Studies in myasthenia gravis. Transcervical total thymectomy," *JAMA* 209 (1969): 906–10.

28. R. A. Jurado, H. L. Fitzkee, R. A. de Asla, et al., "Reduction of unexpected, life-threatening events in postoperative cardiac surgical patients; the role of computerized surveillance," *Circulation* 56, Suppl II (1977): 44-9.

29. R. S. Litwak, R. M. Koffsky, S. B. Lukban, et al., "Implanted heart assist device after intracardiac surgery," *N Engl J Med* 291 (1974): 1341–43.

NOTES TO CHAPTER 16

1. G. Fischer and H. Heuser, *The Early Days of Local Anaesthesia in Dentistry [motion picture]: The Story of Injection Analgesia: Illustrated by Extracts from a Film Made by and Showing Prof. Dr. Guido Fischer in 1914* (Frankfurt-am-Main: Farbwerke Hoechst, 1914).

2. L. Stern, "Putrid abscess of lung following dental operations," *J Thor Surg* 4 (1935): 547–57; L. Stern, "Two pulmonary abscesses in a patient with a fourteen-year interval," *J Mt Sinai Hosp* 3 (1936): 118–20; L. Stern, "Etiologic factors in the pathogenesis of putrid abscess of the lung," *J Thor Surg* 6 (1936): 202–11.

3. See the chapter on the Division of Pulmonary Medicine for earlier work on the subject by Harry Wessler.

4. L. Stern and L. Eisenbud, "Giant hyperplasia of the gums from dilantin sodium," *J Mt Sinai Hosp* 9 (1942): 100–3.

5. L. Stern, L. Eisenbud, and J. Klatell, "Analysis of oral reactions to dilantin sodium," *J Dent Res* 22 (1943): 157–64.

6. L. Stern and M. Gottlieb, "Metastatic tumor of the maxilla derived from carcinoma of the lung," *J Mt Sinai Hosp* 4 (1938): 452–56.

7. *Minutes of the Medical Board*. Mount Sinai Archives, 1946, p. 199.

8. Ibid.

9. L. Stern, "Preliminary report on penicillin in dentistry," *Ann Dent* 3 (1944): 1–4.

10. J. A. Salzmann, "General growth acceleration and retardation in relation to dentofacial development," *Am J Orthod* 40 (1954): 243.

11. J. A. Salzmann and D. B. Ast, "The Newburgh-Kingston fluorine study. IX. Dentofacial growth and development cephalometric study," *Am J Orthod* 41 (1955): 674.

12. L. Stern, Jr., "The diagnosis of pemphigus by its oral signs," *Oral Surg Oral Med Oral Pathol* 2 (1949): 1447–53.

13. L. Stern, Jr., "Conservative surgery of the mandible," *J Mt Sinai Hosp* 18 (1951): 103–18.

14. L. Stern, Jr., and S. Lane, "The Hospital Cleft Palate Center: Surgical problems and procedures," *NY State Dent J* 23 (1957): 245–50.

15. L. Stern, Jr., and P. Stern, "Cleft palate rehabilitation: A community service," *NY State Dent J* 37 (1972): 407–12.

16. J. A. Markowitz, R. G. Gerry, and R. Fleishner, "Immediate obturation of neonatal cleft palates," *Mt Sinai J Med* 46 (1979): 123–29.

17. B. E. Evans, L. M. Aledort, J. Klatell, et al., "Dental Care for Hemophiliacs," *J Hosp Dent Pract* 11 (1977): 10–12.

18. J. Klatell, M. Rubin, and B. E. Evans, "Dental care for the cardiac patient," *Primary Cardiology Publication* 4 (1978): 56–59.

19. J. Klatell and A. S Kaplan, "Dental complications of pregnancy," in *Rovinsky and Guttmacher's Medical, Surgical, and Gynecological Complications of Pregnancy*, ed. S. H. Cherry, R. L. Berkowitz, and N. G. Kase (Baltimore: Williams and Wilkins, 1985), pp. 820–25.

20. J. Klatell, J. Hirsch, W. Heilbut, and D. Rosenman, "A new approach to hospital dentistry," *NY State Dent J* 38 (1972): 473–76.

21. A. S. Kaplan and L. A. Assael, *Temporomandibular Disorders: Diagnosis and Treatment* (Philadelphia: W. B. Saunders, 1991).

22. J. Klatell, A. Kaplan, and G. Williams, Jr., *The Mount Sinai Medical Center Family Guide to Dental Health* (New York: Macmillan, 1991).

23. M. L. Urken, D. Buchbinder, P. D. Costantino, et al., "Oromandibular reconstruction using microvascular composite flaps: Report of 210 cases," *Arch Otolaryngol Head Neck Surg* 124 (1998): 46–55.

24. K. E. Blackwell, D. Buchbinder, and M. L. Urken, "Lateral mandibular reconstruction using soft-tissue free flaps and plates," *Arch Otolaryngol Head Neck Surg* 122 (1996): 672–78.

25. K. E. Blackwell, D. Buchbinder, H. F. Biller, and M. L. Urken, "Reconstruction of massive defects in the head and neck: The role of simultaneous distant and regional flaps," *Head Neck* 19 (1997): 620–28.

NOTES TO CHAPTER 17

1. G. H. Fox, *Photographic Illustrations of Skin Diseases* (New York: E. B. Treat, 1881).

2. Interview with Richard Hoffman, M.D., May 5, 1939. In Historian's Office Files, 1852–1952, Box 2: "Depts.: Dermatology," Mount Sinai Archives.

3. Ibid.

4. Interview with Isadore Rosen, M.D., January 10, 1939, Historian's Office Files. Mount Sinai Hospital. Box 2, Folder 4. Mount Sinai Archives.

5. Ibid.

6. Hoffman interview, 1939.

7. W. G. Highman, *Dermatology: The Essentials of Cutaneous Medicine* (New York: Macmillan, 1921).

8. F. J. Szymanski, *Centennial History of the American Dermatological Association 1876–1976* (Chicago: American Dermatological Association, 1976).

9. S. Rosen, H. Rosenfeld, and F. Krasnow, "Effect of hyperpyrexia in the treatment of chronic recurrent dermatoses," *Arch Derm and Syph* 33 (1936): 518–31.

10. Hoffman interview, 1939.

11. The five-day treatment of syphilis by means of the continuous slow intravenous drip method was announced at The New York Academy of Medicine, April 12, 1940. This was a result of work begun five years before. See L. Chargin, W. Leifer, and H. T. Hyman, "Studies in velocity and response to intravenous injections: Application of intravenous drip method to chemotherapy as illustrated by massive doses of arsphenamine in treatment of early syphilis," *JAMA* 104 (1935): 878–83.

12. H. Koplik, "The diagnosis of the invasion of measles from a study of the exanthema as it appears on the buccal mucous membranes," *Arch Pediatr* 13 (1896): 918–22.

13. J. Churg and L. Strauss, "Allergic granulomatosis, allergic angiitis, and periarteritis nodosa," *Am J Path* 27 (1951): 277–301.

14. L. Siltzbach, "An International Kveim Test study," *Acta Med Scand* 176, Suppl 425 (1964): 178–90.

15. L. Siltzbach, "Significance and specificity of the Kveim reaction," *Acta Med Scand* 176, Suppl. 425 (1964): pp. 74–8.

16. S. M. Peck, "Attempts at treatment of hemorrhagic diathesis by injections of snake venom," *Proc Soc Exper Bio and Med* 29 (1932): 579–81.

17. S. M. Peck and H. Rosenfeld, "The effects of hydrogen ion concentration, fatty acids and vitamin C on the growth of fungi," *J Invest Derm* 1 (1938): 237–65.

18. L. Schwartz, L. Tulipan, and S. M. Peck, *Occupational Diseases of the Skin* (Philadelphia: Lea and Febiger, 1947).

19. O. Canizares, *Clinical Tropical Dermatology* (Philadelphia: J. B. Lippincott, 1975).

20. R. Fleischmajer, T. Krieg, M. Dziadek, et al., "Ultrastructure and composition of connective tissue in hyalinosis cutis et mucosae skin," *J Invest Derm* 82 (1984): 252–58.

21. M. G. Lebwohl, *Atlas of the Skin and Systemic Disease* (New York: Churchill Livingstone, 1995).

22. M. G. Lebowhl, ed., *Difficult Diagnoses in Dermatology* (New York: Churchill Livingstone, 1988).

23. M. G. Lebwohl and M. Zanolli, eds., "Psoriasis," *Derm Clin N Am* (Philadelphia: Saunders, 1995).

24. M. G. Lebwohl, R. G. Phelps, L. Yannuzzi, et al., "Diagnosis of pseudoxanthoma elasticum by scar biopsy in patients without characteristic skin lesions," *N Engl J Med* 317 (1987): 347–50.

25. M. G. Lebwohl, J. Halperin, and R. G. Phelps, "Brief report: Occult pseudoxanthoma elasticum in patients with premature cardiovascular disease," *N Engl J Med* 329 (1993): 1237–39.

26. M. G. Lebwohl, D. Distefano, R. G. Prioleau, et al., "Pseudoxanthoma elasticum and mitral-valve prolapse," *N Engl J Med* 307 (1982): 228–31.

27. M. G. Lebwohl, M. O. Longas, J. Konstadt, et al., "Hyaluronic acid and dermatan sulfate in non-lesional pseudoxanthoma elasticum skin," *Clin Chim Acta* 238 (1995): 101–7.

28. S. C. Poliak, M. G. Lebwohl, A. Parris, and P. G. Prioleau, "Reactive perforating collagenosis associated with diabetes mellitus," *N Engl J Med* 306 (1982): 81–84.

29. M. L. Gordon, M. G. Lebwohl, R. G. Phelps, et al., "Eosinophilic fasciitis associated with tryptophan ingestion. A manifestation of eosinophilia-myalgia syndrome," *Arch Dermatol* 127 (1991): 217–20.

30. H. Wei, "Photoprotective action of isoflavone genistein: Models, mechanisms, and relevance to clinical dermatology," *J Am Acad Dermatol* 39 (1998): 271–72.

31. A. Kurtin, "Corrective surgical planing of skin," *Arch Dermatol Syph* 68 (1953): 389–97.

32. S. Bershad, A. Rubinstein, J. R. Paterniti, et al., "Changes in plasma lipids and lipoproteins during isotretinoin therapy for acne," *N Engl J Med* 313 (1985): 981–85.

NOTES TO CHAPTER 18

1. Board of Directors Minutes, June 3, 1855. Mount Sinai Archives.

2. K. M. Baumlin, M. J. Bessette, C. Lewis, and L. D. Richardson, "EMCyberSchool: An evaluation of computer-assisted instruction on the Internet," *Acad Emerg Med* 7 (2000): 959–62.

3. See the Web site www.mountsinaihistory.org for citations to these and other papers by the faculty.

4. E. Mintz and B. Beirne, "Automated external defibrillator: Understanding today's technology, preparing for wider use." *J Crit Illn* 15 (2000); 621–26.

NOTES TO CHAPTER 19

1. I. L. Nascher, "Longevity and rejuvenescence," *NY Med J* 89 (1909): 795–800.

2. Ibid.

3. I. L. Nascher, *Geriatrics: The Diseases of Old Age and Their Treatment, Including Physiological Old Age, Home and Institutional Care, and Medico-legal Relations*, with an introduction by A. Jacobi, M.D. (Philadelphia: P. Blakiston's Son, 1914).

4. L. Libow, "From Nascher to now, seventy-five years of United States geriatrics," *J Am Geriatr Soc* 38 (1990): 79–83.

5. I. L. Nascher, "A history of geriatrics," *Medical Review of Reviews* 32 (1926): 281.

6. "A Brief History," Gerontological Society of America, www.geron.org/history, 2001.

7. M. Pollack, R. L. Kahn, and A. I. Goldfarb, "Factors related to individual differences in perception in institutionalized aged subjects," *J Gerontol* 13 (1958): 192–97.

8. L. S. Libow, "A fellowship in geriatric medicine," *J Am Geriatr Soc* 20 (1972): 580–84.

9. L. S. Libow, "A geriatric medical residency program. A four-year experience." *Ann Int Med* 80 (1976): 641–47.

10. R. N. Butler, "The teaching nursing home," *JAMA* 245 (1981): 1435–37.

11. Interview with Robert Butler, August 28, 2001.

12. Interview with Leslie Libow, July 31, 2001.

13. See also the chapter on the Department of Psychiatry.

14. Butler interview, 2001.

15. Interview with Christine Cassel, September 8, 2001.

16. R. S. Morrison, S. Wallenstein, D. K. Natale, et al., "'We don't carry that'—failure of pharmacies in predominantly nonwhite neighborhoods to stock opioid analgesics," *N Engl J Med* 342 (2000): 1023–26.

17. D. Meier, C. A. Emmons, S. Wallenstein, et al., "A national survey of physician-assisted suicide and euthanasia in the United States," *N Engl J Med* 338 (1998): 1193–201.

18. Interview with Diane Meier and Sean Morrison, September 4, 2001.

19. Annual report of the Department of Geriatrics and Adult Development, 2000, p. 1.

NOTES TO CHAPTER 20

1. B. Sachs, "On arrested cerebral development with special reference on its cortical pathology," *J Nerv Ment Dis* 14 (1887): 541–53.

2. B. Sachs, "A family form of idiocy, generally fatal, associated with early blindness (amaurotic family idiocy)," *J Nerv Ment Dis* 21 (1896): 475–79.

3. B. Sachs, "Progressive muscular dystrophies: The relation of primary forms to one another and to typical progressive muscular atrophy," *NY Med J* 48 (1888): 620–26.

4. B. Sachs and F. Peterson, "A study of cerebral palsies of early life, based upon analysis of one hundred and forty cases," *J Nerv Ment Dis* 17 (1890): 295–332.

5. B. Sachs, *Nervous Disease of Children* (New York: William Wood, 1895).

6. B. Sachs, "What the law can do to mitigate the evils of medical expert testimony," *NY Med Examiner*, April 11, 1892.

7. New York Neurological Society, "Epidemic poliomyelitis: Report on the New York epidemic of 1907 by the Collective Investigation Committee, Dr. B. Sachs, chairman," *Nervous and Mental Disease Monograph* Series 6 (1910).

8. B. Sachs, "The Wassermann reaction in its relation to disease of the central nervous system," *JAMA* 53 (1909): 929–34.

9. D. Denny-Brown, ed., *Centennial Anniversary Volume of the American Neurological Association, 1875–1975* (New York: Springer, 1975).

10. B. Sachs, "False claims of the psychoanalyst: Review and protest," *Am J Psych* 21 (1933): 725–49.

11. Loewe was a house physician at the time. In 1921, he, Ritter, and Baehr isolated *Rickettsia prowazeki* from the blood for the first time. See the chapters on "The Leadership" and the Division of Infectious Diseases.

12. L. Loewe and I. Strauss, "Etiology of epidemic (lethargic) encephalitis. Preliminary note," *JAMA* 73 (1919): 1056–57.

13. I. Strauss and J. H. Globus, "Spongioblastoma with unusually rapid growth following decompression," *Neurological Bulletin* 1 (1918): 273–81.

14. I. Strauss and N. Savitsky, "Head injury: Neurologic and psychiatric aspects," *Arch Neurol Psychiat* 31 (1934): 893–955.

15. I. Strauss and M. Keschner, "Mental symptoms in cases of tumor of the frontal lobe," *Arch Neurol Psychiat* 33 (1935): 986–1007.

16. I. S. Wechsler, *A Text Book of Clinical Neurology* (New York: W. B. Saunders, 1927).

17. I. S. Wechsler and S. Brock, "Dystonia musculorum deformans," *Arch Neurol Psychiatr* 8 (1922): 538–52.

18. R. Brickner, *The Intellectual Functions of the Frontal Lobes* (New York: Macmillan, 1936).

19. This was a critical event in the future of psychiatry. Having created the department, Joseph Klingenstein and his wife, Esther, contributed the funds to create the Klingenstein Clinical Center to house the new Department. See the chapter on the Department of Psychiatry for more details.

20. M. B. Bender and E. A. Weinstein. "Functional representation in the oculomotor and trochlear nuclei," *Arch Neurol and Psychiat* 49 (1943): 98–106.

21. From *Mount Sinai Medical News*, September 10, 1973.

22. E. A. Weinstein and R. L. Kahn, "Denial of illness: Symbolic and physiological aspects," *American Lecture Series, No. 249. The Bannerstone Division of American Lectures in Neurology* (Springfield, Ill.: Charles C. Thomas, 1955).

23. E. A. Weinstein, *Woodrow Wilson, a Medical and Psychological Biography* (Princeton, N.J.: Princeton University Press, 1981).

24. M. B. Bender and H. L. Teuber, "Spatial organization of visual perception following injury to the brain," *Arch Neurol and Psychiat* 58 (1947): 721–39; 59 (1948): 39–62.

25. M. B. Bender, "Disorders in perception, with particular reference to the phenomena of extinction and displacement," *American Lecture Series, No. 120. American Lectures in Neurology* (Springfield, Ill: Charles C. Thomas, 1952).

26. M. B. Bender and S. Shanzer, "Oculomotor pathways defined by electric stimulation and lesions in the brainstem of monkey." In *The Oculomotor System*, ed. M. B. Bender (New York: Paul B. Hoeber, 1964), pp. 81–140.

27. M. B. Bender, "Resolution of subdural hematoma," *Trans Am Neurol Assoc* 58 (1960): 192–94.

28. M. B. Bender, "Syndrome of isolated episode of confusion with amnesia," *J Hillside Hosp* 5 (1956): 212–15.

29. M. D. Yahr, personal communication, September 2001.

30. M. D. Yahr and M. M. Hoehn, "Parkinsonism: Onset, progression, and mortality," *Neurology* 17 (1967): 427–42.

31. M. D. Yahr, R. C. Duvoisin, M. J. Schear, et al., "Treatment of parkinsonism with levodopa," *Arch Neurol* 21 (1969): 343–54.

32. P. Pasik and T. Pasik. "Visual functions in monkeys after total removal of visual cerebral cortex," in *Contributions to Sensory Physiology*, ed. W. D. Neff (New York: Academic Press, 1982), pp. 147–200.

33. P. Pasik, T. Pasik, and J. Martinez, "The neurobiology of non-fetal implants into the dopamine-derived neostriatum, with reference to sympathetic ganglia," *Int J Neurol* 23–24 (1989–1990): 108–31.

34. B. Cohen, J. Suzuki, and M. B. Bender, "Eye movements from semicircular canal nerve stimulation in the cat," *Ann Otol Rhin Laryn* 73 (1964): 153–69.

35. B. Cohen, V. Matsuo, and T. Raphan, "Quantitative analysis of the velocity characteristics of optokinetic nystagmus and optokinetic after-nystagmus," *J Physiol* 270 (1977): 321–44.

36. S. T. Moore, G. Clement, T. Raphan, and B. Cohen, "Ocular counter-rolling (OCR) induced by centrifugation during space flight," *Exp Brain Res* 137 (2001): 323–35.

37. C. E. Morrison, J. C. Borod, M. F. Brin, et al., "A program for neuropsychological investigation of deep brain stimulation (PNIDBS) in movement disorder patients: Development, feasibility, and preliminary data," *Neuropsychiatry Neuropsychol Behav Neurol* 13 (2000): 204–19.

38. M. F. Brin, S. Fahn, C. Moskowitz, et al., "Localized injections of botulinum toxin for the treatment of focal dystonia and hemifacial spasm," *Mov Disord* 2 (1987): 237–54.

39. D. M. Simpson, P. Slasor, U. Dafni, et al., "Analysis of myopathy in a placebo-controlled zidovudine trial," *Muscle Nerve* 20 (1997): 382–85.

NOTES TO CHAPTER 21

1. W. Fluhrer, "A successful operation for the extraction of a pistol-ball from the brain through a counter-opening in the skull," *Quart Bull Clin Soc NY Postgrad Med Sch and Hosp* 1 (1885–86): 209–34.

2. A. Gerster and B. Sachs, "The surgical treatment of epilepsy," *Am J Med Sci* 104 (1892): 503–8.

3. B. Sachs and A. Gerster, "The surgical treatment of focal epilepsy: A critical analysis of the result in nineteen cases," *Am J Med Sci* 112 (1896): 377–93.

4. L. Stieglitz, A. Gerster, and H. Lilienthal, "A study of three cases of tumors of the brain in which operation was performed; one recovery, two deaths," *J Nerv Ment Dis* 22 (1895): 730–33.

5. W. Van Arsdale, "The technique of temporary resection of the skull with demonstration of a new set of instruments," *Ann Surg* 24 (1896): 465–80.

6. See the chapter on the Department of Pathology.

7. C. A. Elsberg, J. Frankel, and J. Hunt, "Report of two cases of tumor of the ponto-medullo-cerebellar space (acoustic neuroma) with operation," *J Nerv Ment Dis* 31 (1904): 468–73.

8. C. A. Elsberg, "A simple cannula for the direct transfusion of blood," *JAMA* 52 (1909): 887–88.

9. C. A. Elsberg, "Clinical experiences with intratracheal insufflation (Meltzer) with remarks upon the value of the method for thoracic surgery," *Ann Surg* 52 (1910): 23–29. See also the chapter on the Department of Anesthesiology.

10. C. A. Elsberg, "The extrusion of intra-spinal tumors: Preliminary report of the application of a new principle to operations for localized extramedullary and intra-medullary growths of the spinal cord," *JAMA* 54 (1910): 1308–9.

11. C. A. Elsberg, "Observations upon a series of fifty-three laminectomies," *Ann Surg* 55 (1912): 217–26.

12. C. A. Elsberg, "Surgery of intramedullary affections of the spinal cord: Anatomic basis and technic," *JAMA* 59 (1912): 1532–36.

13. P. Bailey, discussion of Elsberg, "Surgery of intramedullary affections of the spinal cord," *JAMA* 59 (1912): 1536.

14. Ibid.

15. C. A. Elsberg, "Mount Sinai in the late nineties and the beginning of neurosurgery in the hospital," *J Mt Sinai Hosp* 4 (1937): 430–36.

16. C. A. Elsberg, *Tumors of the Spinal Cord and the Symptoms of Irritation and Compression of the Spinal Cord and Nerve Roots: Pathology, Symptomatology, Diagnosis and Treatment* (New York: Paul B. Hoeber, 1925).

17. C. A. Elsberg, *Surgical Diseases of the Spinal Cord, Membranes, and Nerve Roots: Symptoms, Diagnosis, and Treatment* (New York: Paul B. Hoeber, 1941).

18. C. A. Elsberg, *The Story of a Hospital: The Neurological Institute of New York* (New York: Paul B. Hoeber, 1944).

19. C. A. Elsberg, *Diagnosis and Surgical Treatment of Surgical Diseases of the Spinal Cord and Its Membranes* (Philadelphia: W. B. Saunders, 1916).

20. J. Oppenheim, "Neurosurgery at the Mount Sinai Hospital," *J Neurosurg* 80 (1994): 935–38.

21. I. Cohen and J. Turner, "The neurosurgical department in the hospital," *Modern Hosp* 40 (1933): 92–95.

22. S. Gross, "Cerebral angiography by means of a rapidly excreted organic iodide," *Arch Neurol Psych* 44 (1940): 217–22.

23. A. Marti, "The early history of neurosurgery in New York," *Mt Sinai J Med* 64 (1997): 155–59.

24. L. Kruger and A. J. Berman, "Leonard I. Malis: An appreciation," *Mt Sinai J Med* 64 (1997): 166–71.

25. M. Savitz, "Leonard I. Malis, Honoris Causa," *Mt Sinai J Med* 64 (1997): 153–54. Malis published more than one hundred papers. This article and the one that follows are part of a *Festschrift* of the *Mount Sinai Journal of Medicine* 64 (1997): 152–232 honoring Malis. The citations to Malis's publications can be found there and are also available on the Web site www.mountsinaihistory.org.

26. S. I. Savitz, "Leonard I. Malis and prophylactic antibiotics," *Mt Sinai J Med* 64 (1997): 187–88.

27. K. D. Post, M. B. Eisenberg, and P. J. Catalano, "Hearing preservation in vestibular schwannoma surgery: What factors influence outcome?" *J Neurosurg* 83 (1995): 191–96.

28. P. U. Freda, S. L. Wardlaw, and K. D. Post, "Long-term endocrinological follow-up evaluation in 115 patients who underwent transsphenoidal surgery for acromegaly," *J Neurosurg* 89 (1998): 353–58.

29. I. M. Germano, H. Villalobos, A. Silvers, and K. D. Post, "Clinical use of the optical digitizer for intracranial neuronavigation," *Neurosurgery* 45 (1999): 261–69; discussion, 269–70.

30. M. Woloschak, A. Yu and K. D. Post, "Detection of polyomaviral DNA sequences in normal and adenomatous human pituitary tissues using the polymerase chain reaction," *Cancer* 76 (1995): 490–96.

31. M. Woloschak, A. Yu, J. Xiao, and K. D. Post, "Abundance and state of phosphorylation of the retinoblastoma gene product in human pituitary tumors," *Int J Cancer* 67 (1996): 16–19.

32. M. Woloschak, A. Yu, J. Xiao, and K. D. Post, "Frequent loss of the P16INK4a gene product in human pituitary tumors," *Cancer Res* 56 (1996): 2493–96.

33. M. Woloschak, A. Yu, and K. D. Post, "Frequent inactivation of the p16 gene in human pituitary tumors by gene methylation," *Mol Carcinog* 19 (1997): 221–24.

NOTES TO CHAPTER 22

1. *Case Records of the Jews' Hospital, 1855–1856.* Mount Sinai Archives.

2. Ibid.

3. E. Noeggerath and A. Jacobi, *Contributions to Midwifery, and Diseases of Women and Children, with a Report on the Progress of Obstetrics, and Uterine and Infantile Pathology in 1858* (New York: Baillere Brothers, 1859).

4. E. Noeggerath, *Die Latente Gonorrhae im weiblichen Geschlicht* (Bonn: Cohen, 1872).

5. E. Noeggerath, *Beitrage zur Struktur und Entwickelung des Carcinoms* (Wiesbaden: Bergmann, 1892).

6. H. Lilienthal, "The Mount Sinai Hospital and its surgeons of the middle eighties; a few recollections," *J Mt Sinai Hosp* 3 (1937): 240.

7. M. Mayer, *The Gynecological Service.* Personal reminiscences. January 1939. Mount Sinai Archives.

8. P. F. Mundé, "Combined operations in gynecology," *NY Med Jour* 49 (1889): 534–36.

9. Mayer, *Gynecological Service.*

10. P. F. Mundé, *Minor Surgical Gynecology: A Treatise of Uterine Diagnosis and the Lesser Technicalities of Gynecological Practice*, 2d ed., rev. and enl. (New York: Wood, 1885); P. F. Mundé, *The Diagnosis and Treatment of Obstetric Cases by External (Abdominal) Examination and Manipulation* (New York: Wood, 1880); P. F. Mundé, *A Sketch of the Management of Pregnancy, Parturition, and the Puerperal State*, 2d ed. (Detroit: Davis, 1888).

11. P. F. Mundé, *De l'lectricité comme agent thérapeutique en gynécologie.* Tr. et annoté par P. Ménierè (Paris: Doin, 1888).

12. J. Brettauer, "The question of early catharsis after coeliotomy," *NY J Gynaecol Obstet* 4 (1894): 138–46.

13. F. Krug, "Trendelenberg's posture in gynecology with demonstration of a convenient apparatus for obtaining the same," *Ann Gynaecol Paediat* 5 (1891–1892): 609–13.

14. *Journal of the Mount Sinai Hospital* 10 (May–June 1943): 1–333. Vineberg's bibliography is listed on pp. 9–11. See the Web site www.mountsinaihistory.org for the citations of his most important papers.

15. R. T. Frank, "The function of the ovary," *Surg Gynecol Obstet* 13 (1911): 36–53.

16. R. T. Frank and J. Rosenbloom, "Physiologically active substances contained in the placenta and in the corpus luteum," *Surg Gynecol Obstet* 21 (1915): 646–49.

17. R. T. Frank, *Gynecological and Obstetrical Pathology, Including Chapters on the Normal Histology and the Physiology of the Female Genital Tract. Gynecological and Obstetrical Monographs* (New York: D. Appleton, 1922).

18. R. T. Frank and R. G. Gustavson, "The female sex hormone and the gestational gland," *JAMA* 84 (1925): 1715–19.

19. R. T. Frank, M. Frank, R. G. Gustavson, and W. W. Weyerts, "Demonstration of the female sex hormone in the circulating blood. I. Preliminary report," *JAMA* 85 (1925): 510.

20. R. T. Frank, "The ovary and the endocrinologist," *JAMA* 78 (1922): 181–85.

21. L. Lapid, "Retrospective of Dr. Robert Tilden Frank (1875–1949)," presented at The Mount Sinai Hospital and Medical Center Alumni Day, April 17, 1993.

22. Diary of Robert T. Frank. Quoted in L. Lapid, "Retrospective of Dr. Robert Tilden Frank (1875–1949)."

23. R. T. Frank and M. A. Goldberger, "The female sex hormone: IV. Its occurrence in the circulating and menstrual blood: Preliminary report," *JAMA* 86 (1926): 1686–87.

24. R. T. Frank and M. A. Goldberger, "Clinical data obtained with the female sex hormone test," *JAMA* 90 (1928): 106–10.

25. R. T. Frank and S. H. Geist, "The formation of an artificial vagina by a new plastic technic," *Am J Obstet Gynecol* 14 (1927): 712–18.

26. R. T. Frank, "The hormonal causes of premenstrual tension," *Arch Neurol Psych* 26 (1931): 1053–57.

27. I. C. Rubin, "X-ray diagnosis in gynecology with the aid of intrauterine collargol injection," *Surg Gynecol Obstet* 20 (1915): 435–43.

28. I. C. Rubin, "The nonoperative determination of patency of Fallopian tubes by means of intra-uterine insufflation with oxygen and the production of an artificial pneumoperitoneum," *JAMA* 75 (1920): 661–66.

29. I. C. Rubin, "Rhythmic contractions and peristaltic movement in the intact fallopian tube as determined by periuterine gas insufflation and the kymograph (an experimental and clinical study)," *Am J Obstet Gynecol* 14 (1927): 557–72.

30. I. C. Rubin, "Sudden acute pain in the shoulders associated with acute pelvic pain in women. A symptom of ruptured ectopic pregnancy, indicating subphrenic blood extravasation (subphrenic hemoperitoneum)," *JAMA* 80 (1923): 1050–52.

31. *Journal of the Mount Sinai Hospital* 14 (1947): 133–826. Rubin's bibliography is listed on p. 135–142. More citations are listed on the Web site www.mountsinaihistory.org.

32. S. H. Geist, *Ovarian Tumors* (New York: Hoeber, 1942).

33. I. C. Rubin, "The maternity service of the future with special reference to the Mount Sinai Institute of Biogenetics," *J Mt Sinai Hosp* 10 (1944): 773–81.

34. L. Lapid, personal communication.

35. Ibid.

36. J. J. Rovinsky and A. F. Guttmacher, *Medical, Surgical, and Gynecological Complications of Pregnancy*, 1st ed. (Baltimore: Williams and Wilkins, 1960). Rovinsky and Guttmacher produced a second edition in 1965. Sheldon Cherry was the senior editor of the third (1985) and fourth (1991) editions.

37. The work noted was done while Gusberg was on the faculty at P&S. The citations can be found on the Web site www.mountsinaihistory.org.

38. S. B. Gusberg, S. Chen, and C. J. Cohen, "Endometrial cancer. Factors influencing the choice of treatment," *Gynecol Oncol* 2 (1974): 308–13.

39. C. J. Cohen, S. B. Gusberg, and D. Koffler, "Histologic screening for endometrial cancer," *Gynecol Oncol* 2 (1974): 279–86.

40. S. Chen, D. Koffler, and C. J. Cohen, "Cell-mediated immunity in patients with ovarian carcinoma," *Am J Obst Gynecol* 115 (1973): 467–70; S. Chen, D. Koffler, and C. J. Cohen, "Cellular hypersensitivity in patients with squamous cell carcinoma of the cervix," *Am J Obstet Gynecol* 121 (1975): 91–95.

41. H. Bruckner, C. J. Cohen, G. Deppe, et al., "Chemotherapy of gynecologic tumors with platinum II," *J Clin Hemat Oncol* 7 (1977): 619–32.

42. C. J. Cohen, G. Deppe, C. A. Castro-Marin, and H. W. Bruckner, "Treatment of advanced squamous cell carcinoma of the cervix with cisplatinum (II) diamminedichloride," *Am J Obstet Gynecol* 130 (1978): 853–54.

43. C. J. Cohen, J. D. Goldberg, J. F. Holland, et al., "Improved therapy with cis-platin regimens for patients with ovarian carcinoma (FIGO stages III and IV) as measured by surgical end-staging (second-look operation)," *Am J Obstet Gynecol* 145 (1983): 955–67.

44. S. H. Cherry, S. Kochwa, and R. E. Rosenfield, "Bilirubin-protein ratio in amniotic fluid as an index of the severity of erythroblastosis fetalis," *Obst Gynecol* 26 (1965): 826–32.

45. S. H. Cherry and R. E. Rosenfield, "Intrauterine fetal transfusions for the management of erythroblastosis," *Am J Obstet Gynecol* 98 (1967): 275–82.

46. E. Gurpide, "A tracer superfusion method to measure rates of entry, exit, and metabolism and synthesis of steroids in cells," *Methods in Enzymology* 36 (1975): 75–88; E. Gurpide and L. Tseng, "Factors controlling intracellular levels of estrogens in human endometrium," *Gynecol Oncol* 2 (1974): 221–27.

47. E. Gurpide, "Hormones and gynecologic cancer," *Cancer* 38 (1976): 503–8.

48. E. Gurpide, L. Tseng, and S. B. Gusberg, "Estrogen metabolism in normal and neoplastic endothelium," *Am J Obstet Gynecol* 129 (1977): 809–16; E. Gurpide, "Endometrial cancer in postmenopausal estrogen users, a rationale for uterine protection with progestins," in *Steroid Receptors and Hormone-Dependent Neoplasia*, ed. J. L. Wittliff and O. Dapunt (New York: Masson, 1980).

49. N. G. Kase, E. Forchielli, and R. Dorfman, "In vitro production of testosterone and andros-4-ene, 3, 17-dione in a human ovarian homogenate," *Acta Endocrinol* 37 (1961): 19–23.

50. N. G. Kase and G. I. Cohn, "Clinical implications of extragonadal estrogen production," *New Engl J Med* 276 (1967): 28–31.

51. N. G. Kase, A. Mroueh, and L. Olson, "Clomid therapy of anovulatory infertility," *Am J Obstet Gynecol* 989 (1967): 1037–42.

52. N. G. Kase and A. Mroueh, "Pergonal therapy of anovulatory infertility," *Am J Obstet Gynecol* 100 (1968): 176–84.

53. L. Speroff, R. H. Glass, and N. G. Kase, *Clinical Gynecologic Endocrinology and Infertility*, 1st ed. (Baltimore: Williams and Wilkins, 1973).

54. R. L. Berkowitz, U. Chitkara, J. D. Goldberg, et al., "Intravascular transfusion in utero: The percutaneous approach," *Am J Obstet Gynecol* 154 (1986): 622–23.

55. C. Lockwood, A. E. Senyei, M. R. Dische, et al., "Fetal fibronectin in cervical and vaginal secretions as a predictor of preterm delivery," *New Engl J Med* 325 (1991): 669–674.

56. E. M. Connor, R. S. Sperling, R. Gelber, et al., "Reduction of maternal-infant transmission of human immunodeficiency virus type 1 with zidovudine treatment. Pediatric AIDS Clinical Trials Group Protocol 076 Study Group," *N Engl J Med* 331 (1994): 1173–80.

57. J. Gordon, G. A. Scangos, D. J. Plotkin, et al., "Genetic transformation of mouse embryos by microinjection of purified DNA," *Proc Natl Acad Sci USA* 77 (1980): 7380–4.

58. J. Gordon and F. Ruddle, "Integration and stable germ line transmission of genes injected into mouse pronuclei," *Science* 214 (1981): 1244–46.

59. J. W. Gordon and B. E. Talansky, "Assisted fertilization by zona drilling: A mouse model for correction of oligospermia," *J Exp Zoology* 239 (1986): 347–54.

60. J. Gordon, L. Grunfeld, G. J. Garrisi, et al., "Fertilization of human oocytes by sperm from infertile males after zona pellucida drilling," *Fertl Steril* 50 (1988): 68–73.

61. M. Bradbury, L. Isola, and J. Gordon, "Enzymatic amplification of a repeated DNA sequence from the mouse Y chromosome allows the determination of sex in a single blastomere," *Proc Natl Acad Sci USA* 87 (1989): 4053–57.

62. M. E. Ripps, G. W. Huntley, P. R. Hof et al., "Transgenic mice expressing an altered murine superoxide dismutase gene provide an animal model of amyotrophic lateral sclerosis," *Proc Natl Acad Sci USA* 92 (1995): 689–93.

NOTES TO CHAPTER 23

1. *Case Book of the Jews' Hospital, 1855–1856.* Mount Sinai Archives.

2. See the chapter on the Department of Otolaryngology for more on Gruening.

3. H. Lilienthal, "The Mount Sinai Hospital and its surgeons of the middle eighties; a few recollections," *J Mt Sinai Hosp* 3 (1937): 229–40.

4. P. Fridenberg, "Astigmatism cured by corneal trauma," *NY Med* 77 (1903): 837–38.

5. C. Koller, "Preliminary report on local anesthesia of the eye," *Wiener Medizinische Wochenschaft* (October 25, 1884). Translated in *Arch Ophthalmol* (1934): 473–74. See also the chapter on the Department of Anesthesiology.

6. C. H. May, "Enucleation with transplantation and reimplantation of eyes," *Med Rec* 29 (1886): 613–21.

7. C. H. May, "Transplantation of a rabbit's eye into the human orbit," *Arch Ophthalmol* 16 (1887): 47–53.

8. C. H. May, "A new electric ophthalmoscope," *Ophth Rev* 23 (1914): 386–89.

9. C. H. May, *Manual of Diseases of the Eye* (New York: Williams and Wilkins, 1900).

10. C. Barnert, *The Mount Sinai Unit in the World War* (New York: The Mount Sinai Hospital, 1919).

11. C. Simon and I. Goldstein, "A new scientific method of identification," *NYS J Med* 35 (1935): 901–6.

12. H. Minsky, "Surgical repair of recent lid lacerations: Intramarginal splinting suture," *Surg Gynecol Obstet* 75 (1946): 449–56.

13. H. Minsky, "The surgical limbus," in *Proceedings of the XVI International Congress of Ophthalmology* (London: Brittania, 1950), pp. 928–37.

14. H. Minsky, "Correlation of ocular changes in essential hypertension with diastolic blood pressure," *Arch Ophthalmol* 51 (1954): 863–74.

15. F. A. Bassen and A. L. Kornzweig, "Malformation of the erythrocytes in a case of atypical retinitis pigmentosa," *Blood* 5 (1950): 381–87.

16. F. H. Theodore and A. Schlossman, *Ocular Allergy* (Philadelphia: Williams and Wilkins, 1958).

17. F. H. Theodore, "Superior limbic keratoconjunctivitis," *Eye Ear Nose Throat Mon* 42 (1963): 25–28.

18. F. H. Theodore, "Conjunctival carcinoma masquerading as chronic conjunctivitis," *Eye Ear Nose Throat Mon* 46 (1967): 1419–20.

19. A. Safir and L. Hyams, "Distribution of cone orientations as an explanation of the Stiles-Crawford effect," *J Opt Soc Am* 59 (1969): 757–65.

20. A. P. Ferry and A. H. Barnert, "Granulomatous keratitis resulting from use of cyanoacrylate adhesive for closure of perforated corneal ulcer," *Am J Ophthalmol* 72 (1971): 538–41.

21. S. M. Podos, "Prostaglandins, nonsteroidal anti-inflammatory agents and eye disease," *Trans Am Ophthalmol Soc* 74 (1977): 637–60.

22. A. Stein, R. Pinke, T. Krupin, et al., "The effect of topically administered carbonic anhydrase inhibitors on aqueous humor dynamics in rabbits," *Am J Ophthalmol* 95 (1983): 222–28.

23. R. A. Schumer and S. M. Podos, "The nerve of glaucoma!" *Arch Ophthalmol* 112 (1994): 37–44.

24. S. M. Podos and M. Yanoff, *Textbook of Ophthalmology*, 10 vols. (New York: Gower Medical Publishers, 1991), vol. 1.

25. T. Mittag, P. Kornfeld, A. Tormay, and C. Woo, "Detection of anti-acetylcholine receptor factors in serum and thymus from patients with myasthenia gravis," *N Engl J Med* 294 (1976): 691–94.

26. E. Kaplan and R. M. Shapley, "X and Y cells in the lateral geniculate nucleus of macaque monkeys," *J Physiol* 330 (1982): 125–43.

27. S. K. Masur, J. K. Cheung, and S. Antohi, "Identification of integrins in cultured corneal fibroblasts and in isolated keratocytes," *Invest Ophthalmol Vis Sci* 34 (1993): 2690–98.

28. S. K. Masur, H. S. Dewal, T. T. Dinh, et al., "Myofibroblasts differentiate from fibroblasts when plated at low density," *Proc Natl Acad Sci USA* 93 (1996): 4219–23.

NOTES TO CHAPTER 24

1. *Case Records of the Jews' Hospital, 1855–56.* Mount Sinai Archives.

2. Ibid.

3. Ibid.

4. P. W. Nathan, "Osteoarthritis: Etiology, pathology, and classification," *Am J Med Sci* 131 (1906): 636–48.

5. P. W. Nathan, "The biology of bone development and its relation to transplantation," *NY Med J* 114 (1922): 454–56.

6. P. W. Nathan, "The mechanical and operative treatment of poliomyelitis anterior," *Am J Orthop Surg* 12 (1914–1915): 430–46.

7. P. W. Nathan, "Mechanisms and pathology of tuberculous hip disease in their relation to its diagnosis and treatment," *JAMA* 64 (1915): 1732–34.

8. P. W. Nathan, "Differential diagnosis and the treatment of acute osteomyelitis of the upper femur, involving the hip joint," *Surg Gynecol Obstet* 54 (1932): 52–80.

9. Ibid.

10. P. W. Roberts, "A new traction frame," *JAMA* 58 (1912): 1192.

11. P. W. Roberts, "Reconstruction of ball and socket joints," *JAMA* 59 (1912): 1439–40.

12. S. Selig, "Interinnomino-abdominal (hind-quarter) amputation," *J Bone Joint Surg* 23 (1941): 929–34.

13. S. Selig, "Surgical approach to obturator foramen," *J Bone Joint Surg* 16 (1934): 1950–52.

14. S. Selig, "Hammer toe," *Surg Gynecol Obstet* 72 (1941): 101–5.

15. R. K. Lippmann, "Corkscrew-bolt for compression fixation of femoral neck fractures," *Am J Surg* 37 (1937): 79–87.

16. R. K. Lippmann, "Depressed fracture of the tibial plateau," *J Mt Sinai Hosp* 17 (1951): 761–68.

17. R. K. Lippmann, "Frozen shoulder; periarthritis; bicipital tenosynovitis," *Arch Surg* 47 (1943): 283–96.

18. E. Bick, *Source Book of Orthopaedics* (Baltimore: Williams and Wilkens, 1937).

19. R. K. Lippmann, "The use of auscultatory percussion for the examination of fractures," *J Bone Joint Surg* 14 (1932): 118–26.

20. R. S. Siffert, "Robert K. Lippmann," *J Mt Sinai Hosp* 36 (1969): 447–50.

21. E. M. Bick, "Fibroblastic tumor of the extremities," *Arch Surg* 35 (1937): 841–53.

22. E. M. Bick and J. W. Copel, "Longitudinal growth of human vertebrae," *J Bone Joint Surg* 32A (1950): 803–14.

23. E. M. Bick, *Trauma in the Aged* (New York: McGraw-Hill, 1960).

24. E. M. Bick, "Common degenerative disease of the aging spine," *Geriatrics* 19 (1964): 35–40.

25. E. M. Bick, *Source Book of Orthopaedics.*

26. E. M. Bick, *Classics of Orthopaedics* (Philadelphia: J. B. Lippincott, 1976).

27. A. M. Arkin, "Mechanism of structural change in scoliosis," *J Bone Joint Surg* 31A (1949): 519–28.

28. A. M. Arkin, "Effects of pressure on epiphyseal growth: Mechanism of plasticity of growing bone," *J Bone Joint Surg* 38A (1952): 1056–76.

29. J. Hartley, S. S. Tan, and M. Schneider, "Ontogenesis produced by a chemical extract of bone," *J Mt Sinai Hosp* 15 (1949): 383–87.

30. J. Hartley, *New Ways in First Aid* (New York: Hart, 1971).

31. J. Hartley, *First Aid without Panic* (New York: Hart, 1975).

32. R. S. Siffert, "Robert K. Lippman."

33. R. S. Siffert and A. M. Arkin, "Trephine biopsy of bone with special reference to the lumbar vertebral bodies," *J Bone Joint Surg* 31A (1949): 146–49.

34. R. S. Siffert, "Role of alkaline phosphatase in Osteogenesis," *J Exp Med* 93 (1950): 415–26.

35. R. N. Levy, C. M. Levy, J. Snyder, and J. Digiovanni, "Outcome and long-term results following total hip replacement in elderly patients," *Clin Orthop* 54 (1995): 25–30.

36. A. J. Schein and A. M. Arkin, "Hip joint involvement in Gaucher's disease," *J. Bone and Joint Surg* 24 (1942): 396–410.

37. R. S. Siffert and J. F. Katz, "Experimental intra-epiphyseal osteotomy," *Clin Orthop* 82 (1972): 234–45.

38. J. F. Katz, "Alternative treatments in Legg-Calve-Perthes disease," *Bull NY Acad Med* 53 (1977): 605–14.

39. R. S. Siffert, R. I. Forster, and B. Nachamie, "Beak triple arthrodesis for correction of severe cavus deformity," *Clin Orthop* 45 (1966): 101–6.

40. R. S. Siffert, "Intraepiphyseal osteotomy for progressive tibia vara: Case report and rationale of management," *J Pediatr Orthop* 2 (1982): 81–85.

41. J. F. Katz and R. S. Siffert, *Management of Hip Disorders in Children* (Philadelphia: J. B. Lippincott, 1983); J. Katz, *Legg-Calve-Perthes Disease* (New York: Praeger, 1984).

42. R. S. Siffert, *See How They Grow: A Parent's Guide to Normal and Abnormal Physical Growth from Birth through Adolescence* (New York: Raven Press, 1985).

43. M. S. Gilbert and K. Glass, "Hemophilic arthropathy in the elbow," *Mt Sinai J Med* 44 (1977): 389–96.

44. G. Hermann, H. C. Yeh, and M. S. Gilbert, "Computed tomography and ultrasonography of the hemophilic pseudotumor and their use in surgical planning," *Skeletal Radiol* 15 (1986): 123–28.

45. A. A. Pilla, M. A. Mont, P. R. Nasser, et al., "Non-invasive low-intensity pulsed ultrasound accelerates bone healing in the rabbit," *J Orthop Trauma* 4 (1990): 246–53.

46. S. Lichtblau, "A medial and lateral release operation for clubfoot," *J Bone Joint Surg* 55A (1973): 1377–84.

47. M. M. Lewis, "The use of an expandable and adjustable prosthesis in the treatment of childhood malignant bone tumors of the extremity," *Cancer* 57 (1986): 499–502.

48. M. M. Lewis, *Bone Tumor Surgery: Limb-Sparing Techniques* (Philadelphia: J. B. Lippincott, 1988).

49. T. A. Einhorn, "Evaluation and treatment methods of metabolic bone disease," *Contemp Orthop* 14 (1987): 21–34.

50. T. A. Einhorn and R. J. Majeska, "Neutral proteases in regenerating bone," *Clin Orthop* 262 (1991): 286–97.

51. R. S. Siffert, G. M. Luo, S. C. Cowin, and J. J. Kaufman, "Dynamic relationships of trabecular bone density, architecture, and strength in a computational model of osteopenia," *Bone* 18 (1996): 197–206.

NOTES TO CHAPTER 25

1. E. Gruening, "Notes on operations on the mastoid process," *Trans Am Otol Soc* 5 (1892): 66–69.

2. E. Gruening, "Six cases of thrombosis of the lateral sinus operated upon in the ear ward of the Mount Sinai Hospital in the course of the past year," *Trans Am Otol Soc* 9 (1906): 304–18.

3. Gruening was equally well known for his work in ophthalmology and had a reputation as a fine ophthalmic surgeon. See the chapter on the Department of Ophthalmology for more on Gruening.

4. A. G. Gerster, *Recollections of a New York Surgeon* (New York: Paul B. Hoeber, 1917), p. 204.

5. Ibid.

6. F. Whiting, *The Modern Mastoid Operation* (Philadelphia: P. Blakiston's Son, 1905).

7. A. Braun and I. Freisner, *The Labyrinth: An Aid to the Study of Inflammations of the Internal Ear* (New York: Rebman, 1913).

8. J. L. Maybaum, "An operative procedure suggested for sinus thrombosis," *Arch Otolaryngol* 8 (1928): 75–77.

9. I. Friesner, "Invasion of internal ear by tympanic suppuration," *Am J Surg* 34 (1920): 138–40.

10. J. Maybaum, E. Snyder, and L. Coleman, "The value of sulfanilamide in otogenous infections," *JAMA* 112 (1939): 2589–92.

11. H. Rosenwasser, "Carotid body tumor of the middle ear and mastoid," *Arch Otolaryngol* 41 (1945): 64–67.

12. S. Yankauer, "Foreign body in the bronchus; removal with the aid of the bronchoscope; recovery," *Med Rec NY* 67 (1905): 217.

13. S. Yankauer, "A speculum for the direct examination and treatment of the naso-pharynx and Eustachian tubes," *Laryngoscope* 21 (1911): 173–175.

14. S. Yankauer, "The isthmus of the Eustachian tube. A contribution to the pathology and treatment of middle-ear diseases," *Laryngoscope* 20 (1909): 675–718.

15. H. Lilienthal, "War memories of Dr. Yankauer," *The Mount Sinai Hospital Bulletin* October (1932): pp. 9–10

16. The Mount Sinai Hospital, *Annual Report for 1920*, p. 42.

17. S. Yankauer, "Bronchoscopy in treatment of lung abscess," *Surg Clin North Am* 5 (1925): 525–30.

18. S. Yankauer, "Radium in carcinoma of the esophagus: A method of application," *Arch Surg* 12 (1926): 247–56.

19. R. Kramer and S. Yankauer, "Hemangioma of the larynx," *Laryngoscope* 34 (1924): 405–25; R. Kramer and S. Yankauer, "Lymphangioma of the larynx," *Laryngoscope* 34 (1924): 621–29.

20. R. Kramer and A. Glass, "Bronchoscopic localization of lung abscess," *Am J Otol Rhinol Laryngol* 41 (1932): 1210–20.

21. S. Rosen, "Observations on surgical anatomy in the fenestration operation," *Ann Otol Rhinol Laryngol* 57 (1948): 1007–17.

22. S. Rosen, "Effect of stimulation and section of the chorda tympani nerve," *Neurology* 2 (1952): 244–47; S. Rosen, "A new nervous pathway for Meniere's disease," *NYS J Med* 53 (1953): 1095–97.

23. S. Rosen, "Mobilization of the stapes to restore hearing in otosclerosis," *NYS J Med* 53 (1953): 2650–53.

24. R. L. Simons and T. S. Hill, "History, Coming of Age . . . The History of the AAFPRS," *Web site of the American Academy of Facial Plastic and Reconstructive Surgery,* www.facial-plastic-surgery.org, accessed January 2002.

25. J. L. Goldman and C. Herschberger, "Prophylactic vaccination against intracranial complications," *JAMA* 109 (1937): 1254–56.

26. J. L. Goldman, "Boundaries of otolaryngology," *JAMA* 187 (1964): 604–5.

27. R. L. Simons and T. S. Hill, *Web site of the American Academy of Facial Plastic and Reconstructive Surgery,* www.facial-plastic-surgery.org.

28. M. L. Som and S. H. Klein, "Extensive segmental resection of the trachea with primary suture anastomosis: An experimental study," *Surgical Forum* 9

(1958): 353–56; M. L. Som and L. Arnold, "Esophagoscopy in the diagnosis and treatment of esophageal disease," *Am J Surg* 93 (1957): 183–95.

29. J. L. Goldman, S. M. Silverstone, J. D. Roffman, and E. A. Birken, "High dosage pre-operative radiation and surgery for carcinoma of the larynx and laryngopharynx: a 14-year program," *Laryngoscope* 82 (1972): 1869–82.

30. A comprehensive listing of all of the important papers by Biller and the faculty is beyond the scope of this work. They can, however, be found on the Web site www.mountsinaihistory.org.

31. A. Blitzer, W. Lawson, and W. Friedman, *Surgery of the Paranasal Sinuses* (Philadelphia: W. B. Saunders, 1985).

32. F. Zak and W. Lawson, *The Paraganglionic Chemoreceptor System* (New York: Springer-Verlag, 1982).

33. J. L. Goldman, *The Principles and Practice of Rhinology: A Text on the Diseases and Surgery of the Nose and Paranasal Sinuses* (New York: Wiley, 1987).

34. K. Remsen, W. Lawson, N. Patel, and H. F. Biller, "Laser lateralization for bilateral vocal cord abductor paralysis," *Otolaryngol Head Neck Surg* 93 (1985): 645–49; J. Shugar, P. Som, and H. Biller, "An evaluation of the carbon dioxide laser in the treatment of traumatic laryngeal stenosis," *Laryngoscope* 92 (1982): 23–26.

35. B. Bailey and H. F. Biller, *Surgery of the Larynx* (Philadelphia: W. B. Saunders, 1985).

36. Y. Han, J. Wang, D. A. Fischman, H. F. Biller, and I. Sanders, "Slow tonic muscle fibers in the thyroarytenoid muscles of human vocal folds; a possible specialization for speech," *Anat Rec* 256 (1999): 146–57.

37. H. F. Biller, J. M. Shugar, and Y. P. Krespi, "A new technique for wide-field exposure of the base of the skull," *Arch Otolaryngol* 107 (1981): 698–702.

38. M. Babajanian, W. X. Zhang, J. B. Turk, et al., "Temporal factors affecting the secondary critical ischemia of normothermic experimental skin flaps," *Arch Otolaryngol Head Neck Surg* 117 (1991): 1360–64; B. T. Ho, H. Weinberg, W. X. Zhang, et al., "Hemodynamics of the rodent abdominal skin flap following primary ischemia," *Laryngoscope* 103 (1993): 981–84; J. F. Moscoso, J. Keller, E. Genden, et al., "Vascularized bone flaps in oromandibular reconstruction," *Arch Otolaryngol Head Neck Surg* 129 (1994): 36–43; H. Weinberg, W. X. Zhang, and M. L. Urken, "UW solution as an experimental microvascular skin flap perfusate," *Microsurgery* 14 (1993): 537–40.

39. The following papers are representative of the work produced by the liaison group. For others, see the Web site www.mountsinaihistory.org. See also the chapter on the Department of Psychiatry for more on liaison psychiatry. J. Wallack, F. Lucente, H. F. Biller, and J. Strain, "Liaison psychiatry—Otolaryngology rounds," *Laryngoscope* 92 (1982): 125–28; B. I. Ginsberg, J. J. Wallack, J. J. Strain, and H. F. Biller, "Defining the psychiatric role in spastic dysphonia," *Gen Hosp Psych* 10 (1988): 132–37; H. Bronheim, J. J. Strain, H. F. Biller, and G. Fulop,

"Psychiatric consultation on an otolaryngology liaison service," *Gen Hosp Psych* 11 (1989): 95–102.

40. M. L. Urken, H. Weinberg, C. Vickery, and H. F. Biller, "The neurofasciocutaneous radial forearm flap in head and neck reconstruction: A preliminary report," *Laryngoscope* 100 (1990): 161–73.

41. M. L. Urken, D. Buchbinder, H. Weinberg, et al., "Functional evaluation following microvascular oromandibular reconstruction of the oral cancer patient: A comparative study of reconstructed and nonreconstructed patients," *Laryngoscope* 101 (1991): 935–50.

42. M. L. Urken, *Atlas of Regional and Free Flaps for Head and Neck Reconstruction* (New York: Raven Press, 1995).

NOTES TO CHAPTER 26

1. The Jews' Hospital, *Annual Report for 1855–1856*. Mount Sinai Archives.

2. Ibid.

3. The Mount Sinai Hospital, Board of Directors' minutes, April 28, 1895. Mount Sinai Archives.

4. F. S. Mandlebaum, "The diagnosis of malignant tumors by paraffin sections of centrifuged exudates," *J Lab Clin Med* 2 (1917): 580.

5. C. A. Elsberg, "The serum diagnosis of typhoid fever," *Med Record NY* 51 (1897): 510–14.

6. C. A. Elsberg, "An experimental investigation of the treatment of wounds of the heart by means of suture of the heart muscle," *J Exp Med* 4 (1899): 479–520.

7. See the chapter on the Department of Neurosurgery.

8. See the chapter on the Department of Anesthesiology.

9. C. A. Elsberg, "Mount Sinai in the late nineties and the beginning of neurosurgery in the hospital," *J Mt Sinai Hosp* 4 (1937): 430–36.

10. See the comments by Crohn and Dolger in The Afterword.

11. L. Buerger, "Thromboangiitis obliterans: A study of the vascular lesions leading to presenile spontaneous gangrene," *Am J Med Sci* 136 (1908): 567–80. See also the chapter on the Department of Surgery.

12. N. E. Brill, "An acute infectious disease of unknown origin: A clinical study based on 221 cases," *Am J Med Sci* 139 (1910): 484–502.

13. N. E. Brill, "Primary splenomegaly. With a report of three cases occurring in one family," *Am J Med Sci* 121 (1901): 377–92.

14. F. S. Mandlebaum, "A contribution to the pathology of primary splenomegaly (Gaucher type), with the report of an autopsy on a male child four and one half years of age," *J Exp Med* 16 (1912): 797–821.

15. N. E. Brill and F. S. Mandlebaum, "Large cell splenomegaly (Gaucher's Disease): A clinical and pathological study," *Am J Med Sci* 146 (1913): 863–83.

16. P. C. E. Gaucher, *De l'epithélioma primitif de la rate*, thèse pour le Doctorat en Medecine (Paris: Doin, 1882).

17. N. E. Brill, G. Baehr, and N. Rosenthal, "Generalized giant lymph follicle hyperplasia of lymph nodes and spleen: A hitherto undescribed type," *JAMA* 84 (1925): 668–71. See the chapter on "The Leadership" for more on Brill.

18. E. Libman, "On some experience with blood-cultures in the study of bacterial infections," *Johns Hopkins Hosp Bull* 17 (1906): 215–28.

19. E. Libman, "A study of the endocardial lesions of subacute bacterial endocarditis: With particular reference to healing or healed lesions; with clinical notes," *Am J Med Sci* 144 (1912): 313–27.

20. E. Libman and B. Sacks, "A hitherto undescribed form of valvular and mural endocarditis," *Arch Int Med* 33 (1924): 701–37.

21. See the chapter on "The Leadership" for more on Libman.

22. G. Baehr, "Glomerular lesions of subacute bacterial endocarditis," *J Exp Med* 15 (1912): 330–47. See also the chapter on the Division of Nephrology.

23. G. Baehr, P. Klemperer, and A. Schifrin, "A diffuse disease of the peripheral circulation (usually associated with lupus erythematosus and endocarditis)," *Tr Assoc Am Physicians* 50 (1935): 139–55.

24. G. Baehr, P. Klemperer, and A. Schifrin, "Acute febrile anemia and thrombocytopenic purpura with diffuse platelet thromboses of capillaries and arterioles," *Tr Assoc Am Physicians* 51 (1936): 43–58.

25. G. Baehr and P. Klemperer, "Giant follicle lymphoblastoma; benign variety of lymphosarcoma," *NYS J Med* 40 (1940): 7–11.

26. E. Moschcowitz, "Eosinophilia and anaphylaxis," *NY Med J* 93 (1911): 15–19.

27. E. Moschcowitz and A. O. Wilensky, "Non-specific granulomata of the intestine," *Am J Med Sci* 166 (1923): 48–66.

28. B. B. Crohn, L. Ginzburg, and G. D. Oppenheimer, "Regional ileitis," *JAMA* 99 (1932): 1323–28.

29. E. Moschcowitz, "An acute febrile pleiochromic anemia with hyaline thrombosis of the terminal arterioles and capillaries: an undescribed disease," *Arch Int Med* 36 (1925): 89–93.

30. E. Moschcowitz, "Hypertension of the pulmonary circulation," *Am J Med Sci* 174 (1927): 388–406.

31. I. Strauss and J. Globus, "Spongioblastoma with unusually rapid growth following decompression," *Neurol Bull* 1 (1918): 273–81; J. Globus and I. Strauss, "Spongioblastoma multiforme," *Arch Neurol Psych* 14 (1925): 139–91. See also the chapter on the Department of Neurology.

32. L. Gross, *The Blood Supply to the Heart in Its Anatomical and Clinical Aspects* (New York: Paul B. Hoeber, 1921).

33. L. Gross, "The cardiac lesions in Libman-Sacks disease. With a consideration of its relationship to acute diffuse lupus erythematosus," *Am J Path* 16 (1940): 375–405 (plus multiple plates).

34. E. Moschcowitz, "Paul Klemperer—an appreciation," *J Mt Sinai Hosp* 24 (1957): 648–51.

35. J. C. Ehrlich, "Sadao Otani, 1892–1969: A brief memoir," in *Dr. Sadao Otani: His Contribution to American Pathology*, ed. J. Churg and L. Strauss (New York: The Mount Sinai Hospital, 1972).

36. P. Klemperer, "Cavernomatous transformation of the portal vein; its relation to Banti's Disease," *Arch Path* 6 (1928): 353–77.

37. P. Klemperer and S. Otani, "Malignant nephrosclerosis (Fahr)," *Arch Path* 11 (1931): 60–117.

38. P. Klemperer, A. D. Pollack, and G. Baehr, "Pathology of disseminated lupus erythematosus," *Arch Path* 32 (1941): 569–631.

39. P. Klemperer, A. D. Pollack, and G. Baehr, "Diffuse collagen disease: Acute disseminated lupus erythematosus and diffuse scleroderma," *JAMA* 119 (1942): 331–32.

40. J. C. Ehrlich, "Sadao Otani, 1892–1969."

41. S. Otani and J. C. Ehrlich, "Solitary granuloma of bone simulating primary neoplasm," *Am J Path* 16 (1940): 479–90.

42. H. Rosenwasser, "Carotid body tumor of the middle ear and mastoid," *Arch Otolaryngol* 41 (1945): 64–67.

43. A. Penner and A. I. Bernheim, "Acute postoperative enterocolitis: A study on the pathologic nature of shock," *Arch Path* 27 (1939): 966–83; A. Penner and A. I. Bernheim, "Acute postoperative esophageal, gastric, and duodenal ulcerations," *Arch Path* 28 (1939): 129–40.

44. A. Penner and A. I. Bernheim, "Experimental production of digestive tract ulcerations," *Exper Med* 70 (1939): 453–60.

45. J. Churg and L. Strauss, "Allergic granulomatosis, allergic angiitis and periarteritis nodosa," *Am J Path* 27 (1951): 277–301.

46. J. Churg, L. Strauss, and R. L. Sherman, "Electron microscopic studies in hereditary nephritis," *Birth Defects Orig Arctic Ser* 10 (1974): 89–92.

47. I. J. Selikoff, J. Churg, and E. C. Hammond, "Asbestos exposure and neoplasia," *JAMA* 188 (1964): 22–26; I. J. Selikoff, E. C. Hammond, and J. Churg, "Asbestos exposure, smoking, and neoplasia," *JAMA* 204 (1968): 106–12. See also the chapter on the Division of Pulmonary Medicine. More of Churg's papers are cited on the Web site www.mountsinai history.org.

48. H. Popper and F. Schaffner, *Liver: Structure and Function* (New York: Blakiston Division, 1957).

49. The Mount Sinai Hospital, *Annual Report for 1873*. Mount Sinai Archives.

50. B. J. Niss and N. G. Kase, "An overview of the history of the Mount Sinai School of Medicine of the City University of New York, 1963–1988," *Mt Sinai J Med* 56 (1989): 356–66.

51. P. D. Berk, F. Schaffner, and R. Schmid, *Hans Popper: A Tribute* (New York: Raven Press, 1992), p. 6.

52. A partial list of Popper's most important contributions are cited on the Web site www.mountsinaihistory.org. See also P. D. Berk, F. Schaffner, and R. Schmid, *Hans Popper: A Tribute.*

53. "Hans Popper" (obituary), *Lancet* 1 (1988): 1176.

54. As quoted by R. Schmid and S. Schenker, in P. D. Berk, F. Schaffner, and R. Schmid, *Hans Popper: A Tribute*, p. 154.

55. See the Web site www.mountsinaihistory.org for citations of recent work by the members of the department.

56. J. D. Appel, T. M. Fasy, D. S. Kohtz, et al., "Asbestos fibers mediate transformation of monkey cells by exogenous plasmid DNA," *Proc Natl Acad Sci U S A* 85 (1988): 7670–74; K. Lezon-Geyda, C. M. Jaime, J. H. Godbold, et al., "Chrysotile asbestos fibers mediate homologous recombination in Rat2 lambda fibroblasts: implications for carcinogenesis," *Mutat Res* 361 (1996: 113–20.

NOTES TO CHAPTER 27

1. R. Viner, "Abraham Jacobi and German medical radicalism in antebellum New York," *Bull Hist Med* 72 (1998): 434–63.

2. A. Jacobi, *Dr. Jacobi's Works. Collected Essays, Addresses, Scientific Papers, and Miscellaneous Writings of A. Jacobi*, ed. W. J. Robinson, M.D. (New York: Critic and Guide Company, 1909), p. 8 (Author's preface).

3. E. Noeggerath and A. Jacobi, *Contributions to Midwifery and Diseases of Women and Children, with a Report on the Progress of Obstetrics, and Uterine and Infantile Pathology in 1858* (New York: Baillere Brothers, 1859).

4. This is not the New York Medical College of today.

5. A. Jacobi and M. P. Jacobi, *Infant Diet* (New York: Putnam, 1874).

6. A. Jacobi, *Dr. Jacobi's Works.*

7. L. Thomas, "Medicine without science," *Atlantic Monthly* (April 1981): 40–42.

8. See the Afterword. See Appendix A for a list of the recipients through 2002.

9. A. G. Gerster, *Recollections of a New York Surgeon* (New York: Paul B. Hoeber, 1917), p. 212.

10. H. Koplik, "The history of the first milk depot or *gouttes de lait* with consultations in America," *JAMA* 50 (1914): 1574–75.

11. H. Koplik, "The diagnosis of the invasion of measles from a study of the exanthem as it appears on the buccal mucous membranes," *Arch Pediatr* 13 (1896): 918–22.

12. M. H. Bass, "Henry Koplik (1858–1927)," *J Pediatr* 46 (1955): 119–25.

13. See the chapter on the Department of Neurology for more details.

14. A. A. Epstein, "Concerning the causation of edema in chronic parenchymatous nephritis: Method for its alleviation," *Am J Med Sci* 154 (1917): 638–47.

15. See the chapter on the Department of Urology for more on Beer and Hyman and for the citations.

16. I. S. Wile, "Physical problems of abnormal behavior," paper presented to New York Physicians Association Section of The New York Academy of Medicine, October 20, 1927. See also the chapter on the Department of Psychiatry.

17. Wile, "Physical problems of abnormal behavior."

18. C. Frh. Von Pirquet and B. Schick, *Die Serumkrankheit* (Leipzig: Deuticke, 1905).

19. B. Schick, "Die Diphtherietoxin-Hautreaktion des Menschen als Vorprobe der Prophylaktischen Diphtherie-heilserum Injektion," *Munchen med Wchnschr* 60 (1913): 2608–10.

20. A. Gronowicz, *Bela Schick and the World of Children* (New York: Abelard and Schuman, 1954), p 2.

21. M. M. Peshkin, "Postscript," in I. J. Wolf, *Aphorisms and Facetiae of Bela Schick.* (Orange, N.J.: Knoll Pharmaceutical Co., 1965), p. 45.

22. Director's Office, The Mount Sinai Hospital. (Turner) Papers, 1871–1950: Pediatrics files, Box 3, f.5.

23. J. Pakter and H. Jacobziner, "A five-year review of the premature infant program, New York City Department of Health," *NY State J Med* 54 (1954): 3207–14; J. Pakter and F. Nelson, "Factors in the unprecedented decline in infant mortality in New York City," *Bull NY Acad Med* 50 (1974): 839–68; A. Steele and J. Pakter, "SIDS, apnea, and home monitoring," Policy Statement #9021, *J Am Public Health Asso* 81 (1991): 254–56.

24. M. H. Bass and S. Blumenthal, "Fatal lead poisoning in nursing infant due to prolonged use of lead nipple shields," *J Pediatr* 15 (1939): 724–32; M. H. Bass, "Periorbital edema as initial sign of infectious mononucleosis," *J Pediatr* 45 (1954): 204–5; M. H. Bass and G. R. Fisch, "Increased intracranial pressure with bulging fontanelle: A symptom of vitamin A deficiency in infants," *Neurology* 2 (1961): 1091–14.

25. S. Karelitz and B. Schick, "Treatment of toxicosis with aid of continuous intravenous drip of dextrose solution," *Am J Dis Child* 42 (1931): 781–802.

26. J. S. Light and H. L. Hodes, "Studies on epidemic diarrhea of the newborn; isolation of filtrable agent causing diarrhea in calves," *Am J Public Health* 33 (1943): 1451–54.

27. D. Gribetz, M.D., personal communication.

28. A. J. Steigman, E. J. Bottone, and B. A. Hanna, "Intramuscular penicillin administration at birth: Prevention of early onset group B streptococcal disease," *Pediatrics* 62 (1978): 842–44.

29. D. Gribetz, M.D., personal communication.

30. E. G. Brown and A. Y. Sweet, "Neonatal necrotizing enterocolitis," *Pediatr Clin North Am* 29 (1982): 1149–70.

31. J. Lin, I. R. Holzman, P. Jiang, and M. W. Babayatsky, "Expression of intestinal trefoil factor in developing rat intestine," *Biol Neonate* 76 (1999): 92–97.

32. A. B. Levine, M. Alvarez, J. Wedgewood, et al., "Contemporary management of a potentially lethal fetal anomaly: A successful perinatal approach to epignathus," *Obstet Gynecol* 76 (1990): 962–68.

33. K. Hirschhorn, H. L. Cooper, and I. L. Firschein, "Detection of short arms of chromosome 4 and 5 in a child with defects of midline fusion," *Humangenetik* 1 (1965): 479–82; V. Wolf, H. Reinwein, R. Porsch, et al., "Defizienz an den kurzen Armen eines Chromosoms Nr. 4," *Humangenetik* 1 (1965): 397–413.

34. K. Hirschhorn, F. Bach, R. L. Kolodny, et al., "Immune response and mitosis of human peripheral blood lymphocytes in vitro," *Science* 142 (1963): 1185–87 [Citation Classic, Current Contents, 30 (1983): 20]; F. Bach and K. Hirschhorn, "Lymphocyte interaction: A potential histocompatibility test *in vitro*," *Science* 143 (1964): 813–14 [Citation Classic, Current Contents, 35 (1992): 10].

35. M. R. Swift and K. Hirschhorn, "Fanconi's anemia: Inherited susceptibility to chromosome breakage in various tissues," *Ann Int Med* 65 (1966): 496–503 [Citation Classic, Current Contents, 35 (1992): 10].

36. F. J. Suchy, *Liver Disease in Children* (St. Louis: Mosby, 1994).

37. See the Web site www.mountsinaihistory.org for recent citations.

NOTES TO CHAPTER 28

1. The Mount Sinai Hospital, *Annual Report for 1920*, p. 43.

2. The Mount Sinai Hospital, *Annual Report for 1942–1943*, p. 78.

3. The Mount Sinai Hospital, *Annual Report for 1945*, p. 92.

4. S. Feitelberg, P. E. Kaunitz, L. R. Wasserman, and S. B. Yohalem, "Use of radioactive iodine in diagnosis of thyroid disease," *Am J Med Sci* 216 (1948): 129–35.

5. See the chapter on the Division of Endocrinology.

6. S. Silver, S. B. Yohalem, and M. H. Fieber, "Blood iodine and I-131 excretion in diagnostic problems of hyperthyroidism," *J Mt Sinai Hosp* 17 (1951): 781–86.

7. S. Silver and M. H. Fieber, "Blood levels of I-131 after tracer doses in the diagnosis of hyperthyroidism," *Proc Soc Exp Biol Med* 75 (1950): 570–73.

8. S. Silver, P. Poroto, and E. B. Crohn, "Hypermetabolic states without hyperthyroidism (nonthyrogenous hypermetabolism)," *Arch Int Med* 85 (1950): 479–82.

9. E. H. Quimby, S. Feitelberg, and S. Silver, *Radioactive Isotopes in Clinical Practice* (Philadelphia: Lea and Febiger, 1958).

10. M. Eller, S. Silver, S. B. Yohalem, and R. L. Segal, "The treatment of toxic nodular goiter with I-131: 10 years' experience with 436 cases," *Ann Int Med* 52 (1960): 976–1013.

11. H. Popper, "In Memoriam: Sergei Feitelberg," *J Mt Sinai Hosp* 35 (1968): 108–10.

12. J. Meller, S. J. Goldsmith, A. Rudin, et al., "Spectrum of exercise thallium-201 myocardial perfusion imaging in patients with chest pain and normal coronary angiograms," *Am J Cardiol* 43 (1979): 717–23.

13. D. S. Fineman, C. J. Palestro, C. K. Kim, et al., "Detection of abnormalities in febrile AIDS patients with In-111-labeled leukocyte and Ga-67 scintigraphy," *Radiology* 170 (1989): 677–80.

14. C. J. Palestro, C. K. Kim, A. J. Swyer, et al., "Total-hip arthroplasty: Periprosthetic indium-111-labeled leukocyte activity and complementary technetium-99m-sulfur colloid imaging in suspected infection [see comments]," *J Nucl Med* 31 (1990): 1950–55.

NOTES TO CHAPTER 29

1. J. Hirsh and M. Kaufman, "The Jews' Hospital and psychological medicine," *J Mt Sinai Hosp* 19 (1952): 481–89.

2. B. Blustein, "A hollow square of psychological science: American neurologists and psychiatrists in conflict," in *Madhouses, Mad-doctors, and Madmen,* ed. A. Scull (Philadelphia: University of Pennsylvania Press, 1981), pp. 241–70.

3. C. Oberndorf, "The psychiatric clinic and the general hospital," *Med J Rec* 121 (1925): 424–27.

4. J. Hirsh and B. Doherty, *The First Hundred Years of the Mount Sinai Hospital of New York 1852–1952* (New York: Random House, 1952).

5. A. Stern, "Neurotic manifestations in children," *Med Record* 89 (1916): 361–63; W. Bromberg, *Psychiatry between the Wars 1918–1945. A recollection* (Westport, Conn.: Greenwood Press, 1982).

6. P. Lehrman, "Clarence Paul Oberndorf 1882–1954," *Psychoanalytic Quarterly* 23 (1954): 424–33.

7. I. Sands, "The first twenty-five years of Hillside Hospital," *J Hillside Hosp* 2 (1953): 199–206.

8. L. Kolb and S. Lorand. Oral history interview by Lawrence Kolb. Brill Archives of the New York Psychoanalytic Institute. Original in the Library of Congress.

9. Interview with Sandor Lorand, September 22, 1941. Historian's Office Folder, Mount Sinai Hospital, Folder 2–7. Mount Sinai Archives.

10. I. Wechsler, *Textbook of Clinical Neurology*, 9th ed. (Philadelphia: W. B. Saunders, 1962).

11. Minutes of the Joint Conference Committee of The Mount Sinai Hospital, May 1939. Mount Sinai Archives.

12. The Mount Sinai Hospital, *Annual Report for 1939*. Mount Sinai Archives.

13. L. Kubie, "The organization of a psychiatric service in a general hospital," *Psychosomatic Medicine* 4 (1942): 252–72.

14. L. Kubie, letter to the President of the Board of Trustees, The Mount Sinai Hospital, May 4, 1943. Folder, Psychiatry Department of The Mount Sinai Hospital. Mount Sinai Archives.

15. M. R. Kaufman and S. Margolin, "Theory and practice of psychosomatic medicine in a general hospital," *Med Cl N Amer* 32 (1948): 611–16; M. R. Kaufman, "Role of the psychiatrist in the general hospital," *Psych Quart* 27 (1953): 367–81.

16. L. Linn, *A Handbook of Hospital Psychiatry* (New York: International Universities Press, 1955).

17. C. Fisher, J. Gross, and J. Zuch, "Cycle of penile erection synchronous with dreaming (REM)," *Arch Gen Psych* 12 (1965): 29–45.

18. A. Richards, eulogy at memorial service for Charles Fisher, November 1988. Brill Archives of the New York Psychoanalytic Institute.

19. W. Dement, "The effect of dream deprivation," *Science* 131 (1960): 1705–7.

20. C. Fisher, R. Schiavi, A. Edwards, et al., "Evaluation of nocturnal penile tumescence (NPT) in the differential diagnosis of sexual impotence: A quantitative study," *Arch Gen Psych* 36 (1979): 431–37.

21. R. Schiavi, A. Theilgard, D. Owen, and D. White, "Sex chromosome anomalies, hormones, and sexuality," *Arch Genl Psych* 45 (1988): 19–24.

22. R. Schiavi, *Aging and Male Sexuality* (New York: Cambridge University Press, 1999).

23. K. Davis, R. Mohs, J. Tinklenberg, et al., "Physostigmine: Improvement of long-term memory processes in normal humans," *Science* 201 (1978): 272–74.

24. K. Davis, M. Davidson, R. Mohs, et al., "Plasma homovanilic acid concentration and the severity of schizophrenic illness," *Science* 227 (1985): 1601–2.

25. K. Davis, R. Kahn, G. Ko, and M. Davidson, "Dopamine in schizophrenia: A review and reconceptualization," *Am J Psych* 148 (1991): 1474–86.

26. R. Mohs, W. Rosen, and K. Davis, "The Alzheimer's Disease Assessment Scale: An instrument for assessing treatment efficacy," *Psychopharmacology Bull* 19 (1983): 448–50.

27. K. Davis and R. Mohs, "Enhancement of memory processes in Alzheimer's disease with multiple-dose intravenous physostigmine," *Am J Psych* 139 (1982): 1421–24.

28. M. Stein, R. Schiavi, and M. Camerino, "Influence of brain and behavior on the immune system," *Science* 191 (1976): 435–40.

29. S. Schleifer, S. Keller, M. Camerino, et al., "Suppression of lymphocyte stimulation following bereavement," *JAMA* 250 (1983): 374–77.

30. J. Naslund, V. Haroutunian, R. Mohs, et al., "Correlation between elevated levels of amyloid beta-peptide in the brain and cognitive decline," *JAMA* 283 (2000): 1571–77.

31. N. K. Robakis, H. M. Wisniewski, E. C. Jenkins, et al., "Chromosome 21q21 sublocalization of the gene encoding the beta amyloid peptide present in cerebral vessels and neuritic (senile) plaques of people with Alzheimer's disease and Down syndrome," *Lancet* 1 (1987): 384–85.

32. K. Davis, R. Mohs, D. Marin, et al., "Cholinergic markers are not decreased in early Alzheimer's disease," *JAMA* 281 (1999): 1401–6.

33. Y. Hakak, J. Walker, C. Li, et al., "Genome-wide expression analysis reveals dysregulation of myelination-related genes in chronic schizophrenia," *Proc Natl Acad Sci USA* 98 (2001): 4746–51.

NOTES TO CHAPTER 30

1. W. M. Brickner and E. Eising, "Report of the X-Ray Department," *Mount Sinai Hospital Reports, 1901–1902*, p. 557.

2. R. Frank, "The early history of the X-Ray Department of Mount Sinai Hospital." Mount Sinai Archives, c. 1939.

3. S. Stern, "Practical results accomplished with radiant energy," *NY Med J* 33 (1906): 493–97.

4. S. Stern, "Report of 800 dermatological cases treated with x-ray and high-frequency currents at the Mount Sinai Hospital," *Am J Dermatol* 12 (1908): 163–64.

5. S. Stern, "Hypertrichosis: Its treatment with the x-ray," *NY Med J* 95 (1912): 21–23.

6. S. Stern, "The value of prophylactic x-ray treatments," *Am J Roentgenol* 8 (1921): 199–202.

7. R. Brecher and E. Brecher, *The Rays* (Baltimore: Williams and Wilkins, 1969).

8. The Mount Sinai Hospital, *Annual Report for 1920*, p. 43.

9. S. Stern, "Practical results accomplished with radiant energy."

10. W. Harris, "Neoplasms of the oral and upper respiratory tracts treated by protracted roentgen therapy," *Am J Roentgenol* 34 (1935): 482–90.

11. W. Harris, S. M. Silverstone, and R. Kramer, "Roentgen therapy for cancer of the larynx and laryngopharynx," *Am J Roentgenol Radium Ther Nucl Med* 71 (1954): 813–25.

12. M. Berck and W. Harris, "Roentgen therapy for bronchiectasis," *JAMA* 108 (1937): 517–22.

13. S. H. Geist and M. Mintz, "Pituitary radiation for the relief of menopause symptoms," *Am J Obst Gynecol* 33 (1937): 643–45.

14. See the chapter on the Department of Physics for more information.

15. S. M. Silverstone, C. B. Braestrup, and B. S. Wolf, "Isodose charts for fields of special usefulness in the treatment of cancer of the uterine cervix," *Am J Roentgenol* 49 (1943): 819–21.

16. S. M. Silverstone, "Radium therapy for cancer of the cervix uteri: With a new type of colpostat," *Am J Roentgenol* 67 (1952): 294–99.

17. J. L. Goldman, S. M. Silverstone, J. D. Roffman, and E. A. Birken, "High dosage pre-operative radiation and surgery for carcinoma of the larynx and laryngopharynx. A 14-year program," *Laryngoscope* 82 (1972): 1869–82.

18. A. S. Glicksman and J. J. Nickson. "A prospect of computer implementation of radiotherapy," *Int J Biomed Comput* 2 (1971): 39–47.

19. T. D. Sterling, A. S. Glicksman, K. Knowlton, and J. Weinkam, "Three-dimensional treatment plan display on computer-produced films" in *Proceedings of the 3rd International Conference on Computers in Radiotherapy*, ed. A. S. Glicksman, M. Cohen, and J. R. Cunningham (Glasgow: 1970). Published as Special Report No. 5 (1971) by the British Institute of Radiology, London.

20. N. Simon, "Afterloading multiple irradiators for the treatment of cancer of the corpus of the uterus: A preliminary report of a new device," *J Mt Sinai Hosp* 36 (1969): 443–45.

21. N. Simon, "Afterloading and radium substitutes," *Gynecol Oncol* 2 (1974): 324–30.

22. S. M. Silverstone and N. Simon, "Afterloading with miniaturized Cs-137 sources in treatment of cancer of the uterus," *Int J Radiation Oncology, Biology, Physics* 1 (1976): 1017–21.

23. N. Simon, "Iridium-192 as a radium substitute," *Am J Roentgenol Radium Ther Nucl Med* 93 (1965): 170–78.

24. W. D. Bloomer, R. Lipsztein, and J. F. Dalton, "Antibody-mediated radiotherapy," *Cancer* 55 (Suppl.) (1985): 2229–33.

25. T. Garcia, S.Lehrer, W. D. Bloomer, and B. Schachter, "A variant estrogen receptor messenger ribonucleic acid is associated with reduced levels of estrogen binding in human mammary tumors," *Mol Endocrinol* 2 (1988): 785–91.

26. B. Shank, "Total body irradiation for marrow or stem-cell transplantation," *Cancer Invest* 16 (1998): 397–404.

27. S. Lehrer, J. Garey, and B. Shank, "Nomograms for determining the probability of axillary node involvement in women with breast cancer," *J Cancer Res Clin Oncol* 121 (1995): 123–25.

28. B. Shank, J. Moughan, J. Owen, et al., "The 1993–94 patterns of care process survey for breast irradiation after breast-conserving surgery: Comparison with the 1992 standard for breast conservation treatment," *Int J Radiat Oncol Biol Phys* 48 (2000): 1291–99.

29. R. G. Stock, N. N. Stone, M. F. Wesson, and J. K. DeWyngaert, "A modified technique allowing interactive ultrasound-guided three-dimensional transperineal prostate implantation," *Int J Radiat Oncol Biol Phys* 32 (1995): 219–25.

30. R. G. Stock, K. Chan, M. Terk, et al., "A new technique for performing Syed-Neblett template interstitial implants for gynecologic malignancies using transrectal- ultrasound guidance," *Int J Radiat Oncol Biol Phys* 37 (1997): 819–25.

NOTES TO CHAPTER 31

1. W. M. Brickner and E. Eising, "Report of the x-ray department," Mount Sinai Hospital Reports: 1901–1902 pp. 556–59. Mount Sinai Archives.

2. *Minutes of the Medical Board*, The Mount Sinai Hospital, 1905. Mount Sinai Archives.

3. See the chapter on the Department of Physics.

4. Historian's Office Files. Box 2, Folder 20. Mount Sinai Archives.

5. The Mount Sinai Hospital, *Annual Report for 1909*. Mount Sinai Archives. p. 23.

6. H. Wessler and L. Jaches, *Clinical Roentgenology of Diseases of the Chest* (Troy, N.Y.: Southworth, 1923).

7. M. Swick, "Darstellung der niere und harnwege im roentgenbild durch intravenose einbringung eines neuen kontrastoffes, des uroselectans," *Klin Wochenschrift* 8 (1929): 2087–89; M. Swick, "Intravenous urography by means of uroselectan," *Am J Surg* 8 (1930): 405–14. See also the chapter on the Department of Urology.

8. L. Jaches and M. Swick, "Opaque media in urology, with special reference to a new compound sodium ortho-iodohippurate," *Radiology* 23 (1934): 216–22.

9. I. C. Rubin, "The nonoperative determination of patency of Fallopian tubes by means of intra-uterine insufflation with oxygen and the production of an artificial pneumoperitoneum," *JAMA* 75 (1920): 661–66; I. C. Rubin and A. J. Bendick, "Fluoroscopic visualization of tubal peristalsis in women," *JAMA* 87 (1926): 657–58. See also the chapter on the Department of Obstetrics, Gynecology, and Reproductive Sciences.

10. M. L. Sussman, A. J. Gordon, S. A. Brahms, et al., "The technique of cardiac catheterization and angiography as employed at the Mount Sinai Hospital," *J Mt Sinai Hosp* 17 (1951): 272–92.

11. A. Grishman, M. F. Steinberg, and M. L. Sussman, "Contrast roentgen visualization of coarctation of the aorta," *Am Heart J* 21 (1941): 365–70.

12. M. L. Sussman, M. F. Steinberg, and A. Grishman, "A rapid film changer for use in contrast angiography," *Radiol* 28 (1942): 232–33.

13. M. L. Sussman et al., "The technique of cardiac catheterization and angiography."

14. There are at least fifty papers that could and should be cited as "firsts" or as landmark papers written by Wolf, Marshak, and their colleagues on various aspects of gastrointestinal radiology. They have recently been catalogued in articles by E. L. Wolf, "The Esophagus," *Mt Sinai J Med* 67 (2000): 25–31, and D. Maklansky, "Pioneer gastroenterological radiology studies," *Mt Sinai J Med* 67 (2000): 204–7. They may also be viewed on Web site, www.mountsinaihistory.org.

15. J. G. Rabinowitz, "Introduction," in "Gastrointestinal Radiology: A *Festschrift* for Richard H. Marshak, M.D.," *Mt Sinai J Med* 51 (1984): 311.

16. D. Maklansky, "Pioneer gastroenterological radiology studies," *Mt Sinai J Med* 67 (2000): 204–7.

17. Ibid.

18. J. E. Moseley, *Bone Changes in Hematologic Disorders (Roentgen Aspects)* (New York: Grune and Stratton, 1963).

19. J. E. Moseley, "Loculated pneumomediastinum in the newborn: thymic 'spinnaker sail' sign," *Radiology* 75 (1960): 788–90.

20. J. G. Rabinowitz and J. E. Moseley, "The lateral lumbar spine in Down's Syndrome: A new roentgen feature," *Radiology* 83 (1964): 74–79.

21. Y. P. Huang and B. S. Wolf, "The veins of the posterior fossa-superior or galenic draining group," *Am J Roentgenol Radium Ther Nucl Med* 95 (1965): 808–21.

22. J. G. Rabinowitz, M. G. Baron, B. S. Wolf, et al., "Endocardial cushion defects: specific diagnosis by angiocardiography," *Am J Cardiol* 13 (1964): 162–65.

23. J. G. Rabinowitz and B. S. Wolf, "Roentgen significance of the pulmonary ligament," *Radiology* 87 (1966): 1013–20.

NOTES TO CHAPTER 32

1. H. Wolf, "The early days of the Physical Therapy Department," personal notes. December 15, 1938. Historian's Office. Mount Sinai Hospital. Files, 1852–1955. Box 2, f.18. Mount Sinai Archives.

2. Ibid.

3. F. J. Kottke and N. E. Knapp, "The development of physiatry before 1950," *Arch Phys Med Rehabil* 69 (special issue) (1988): 4–14.

4. J. L. Opitz, T. J. Folz, R. Gelfman, and D. J. Peters, "The history of physical medicine and rehabilitation as recorded in the diary of Dr. Frank Krusen. Part 1. Gathering momentum (the years before 1942)," *Arch Phys Med Rehabil* 78 (1997): 442–45.

5. Ibid., p. 444.

6. *J Mt Sinai Hosp* 3 (1938): 121–52.

7. T. J. Folz, J. L. Opitz, D. J. Peters, and R. Gelfman, "The history of physical medicine and rehabilitation as recorded in the diary of Dr. Frank Krusen: Part 2. Forging ahead (1943–1947)," *Arch Phys Med Rehabil* 78 (1997): 446–50.

8. R. Gelfman, D. J. Peters, J. L. Opitz, and T. J. Folz, "The history of physical medicine and rehabilitation as recorded in the diary of Dr. Frank Krusen: Part 3. Consolidating the position (1948–1953)," *Arch Phys Med Rehabil* 78 (1997): 556–61.

9. F. T. Stein, *The Social Service Department: A History*, c. 1957. Mount Sinai Archives.

10. See the Web site www.mountsinaihistory.org for selected citations of Bierman's work.

11. L. H. Wisham, R. S. Yalow, and A. J. Freund, "Consistency of clearance of radioactive sodium from human muscle," *Am Heart J* 41 (1951): 810–18; L. H. Wisham, A. Shaanan, and W. Bierman, "The influence of vibration on temperature and on the clearance of radioactive sodium in human subjects," *Arch Phys Med Rehabil* 37 (1956): 760–65.

12. B. E. Herman, F. F. Dworecka, and L. H. Wisham, "Increase of dermal blood flow after sympathectomy as measured by radioactive sodium uptake," *Vasc Surg* 4 (1970): 161–63.

13. L. H. Wisham, J. F. Katz, and F. F. Dworecka, "The effect of changes in position on the clearance of radioactive sodium from the head of the femur in immature dogs," *Am J Ortho* 8 (1966): 132–35.

14. F. F. Dworecka, L. H. Wisham, and R. Smith, "A new device for the restoration of partially amputated hands," *Mt Sinai J Med* 38 (1971): 462–69.

15. A. A. Fischer, "Tissue compliance meter for objective, quantitative documentation of soft tissue consistency and pathology," *Arch Phys Med Rehabil* 68 (1987): 122–25.

16. E. A. Eastwood, "Functional status and its uses in rehabilitation medicine," *Mt Sinai J Med* 66 (1999): 179–87.

17. NIH Consensus Development Panel on Rehabilitation of Persons with Traumatic Brain Injury (K. T. Ragnarsson, Chairman), "Rehabilitation of persons with traumatic brain injury," *JAMA* 282 (1999): 974–83. Ragnarsson has published extensively on the rehabilitation and comprehensive care of patients with major deficits. Visit the Web site www.mountsinaihistory.org for more citations.

NOTES TO CHAPTER 33

1. *Case Records of the Jews' Hospital, 1855–56.* Mount Sinai Archives.

2. W. H. Van Buren and E. L. Keyes, *A Practical Treatise on the Surgical Diseases of the Genito-Urinary Organs, Including Syphilis, Designed as a Manual for Students and Practitioners* (New York: Appleton, 1874).

3. L. J. T. Murphy, *The History of Urology* (Springfield, Ill.: Charles C. Thomas, 1972).

4. E. G. Ballenger et al., *History of Urology*, 2 vols. (Baltimore: Williams and Wilkins, 1933).

5. H. Lilienthal, "The Mount Sinai Hospital and its surgeons of the middle eighties; a few recollections," *J Mt Sinai Hosp* 3 (1937): 229–40.

6. W. F. Fluhrer, "An improved technique in the operation of external perineal urethrotomy," *NY Med J* 57 (1893): 79–81.

7. W. F. Fluhrer, "A new urethrotome," *NY Med J* 53 (1891): 97–98.

8. W. F. Fluhrer, *An Inquiry into the Principles of Treatment of Broken Limbs, a Philosophico-Surgical Essay with Surgical Notes* (New York: Rebman, 1916).

9. G. E. Brewer, "Some observations upon acute unilateral septic infarcts of the kidney," *Surg Gynecol Obstet* 2 (1906): 485–97.

10. H. Goldenberg, "Polypus of the male urethra," *Med Record* 40 (1891): 600–3.

11. F. T. Brown, "The cystoscope and ureter catheter in the diagnosis of surgical disease of the kidney and ureter," *Medical News* 86 (1905): 442–44.

12. L. Buerger, "A new indirect irrigating observation and double catheterizing cystoscope," *Ann Surg* 49 (1909): 225–37.

13. L. Buerger, "Thromboangiitis obliterans: A study of the vascular lesions leading to presenile spontaneous gangrene," *Am J Med Sci* 136 (1908): 567–80.

14. E. Beer, "Cystoscopy and ureteral catheterization in young children," *Am J Surg* 25 (1911): 79–81.

15. M. Stern, "Minor surgery of the prostate gland; a new cystoscopic instrument employing a current capable of operation in a water medium," *Intl J Med Surg* 39 (1926): 72–77.

16. Appointed in 1910, Stern worked with other members of the staff for a number of years. The papers noted were found in a search of *Index Medicus* for the years 1917–1926. The complete list of citations may be found on the Web site, www.mountsinaihistory.org.

17. E. Beer, "Removal of neoplasms of the urinary bladder: A new method, employing high-frequency (Oudin) current through a catheterizing cystoscope," *JAMA* 54 (1910): 1768–69.

18. Reed Nesbit, quoted in H. Brendler and W. L. F. Ferber, "Early days of urology at Mount Sinai," *Urology* 3 (1974): 246–50.

19. E. Beer, *Collected Papers 1904–1929* (New York: Paul B. Hoeber, 1931).

20. E. Beer, "Essential thrombocytopenic purpura; purpura hemorrhagica and its treatment by splenectomy," *Ann Surg* 84 (1926): 549–60.

21. E. Beer, "Development and progress of surgery of the spleen," *Ann Surg* 88 (1928): 335–46.

22. R. Alessandri, "Experiences with surgery of the spleen; report of 2 unusual cases," *J Mt Sinai Hosp* 4 (1938): 489–500.

23. E. Beer, "Chronic retention of urine in children," *JAMA* 65 (1915): 1709–12.

24. E. Beer and A. Hyman, *Diseases of the Urinary Tract in Children* (New York: Paul B. Hoeber, 1930).

25. E. Beer, "Contribution to the radical operative treatment of carcinoma of the prostate and carcinoma of the neck of the bladder," *Urol and Cutan Rev* Tech Suppl. 3 (1915): 279–83.

26. H. Lilienthal, "Edwin Beer and Base Hospital No. 3," *J Mt Sinai Hosp* 4 (1938): 477–81.

27. M. Swick, "Darstellung der niere und harnwege im roentgenbild durch intravenose einbringung eines neuen kontrastoffes, des uroselectans," *Klin Wochenschrift* 8 (1929): 2087–89.

28. M. Swick, "Intravenous urography by means of uroselectan," *Am J Surg* 8 (1930): 405–14.

29. H. Neuhof, "Fascia transplantation in visceral defects: An experimental and clinical study," *Surg Gyn Obstet* 24 (1917): 383–427.

30. H. Neuhof and S. Hirshfeld, *The Transplantation of Tissues*, 1st ed. (New York: Appleton, 1923).

31. The Mount Sinai Hospital, *Annual Report for 1930*.

32. The Mount Sinai Hospital, *Annual Report for 1939*.

33. R. Colp, "Edwin Beer 1876–1938," *Ann Surg* 110 (1939): 795–96.

34. A. Hyman, "Malignant tumors of the kidney," *Int J Med Surg* 47 (1934): 205–6.

35. A. Hyman and W. H. Mencher, "Causes of death after urological operations: based upon 165 cases with 119 autopsies," *J Urol* 33 (1935): 315–29.

36. B. B. Crohn, L. Ginzburg, G. D. Oppenheimer, "Regional ileitis," *JAMA* 99 (1932): 1323–28.

37. S. S. Rosenak and G. D. Oppenheimer, "An improved drain for peritoneal dialysis," *Surgery* 23 (1948): 832–33. See also the chapter on the Division of Nephrology.

38. A. Saltzman and S. S. Rosenak, "Design of pump suitable for blood," *J Lab Clin Med* 34 (1949): 1561–63.

39. S. S. Rosenak and A. Saltzman, "New dialyzer for use as artificial kidney," *Proc Soc Exper Biol Med* 76 (1951): 471–75.

40. R. M. Nesbit and S. I. Glickman, "The use of glycine solution as an irrigating medium during transurethral resection," *J Urol* 59 (1948): 1212–16.

41. H. J. Goldman and S. I. Glickman, "Ureteral obstruction in regional ileitis," *J Urol* 88 (1962): 616–20.

42. D. Stoll, Executive Director, American Board of Urology, personal communication, 2001.

43. E. Leiter and H. Brendler, "Percutaneous transfemoral renal arteriography," *J Mt Sinai Hosp* 32 (1965): 51–64.

44. E. Leiter, S. Edelman and H. Brendler, "Continuous preoperative intra-arterial perfusion of renal tumors with chemotherapeutic agents," *J Urol* 95 (1966): 169–75.

45. E. Leiter and H. Brendler, "Loss of ejaculation following bilateral retroperitoneal lymphadenectomy," *J Urol* 98 (1967): 375–78.

46. E. Leiter, W. Futterweit, and G. R. Brown, "Gender reassignment: Psychiatric, endocrinologic, and surgical management," in *Reconstructive Urology*, ed. G. D. Webster et al. (Boston: Blackwell Scientific Publications, 1993), pp. 921–32.

47. H. Brendler, "American Urological Association: Dedication to excellence," *J Urol* 132 (1984): 869–71.

48. M. Droller, *Surgical Management of Urologic Disease: An Anatomic Approach* (St. Louis: Mosby Year Book, 1992).

NOTES TO CHAPTER 34

1. H. Sobotka, "Obituary: Samuel Bookman, Ph.D.," *J Mount Sinai Hosp* 14 (1947): 63–66.

2. S. Bookman, "Twenty-five years of physiological chemistry at The Mount Sinai Hospital (1902–1927)," *J Mount Sinai Hosp* 12 (1945): 87–90.

3. H. Sobotka, *The Physiological Chemistry of the Bile* (New York: Williams and Wilkins, 1937); H. Sobotka, *The Chemistry of the Steroids* (New York: Williams and Wilkins, 1938).

4. B. J. Davis, L. Ornstein, "A new high-resolution electrophoresis method." Paper delivered at the Society for the Study of Blood meeting at The New York Academy of Medicine, March 24, 1959.

5. L. Ornstein, "Disc electrophoresis. 1. Background and theory," *Ann NY Acad Sci* 121 (1964): 321–49; B. J. Davis, "Disc electrophoresis. 2. Method and application to human serum proteins," *Ann NY Acad Sci* 121 (1964): 404–27.

6. L. Sarkozi, E. Simson, and L. Ramanathan, "The effects of automated testing, laboratory information systems and automated specimen handling in clinical chemistry." Manuscript prepared for presentation and publication, 2002.

7. E. Libman, "Weitere Mittheilungen uber die Streptokokken-Enteritis bei Sauglingen," *Centralbl fur Bakt* 22 (1897): 376–82.

8. E. Libman, "On some experience with blood-cultures in the study of bacterial infections," *Johns Hopkins Hosp Bull* 17 (1906): 215–28.

9. E. Libman, "A study of the endocardial lesions of subacute bacterial endocarditis: with particular reference to healing or healed lesions; with clinical notes," *Am J Med Sci* 144 (1912): 313–27.

10. L. Loewe, S. A. Ritter, and G. Baehr, "Cultivation of Rickettsia-like bodies in Typhus fever," *JAMA* 77 (1921): 1967–69.

11. J. Cohen, "Bacteriology of abscess of the lung and methods for its study," *Arch Surg* 24 (1932): 171–88.

12. G. Shwartzman, "Studies of bacillus Typhosus toxic substances. I. Phenomenon of local skin reactivity to B. Typhosus culture filtrate," *J Exp Med* 48 (1928): 247–68.

13. G. Shwartzman, *Phenomenon of Local Tissue Reactivity and its Immunological, Pathological and Clinical Significance* (New York: P. B. Hoeber, 1937).

14. L. J. Soffer, G. Shwartzman, S. S. Schneierson, and J. L. Gabrilove, "Inhibition of the Shwartzman phenomenon by adrenocorticotrophic hormone (ACTH) from the adenohypophysis," *Science* 111 (1950): 303–4.

15. The latex agglutination test has become the standard laboratory test to confirm the presence of rheumatoid arthritis. See the chapter on the Division of Rheumatology for more on the subject and for the citations.

16. M. L. Littman and S. S. Schneierson, "Cryptococcus neoformans in pigeon excreta in New York City," *Am J Hyg* 69 (1959): 49–59.

17. *Atlas of Diagnostic Microbiology*. Photographs by S. Stanley Schneierson; text by Alan F. Sewell. (North Chicago, Ill.: Abbott Laboratories, 1971).

18. S. S. Schneierson, "A simple rapid disk-tube method for determination of bacterial sensitivity to antibiotics," *Antibiot Chemother* 4 (1954): 125–32.

19. S. S. Schneierson and D. Amsterdam, "A punch card system for identification of bacteria," *Am J Clin Path* 42 (1964): 328–31; S. S. Schneierson and D. Amsterdam, "A manual punch card system for recording, filing, and analyzing antibiotic sensitivity test results," *Am J Clin Path* 47 (1967): 818–20.

20. E. J. Bottone, B. Chester, M. Malowany, and J. Allerhand, "Unusual Yersinia enterocolitica isolates not associated with mesenteric lymphadenitis," *Appl Microbiol* 27 (1974): 858–61.

21. E. J. Bottone, R. M. Madayag, and M. N. Qureshi, "Acanthamoeba keratitis: Synergy between amebic and bacterial cocontaminants in contact lens care systems as a prelude to infection," *J Clin Microbiol* 30 (1992): 2447–50.

22. E. J. Bottone, personal communication, November 2001.

NOTES TO THE AFTERWORD

1. R. Ottenberg, "An Old Photograph," *J M Sinai Hosp* 14 (September–October 1947): 544.

2. Emanuel Libman Fellowship Fund, Minute Book, 1924–1956. Mount Sinai Archives.

3. The Mount Sinai Alumni, *100 Years . . . A History of the Mount Sinai Alumni* (New York: Mount Sinai Medical Center, 1996), pp. 20–21.

4. See Appendix B for a list of Jacobi Medallion recipients, 1952–2002. Unless otherwise noted, the recipients are physicians.

5. Interview with Percy Klingenstein, M.D., 3/16/67, INT24, Oral History Collection of the Mount Sinai Archives.

6. Interview with Leon Ginzburg, M.D., 7/27/65, INT4, Oral History Collection of the Mount Sinai Archives, p. 19.

7. Klingenstein interview, 1967.

8. Interview with Burrill B. Crohn, M.D., 4/7/65, INT8, Oral History Collection of the Mount Sinai Archives, p. 1.

9. Interview with Samuel Klein, M.D., 10/30/66. INT21, Oral History Collection of the Mount Sinai Archives, pp. 1–2.

10. Interview with Henry Dolger, M.D., 1988. INT37, Oral History Collection of the Mount Sinai Archives, p. 4.

11. Alvin S. Teirstein, "Residency training programs then and now: Medicine," *M Sinai J of Med* 56 (1989): 371–74.

12. Ibid., p. 372.

13. Dolger, interview, p. 13.

14. Interview with Ralph Colp, M.D., 10/23/65. INT25, Oral History Collection of the Mount Sinai Archives, p. 2.

15. Teirstein, "Residency training programs," p. 372.

16. Ginzburg, interview, p. 9.

17. H. Salzstein, "Mount Sinai Sixty Years Ago," *Mount Sinai Spectrum* (spring 1973): 6.

18. E. Libman, "Address delivered by Emanuel Libman as President of the Associated Alumni of the Mount Sinai Hospital, 1911–1912," Alumni Association, Meeting Files, Box 1, f.1. Mount Sinai Archives.

19. Dolger, interview, pp. 2, 4.

20. Teirstein, "Residency training programs," p. 370.

21. Dolger, interview, p. 8.

22. Mrs. Gerson Lesnick to Kristin Wilson, personal communication, 2000.

23. Teirstein, "Residency training programs," 370, 372.

24. Crohn, interview, p. 2.

25. Klein, interview, p. 10.

26. Dolger, interview, p. 10.

27. Klein, interview, pp. 9–10.

28. Dolger, interview, p. 10.

29. Ibid., pp. 17, 19.

30. Crohn, interview, p. 2.

31. Dolger, interview, p. 18.

32. Crohn, interview, p. 2.

33. Dolger, interview, p. 8.
34. Crohn, interview, p. 1.
35. Dolger, interview, p. 12.
36. Bernard Simon, "A Tribute to and remembrances of William M. Hitzig, M.D.," address given at Alumni Day, April 27, 1985. Mount Sinai Archives.
37. Dolger, interview, p. 8.

Index

About the Authors

Born and educated in New York, ARTHUR H. AUFSES, JR., has been affiliated with Mount Sinai for more than forty-five years. He served as Chairman of the Department of Surgery from 1974 to 1996. He has written extensively on surgical topics.

BARBARA J. NISS is the Archivist at The Mount Sinai Medical Center in New York, a program she helped formalize more than fifteen years ago. She has a graduate degree in history from New York University. Ms. Niss is married and has two wonderful children.